Molecular Farming

Molecular Farming

Edited by **Holly Philips**

SYRAWOOD
PUBLISHING HOUSE

New York

Published by Syrawood Publishing House,
750 Third Avenue, 9th Floor,
New York, NY 10017, USA
www.syrawoodpublishinghouse.com

Molecular Farming
Edited by Holly Philips

International Standard Book Number: 978-1-68286-053-3 (Hardback)

The publisher's policy is to use permanent paper from mills that operate a sustainable forestry policy. Furthermore, the publisher ensures that the text paper and cover boards used have met acceptable environmental accreditation standards.

Trademark Notice: Registered trademark of products or corporate names are used only for explanation and identification without intent to infringe.

Printed in the United States of America.

Contents

Preface

Molecular farming also known as pharming, is the application of biotechnology and genetic engineering for using plant and animal proteins and metabolites to produce pharmaceutical substances in large quantities. It is widely used for manufacturing different enzymes, vaccines and hormones at relatively low cost. As this field is emerging at a fast pace, this book will help the readers to better understand the diverse concepts of plant genome, recombinant antibodies, therapeutic medicines and their clinical evaluations, etc. This book is a complete source of knowledge on the present status of this important field. It is appropriate for students seeking detailed information as well as for experts engaged in this field.

This book has been the outcome of endless efforts put in by authors and researchers on various issues and topics within the field. The book is a comprehensive collection of significant researches that are addressed in a variety of chapters. It will surely enhance the knowledge of the field among readers across the globe.

It gives us an immense pleasure to thank our researchers and authors for their efforts to submit their piece of writing before the deadlines. Finally in the end, I would like to thank my family and colleagues who have been a great source of inspiration and support.

Editor

Studies of wine produced from pineapple (*Ananas comosus*)

Idise, Okiemute Emmanuel

Department of Microbiology, Delta State University, Abraka, Nigeria. E-mail: emmaidise@yahoo.com.

Pineapple (*Ananas comosus*) is the common name for a tropical plant with edible fruit, which is actually a multiple fruit, consisting of coalesced berries. The ratio of 1: 4 (pineapple must: sugar) was used to produce wine using recipes A to D. A contained only natural yeast; B contained natural yeast augmented with granulated sugar; C contained natural yeast augmented with baker's yeast and granulated sugar while D (control) contained granulated sugar and baker's yeast. Wines produced after 144 h of fermentation had average values of 3.44, 3.32, 3.46 and 3.50 for pH; 0.583, 0.627, 0.715 and 0.666 for optical density; 0.999, 1.003, 0.998 and 0.993 for specific gravity; 6.67, 6.69, 6.75 and 6.72 for total aerobic count (Log_{10} cfu/ml); 1.355, 1.355, 1.350 and 1.350 for % alcohol and 0.956, 1.246, 0.997 and 0.260 for %.titratable acidity for A to D respectively. The mean values for temperature and R_f were 30.5°c and 0.6 respectively. Malo-lactic fermentation after 48 h was evident. Taste testing showed very little differences in the wines with recipes A to C while statistical analyses at 95% confidence level showed no significant differences. The wine from the control had similar taste and characteristics with natural palm wine. Pineapple wine could thus, be produced for immediate consumption or preservation by refrigeration using recipes A to C. More research is still required to determine the shelf stability of the Pineapple wine.

Key words: Pineapple fermentation, sugar, wine, flavor, yeast.

INTRODUCTION

Pineapple (*Ananas Comosus*), a leading member of the family *Bromeliaceae* comprises about 2,000 species mostly epiphytic and many strikingly ornamental and varies from nearly white to yellow in Color (Morton, 1987). It is an herbaceous perennial plant which grows to 1.0 to 1.5 m tall with 30 or more trough-shaped and pointed leaves, 30 cm long, surrounding a thick stem. It is a multiple fruit, forming what appears to be a single fleshy fruit. Pineapples contain good sugar proportion which makes it suitable for wine making (Adaikan and Ganesan, 2004).

Wine is an alcoholic beverage typically made of fermented fruit juice (Okafor, 2007). Any fruit with good proportion of sugar may be used in producing wine and the resultant wine is normally named after the fruit. The type of wine to be produced dictates the fruit and strain of yeast to be involved (Amerine and Kunkee, 2005). Preservatives used in wine making include sulphur-

dioxide, potassium sorbate, sorbic acid and metabisulphides (Idise and Izuagbe, 1988). High concentration of these preservatives in wine, aside causing off odors, can induce lots of systemic disorderliness such as breathing problems in Asthmatic patients and gastrointestinal disturbances in allergic persons. The effects of bioaccumulation of these chemicals could further compound these situations (Okafor, 2007).

Fermentation is a process of extracting energy from the oxidation of organic compounds such as carbohydrates using an endogenous electron acceptor, usually pyruvate, an organic compound. Before fermentation takes place, one glucose molecule is broken down into two pyruvate molecules during glycolysis. Fermentation is important in anaerobic conditions when there is no oxidative phosphorylation to maintain the production of Adenosine tri-phosphate (ATP) by glycolysis. During

Table 1. The compositions of various fermenting vessels.

Vessel	Composition
A	1.5 liters of Pineapple slurry + 6.0 liters of water.
B	1.5 liters of Pineapple slurry + 6.0 liters of sugar solution.
C	1.5 liters of Pineapple + 6.0 liters of sugar solution + activated baker's yeast
D(control)	7.5 liters of sugar solution + activated baker's yeast

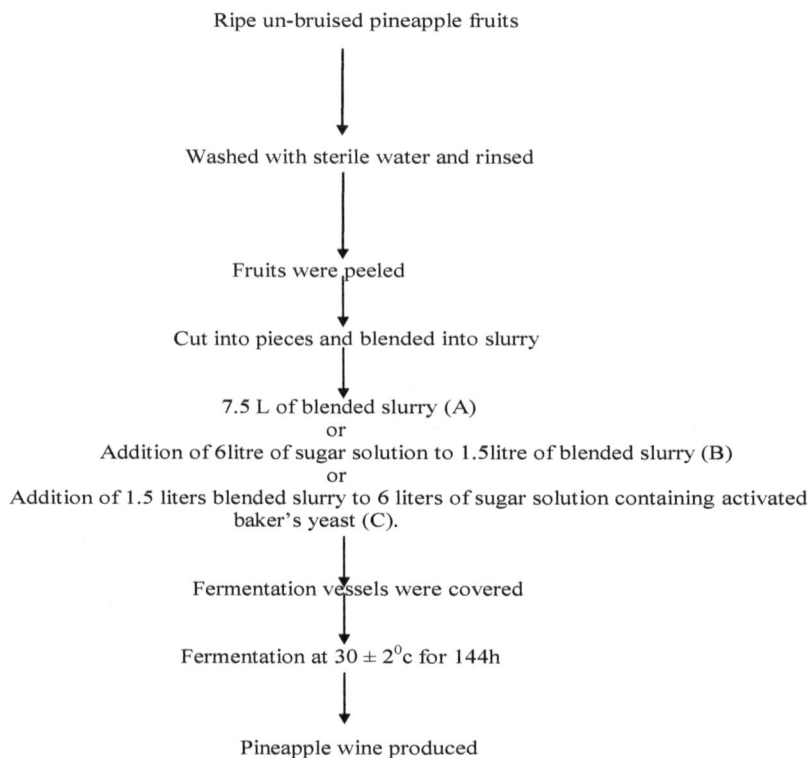

Ripe un-bruised pineapple fruits

↓

Washed with sterile water and rinsed

↓

Fruits were peeled

↓

Cut into pieces and blended into slurry

↓

7.5 L of blended slurry (A)
or
Addition of 6litre of sugar solution to 1.5litre of blended slurry (B)
or
Addition of 1.5 liters blended slurry to 6 liters of sugar solution containing activated baker's yeast (C).

↓

Fermentation vessels were covered

↓

Fermentation at 30 ± 2^0c for 144h

↓

Pineapple wine produced

Figure 1. Flow chart of pineapple wine production.

alcoholic fermentation, usually carried out by yeasts, pyruvate is then converted into ethanol and carbon dioxide thus:

$$C_6H_{12}O_6 \rightarrow 2C_2H_5OH + 2CO_2.$$

During this process, the carboxylic carbon atom is released in the form of carbon-dioxide with the remaining components becoming acetaldehyde. The acetaldehyde in the absence of oxygen will then be further reduced by alcohol dehydrogenase to form ethanol along with carbon-dioxide (Robinson, 2006). This research was aimed at producing wine from pineapple for immediate consumption.

MATERIALS AND METHODS

Collection of materials: Sugar, baker's yeast and ripe un-bruised pineapple were purchased from Abraka market in Delta State,

Nigeria. The fruits were identified at the Botany Department of the Delta State University, Abraka prior to analysis. These were washed with tap water in the laboratory and allowed to air dry.

Preparation of sugar solution

Clean water was boiled for five minutes and allowed to cool. One (1) teacup-full of granulated sugar was dissolved in one liter of water to obtain the sugar solution.

Preparation of must juice

This was carried in accordance with the method of Uraih (2003). The compositions of various fermenting vessels are presented in Table 1.

Fermentation of pineapple juice (must)

This was carried out using a modification of the method of Uraih (2003) using the flowchart in Figure 1.

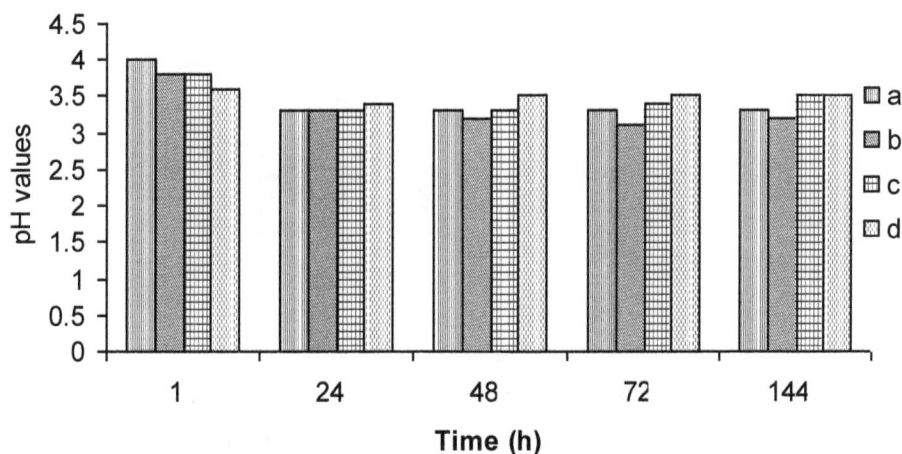

Figure 2. Changes in pH of pawpaw wine.

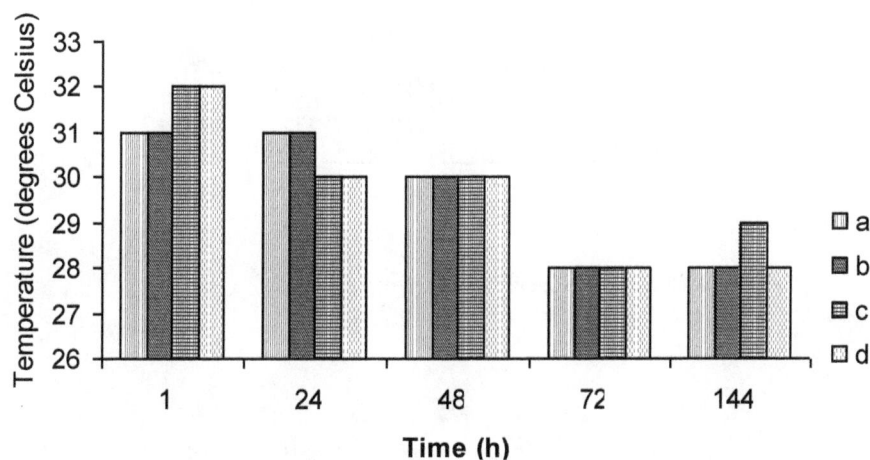

Figure 3. Changes in temperature of pawpaw wine.

Determination of physico-chemical and microbial parameters

These were carried out in accordance with standard methods reported by Ogunkoye and Olubayo (1977), Harrigan and McCane (2001). Kunkee and Amerine (2002), Cowan and Steel (2004) and Fawole and Oso (2008).

Organoleptic evaluation

This was carried out in accordance with the procedure reported by Maragatham and Panneerselvam (2011). The sensory evaluation was done using 8 judge panels after aging for 24 h. Observations recorded for color, clarity, body and taste on a 5 point scale with 5 points for excellent quality and 1 point for bad quality.

Statistical analysis

These were carried out using Microsoft excel 1995-2003 at 95% confidence level.

RESULTS

The pH values of the various wines presented in Figure 2 indicate a reduction after 24 h of fermentation and the values thereafter remained constant. The changes in temperature during orange wine production presented in Figure 3 showed a decrease from 1 to 24 h for recipes C and D and remained constant thereafter for C and increased for D while it decreased to 48 h for recipes A and B and remained constant thereafter. The highest value at 1h was observed for recipe C.

The optical density values presented in Figure 4 showed increases with period of fermentation for all the wines. The specific gravity values are presented in Figure 5. It was observed that there was a decrease from 1 to 72 h and an increase thereafter to 144 h of fermentation for the wines. The percentage alcohol represented in Figure 6 showed constant values till 48 h followed by a decrease

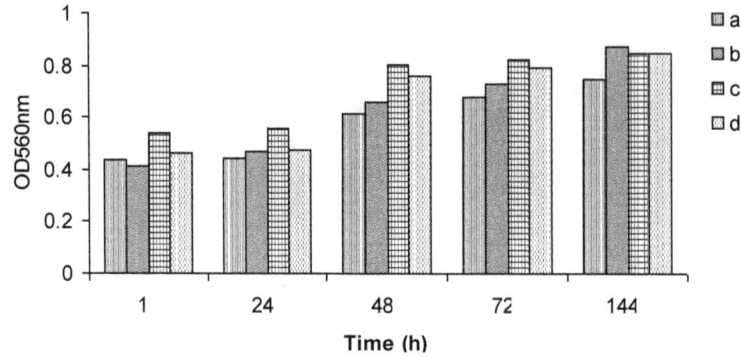

Figure 4. Changes in optical density of pawpaw wine.

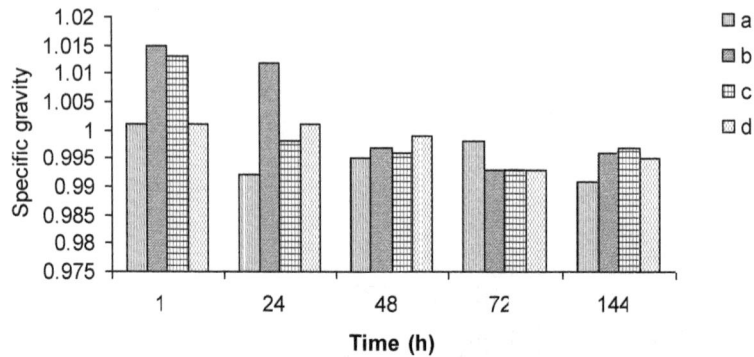

Figure 5. Changes in specific gravity of pawpaw wine.

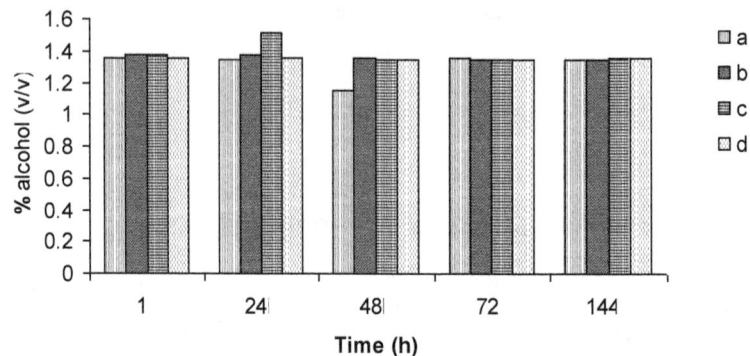

Figure 6. Changes in % alcohol of pawpaw wine.

at 72 h and an increase at 144 h for recipes A and B while constant values were observed for 1and 24 h followed by a decrease at 48 h which was constant till 144 h for recipes C and D.

The changes in % titratable acidity are presented in Figure 7. It was observed to increase with the period of fermentation supporting the occurrence of microbial succession with varying tolerance for the metabolic end products. The total aerobic counts are presented in

Figure 8. It was observed to increase with the period of fermentation supporting the occurrence of microbial succession.

The average values of the tested parameters with period of fermentation presented in Table 2 indicate that there was no appreciable difference in recipes A to C.

The mean values R_f and retardation factor values are presented in Table 3. It was observed that the values indicate the presence of lactic acid in the fermentation

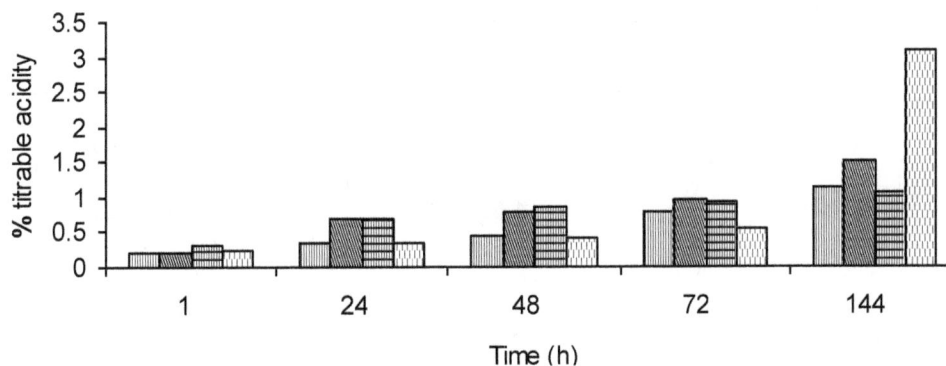

Figure 7. Changes in % titratable acidity of pawpaw wine during production.

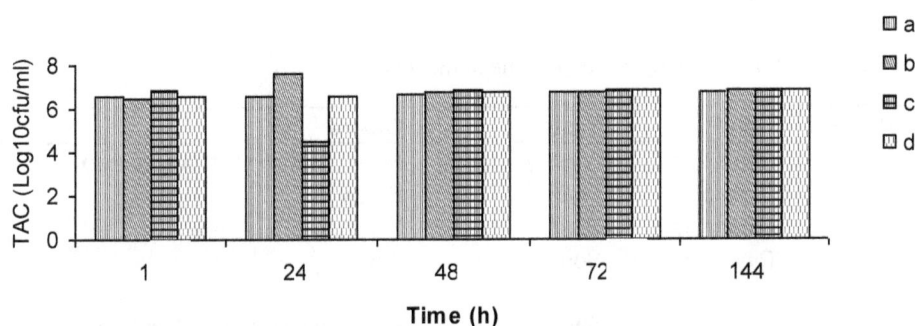

Figure 8. Changes in total aerobic counts of pawpaw wine.

Table 2. Mean values of three determinations.

Parameters	A	B	C	D
pH	3.44 ± 0.06	3.32 ± 0.14	3.46 ± 0.06	3.5 ± 0.14
Temperature	30.4 ± 0.46	30.6 ± 0.17	30.6 ± 0.46	30.6 ± 0.40
Optical density	0.582 ± 0.009	0.627 ± 0.025	0.715 ± 0.0023	0.666 ± 0.054
Specific gravity	0.999 ± 0.0006	1.003 ± 0.002	0.998 ± 0.002	0.993 ± 0.002
Total aerobic count ($\log_{10}$ cfu/ml)	6.67 ± 0.53	6.69 ± 0.052	6.75 ± 0.08	6.72 ± 0.28
Percentage alcohol (v/v)	1.355 ± 0.058	1.355 ± 0.006	1.35 ± 0.098	1.35 ± 0.058
Titratable acidity (%)	0.956 ± 0.019	1.246 ± 0.11	0.997 ± 0.0006	0.26 ± 0.023

medium at the end of 144 h.

The physically observable and taste changes in the wines with period of fermentation are presented in Table 4. It was observed that there were no appreciable changes in the pineapple wines of the different recipes.

DISCUSSION

The observed changes in the pH of the wines could be due to production of acids with period of fermentation probably arising from microbial succession. This result agrees with the reports of previous workers (Amerine and

Kunkee, 2005; Okafor, 2007). The observed changes in the temperature of the wines could be due to microbial succession arising from microbial metabolic activities that made the fermentation medium favor the growth of certain organisms. These results agree with reports of previous workers (Idise and Izuagbe, 1985, 1988; Amerine and Kunkee, 2005; Okafor, 2007).

The observed changes in optical density with period of fermentation could be due to increase in microbial load arising from microbial succession with changes in fermentation end products. These results agree with reports of previous workers (Amerine and Kunkee, 2005; Robinson, 2006; Okafor, 2007).

Table 3. Mean R_f values of three determinations.

Variable	48 h	144 h
A Rfx (cm)	1.9 ±0.017	3 ±0.289
Rfy	0.47 ± 0.012	0.75 ± 0.017
B Rfx (cm)	1.5 ± 0.029	1.8 ± 0.023
Rfy	0.37 ± 0.046	0.45 ± 0.006
C Rfx (cm)	3.8 ± 0.346	2.6 ± 0.058
Rfy	0.95 ± 046	0.65 ± 0.075
D Rfx (cm)	1.95 ± 0.029	3.2 ± 0.19
Rfy	0.48 ± 0.023	0.82 ± 0.214

Table 4. Observed changes during pineapple wine fermentation

Parameters (h)	Color	Taste	Others
A 24	Pineapple	Slightly sweet	Foamy with whitish suspension
48	Pineapple	Sour	Frosty
72	Pineapple	Sour	Flocs
144	Pineapple	Sour	Flocs
B 24	Pineapple	Sweet	Foamy with more whitish suspension than A
48	Pineapple	Sour	Frosty.
72	Pineapple	Sour	Flocs.
144	Pineapple	Sour	Flocs.
C 24	Pineapple	Sweet	Frosty suspension
48	Pineapple	Sour	Sediments
72	Pineapple	Sour	Flocs
144	Pineapple	Sour	Flocs
D 24	Whitish	Sweet	Highly foamy
48	Whitish	Sour	Foamy
72	Whitish	Sour	Flocs
144	Whitish	Sour	Flocs with clear suspension

The observed changes in specific gravity, % alcohol (v/v) and total aerobic counts of the wines with period of fermentation support the occurrence of microbial apparently due to varying tolerance for metabolic end products. These results agree with reports of Idise and Izuagbe (1988), Robinson, (2006) and Okafor (2007). Rf values presented in Table 3 indicate the occurrence of malo-lactic fermentation. There were no appreciably observed changes in the taste of the wines with different recipes presented in Table 4 as well as the statistical analysis which showed no difference at 95% confidence level for f-test. These results agree with reports of Idise and Izuagbe (1988), Kunkee and Goswell (2002),

Robinson, (2006) and Okafor (2007).

CONCLUSION AND RECOMMENDATIONS

Wines were produced from pineapple using its innate micro-organisms, granulated sugar and baker's yeast in varying proportions. There was evidence of Malo-lactic fermentation. The wines produced showed no appreciable differences in the tested parameters – pH, temperature, optical density, specific gravity, total aerobic counts, % alcohol (v/v) and % titratable acidity – taste-testing as well as statistically at 95% confidence level.

They could be consumed within 48 h. No chemical preservatives were required. However, there is the need for further research to ascertain the shelf life of the wines. Production of pineapple wine could be carried out using the flow chart.

REFERENCES

Adaikan P, Ganesan AA (2004). Mechanism of the Oxytoxic activity of Comosus proteinases. J. Pharm. Biol., 42(8): 646-655.

Amerine MA, Kunkee RE (2005). Microbiology of Winemaking. Am. Rev. Microbiol., 22: 232-258.

Cowan ST, Steel KJ (2004). Manual for the Identification of Medical Bacteria (3rded.). Cambridge University Press. London. p. 331.

Fawole MO, Oso BA (2008). Laboratory Manual of Microbiology. Spectrum Books ltd, Nigeria. p. 127.

Harrigan WF, McCane ME (2001). Laboratory Methods in Food and Dairy Microbiology. Academic Press, New York. p. 431.

Idise OE, Izuagbe YS (1985). Effect of preservatives and pasteurization on microorganisms isolated from Nigerian bottled palm wine. Microbios lett., 28(1): 117-121

Idise OE, Izuagbe YS (1988). Microbial and chemical changes in bottled palm wine during storage. Niger. J. Microbiol. 8(1): 175-184.

Kunkee RF, Amerine MA (2002). Yeast in Wine Making. In: Rose, H.A and Harrison, J.S. (Eds). The Yeast-Academic Press, London. pp. 5-71.

Kunkee RF, Goswell RW (2000). Table Wine. In: Alcoholic Beverages. Rose, H.A. (Ed.) Academic Press. London. pp. 315-338.

Maragatham C, Panneerselvam A (2011). Isolation, identification and characterization of wine yeast from rotten papaya fruits for wine production. Adv. Appl. Sci. Res., 2(2): 93-98.

Morton JF (1987). Fruits of warm climates. Miami printing press, Miami. pp. 18-28.

Ogunkoye L, Olubayo O (1977). Basic organic practical. 2nd Ed. University of Ife, Ile-Ife printing press. p. 240.

Okafor N (2007). Microbiology and Biochemistry of Oil Palmwine. Adv. Appl. Microbiol., 24: 237-255.

Robinson J (2006). The Oxford Companion to Wine. 3rd Ed. Oxford University Press. pp. 268-780.

Uraih N (2003). Public Health, Food Industr. Microbiol., (6th Edn.). The Macmillan Press Ltd., London. pp. 196-198.

2

Influence of biofertilizer on essential oil, harvest index and productivity effort of black cumin (*Nigella sativa* L.)

Seyed Alireza Valadabadi and Hossein Aliabadi Farahani

Faculty of Agriculture, Islamic Azad University, Shahr-e-Qods Branch, Tehran, Iran.

In order to investigate the effects of biofertilizer on essential oil harvest index and productivity effort of black cumin (*Nigella sativa L*), an experiment was conducted during the growing season of 2010 at Iran. The experimental design was factorial on the basis of randomized complete block design with three replications. Certain factors including four levels of animal manure (0, 10, 20 and 30 ton/ha, respectively) and two levels of azotobacter (non-application and application) were studied. The final statistical analysis indicated that in the 10 ton/ha animal manure and azotobacter application, essential oil, harvest index and productivity effort were significantly higher.

Key words: Biofertilizer, essential oil, *Nigella sativa*, harvest index.

INTRODUCTION

Nigella sativa is an annual flowering plant, native to southwest Asia. It grows to 20 to 30 cm in height, with finely divided, linear leaves. The flowers are delicate, and usually coloured pale blue and white, with 5 to 10 petals. The fruit is a large and inflated capsule composed of 3 to 7 united follicles, each containing numerous seeds. The seed is used as a spice. It is reported that intact black cumin seeds or their extracts have antidiabetic, anti-histaminic, antihypertensive, anti–inflammatory, antimic-robial, antitumor and insect repellent effects (Riaz et al., 1996; Siddiqui and Sharma, 1996: Worthen et al., 1998). Black cumin oil has been used for many centuries in the Asian, European, Arabian and the Mediterranean coun-tries. It is used for edible and medicinal purposes in Iran. The best method for extraction of black cumin oil is cold press; cold pressed oils are the highest quality oils available. The black cumin seed cake is a by-product obtained from the black cumin seeds with cold pressing and it is used in the production of bio-oil (Sen and Kar, 2012). Some studies show that the black cumin is able to tolerate moderate levels of water stress (Bannayan et al., 2008: Mozzafari et al., 2000). The potential of medicinal and aromatic plants to grow under limited water con-ditions make them suitable alternative crops in such agro-ecosystems (Koocheki and Nadjafi, 2003; Haj, 2011). Chemical fertilizers have several negative impacts on environment and sustainable agriculture. Therefore, bio-fertilizer is recommended in these conditions and growth prompting bacteria uses as a replacement for chemical fertilizers (Wu et al., 2005). Growth promoting bacteria are induced by increasing plant yield as clone in plant root (Gholami et al., 2009). Growth promoting bacteria include *Azotobacter*, *Azospirillum* and *Pseudomonas* (Turan et al., 2006). Tilak reported positive effects of double inoculation of maize and sorghum. *Azotobacter* is an anaerobic, free-living soil microbe which fixes nitrogen from the atmosphere. Beyond *Azotobacter* is used as a model. Organism has biotechnological applications. Examples are its use for alginate production and for nitrogen production in batch fermentations. Biofertilizers

Table 1. The result of soil analysis.

Soil texture	Sand (%)	Silt (%)	Clay (%)	K (mg/kg)	P (mg/kg)	N (mg/kg)	Na (Ds/m)	EC (1:2.5)	pH	Depth of sampling (cm)
Clay loam	35	30	35	142.2	5.2	38.7	0.05	0.18	7.9	0-30

are products containing living cells different types of microorganisms (Vessey, 2003; Chen, 2006) that have an ability to convert nutritionally important elements from unavailable to available form through biological processes (Vessey, 2003) and are known to help with expansion of the root system and better seed germination. Biofertilizers differ from chemical and organic fertilizers in that they do not directly supply any nutrients to crops and are cultures of special bacteria and fungi. Some microorganisms have positive effects on plant growth promotion, including the plant growth promoting rhizobacteria (PGPR) such as *Azospirillum, Azotobacter, Pseudomonas fluorescens* and several gram positive *Bacillus* spp. (Chen, 2006). *Azotobacter* and *Azospirillum* are free-living N_2 fixing-bacteria in the rhizospheric zone that have the ability to synthesize and secret some biologically active substances that enhance root growth. They also increase germination and vigour in young plants, leading to improved crop stands (Chen, 2006). It is well known that a considerable number of bacterial and fungal species possess a functional relationship and constitute a holistic system with plants. They are able to exert beneficial effects on plant growth (Vessey, 2003) and also enhance plant resistance to adverse environmental stresses, such as water and nutrient deficiency and heavy metal contamination (Wu et al., 2005).

Therefore, the objective of this study was to evaluate the biofertilizers influence on essential oil, harvest index) and productivity effort of black cumin *(Nigella sativa* L.

MATERIALS AND METHODS

This study was conducted on experimental field of Islamic Azad University, Shahr-e-Qods Branch at Iran (27°38' N,40°21'E;1417 m above sea level) during 2010, with clay loam soil (Table 1), mean annual temperature of 31°C and rainfall which is distributed with an annual mean of 215 mm. The experimental unit was designed to achieve treatments in factorial on the basis of randomized complete block design with three replications. Certain factors including four levels of animal manure (0, 10, 20 and 30 ton/ha, respectively) and two levels of azotobacter (non-application and application) were studied. The soil consisted of 35% clay, 30% silt and 35% sand (Table 1). Each experimental plot was 3 m long and 2 m wide. Sowing was done manually with 0.5 cm depth and in rows with 25 cm. Weeds were controlled manually. All necessary cultural practices and plant protection measures were followed uniformly for all the plots during the entire period of experimentation. At the end of the growth stage, we collected 10 plants from each plot randomly for determination of seed yield (kg/ha), capsule dry weight (kg/ha) and biological yield (kg/ha) and 100 g seed were selected from each plot for determination of essential oil percentage by were determined using the following formulas:

Clevenger. Finally, harvest index (H.I) and productivity effort (P.E)

H.I = Seed yield / biological yield

P.E=Capsule dry weight / biological yield

Data were subjected to analysis of variance (ANOVA) using Statistical Analysis System (SAS) and followed by Duncan's multiple range tests. Terms were considered significant at p<0.05.

RESULTS

Final results of plants values showed that azotobacter significantly affected essential oil (p≤0.01) harvest index and productivity effort (p≤ 0.05) (Table 2) which indicated that the highest essential oil (21.8 kg/ha), harvest index (22%) and productivity effort (0.36) were obtained by azotobacter application (Table 3). Also, animal manure significantly affected essential oil (p≤0.01), harvest index and productivity effort (p≤0.05). The highest essential oil (17.5 kg/ha) was obtained by application of 20 ton/ha animal manure but the highest productivity effort (0.34) and harvest index (18%) were obtained by application of 30 ton/ha animal manure (Table 3). Interaction of azotobacter and animal manure had significant effect on essential oil and harvest index but productivity effort did not respond to interaction of azotobacter and animal manure (Table 2) and highest essential oil (18.8 kg/ha), harvest index (21.2%) were obtained under application of azotobacter and 10 ton/ha animal manure (Table 4).

DISCUSSION

In this study, increases in agronomic criteria were observed following inoculation with *azotobacter*. This may be due to better utilization of nutrients in the soil through inoculation of efficient microorganisms (Deka et al., 1992; Dixon et al., 2004). A positive effect of *azotobacter* on yield and yield components has been reported in the literature (Migahed et al., 2004).The results showed that application of *azotobacter* and animal manure increased essesntial oil, harvest index and productivity effort of black cumin. It is indicated that using biofertilizers caused increased harvest index due to effect on dry weight and allocating more photosynthetic matters to grain (Kumar et al., 2009; Mandal et al., 2007). It seems that using biofertilizers led to increasing productivity by affecting plant dry weight and allocating more minerals to stems, leaves and grain, so increasing biological and grain yield. Bashan and Levanony (1990) have shown that inoculation of plants with azospirillum can result in a significant change in various plant growth parameters. Another corn study showed that seed inoculation with azotobacter produced

Table 2. Analysis of variance.

S.O.V	df	Mean square		
		Essential oil	Harvest index	Productivity effort
Replication	2	0.005	12.721	0.00422
Azotobacter (A)	1	0.071**	71.542*	0.00912*
Animal manure (M)	3	0.058**	24.372*	0.0139*
A × M	3	0.056**	9.340*	0.00673
Error	18	0.003	6.392	0.00376
CV (%)		2.77	8.08	11.05

*and**:Significant at 5 and 1% levels, respectively.

Table 3. Means comparison.

Treatment		Essential oil (kg/ha)	Harvest index (%)	Productivity effort
Azotobacter (A)	Non-application(A1)	14.8[b]	18.0[b]	0.33[b]
	Application (A2)	20.1[a]	22.0[a]	0.36[a]
Animal manure (M)	Non-application (M1)	16.5[b]	18.3[a]	0.33[b]
	10 ton/ha (M2)	16.6[b]	17.4[ab]	0.32[b]
	20 ton/ha (M3)	17.5[a]	16.6[b]	0.33[b]
	30 ton/ha (M4)	16.2[b]	18.0[a]	0.34[a]

Means within the same column and rows and factors, followed by the same letter are not significantly difference (P<0.05).

Table 4. Means comparison of interaction.

Treatment	Essential oil (kg/ha)	Harvest index (%)
(A1).(M1)	15.6[c]	18.0[c]
(A1).(M2)	15.7[c]	17.8[cd]
(A1).(M3)	16.1[c]	19.0[bc]
(A1).(M4)	15.7[d]	17.7[cd]
(A2).(M1)	18.2[b]	20.4[a]
(A2).(M2)	18.8[a]	21.2[a]
(A1).(M3)	16.3[c]	19.1[b]
(A2).(M4)	15.6[c]	18.2[c]

Means within the same column and row factors followed by the same letter are not significantly difference (P<0.05).

significantly higher dry matter than from non-inoculation (Chela et al., 1993). Manjunatha et al. (2002) conducted a study on the effect of biofertilizer on growth, yield and essential oil content in Patchouli (*Pogostemon cablin* Pellet). The treatments included three levels each of nitrogen (N) and phosphate (P_2O_5) (50, 75 and 100% of recommended) with potash (K_2O) at constant level of 50 kg/ha along with different biofertilizers Azotobacter, Azospirillum, phosphorus solubilising bacteria (PSB) and vesicular arbuscular mycorrhizal fungi (VAM) in combination. The results revealed that the treatments differed significantly; among the treatments, 75% NP + 100 K + *Azotobacter* + *Azospirillum* + VAM recorded

significantly superior values for plant height (80.14 cm), number of branches (22.04) and essential oil yield (71.74 l/ha) as compared to the control (47.5 l/ha). On the whole, the treatment with 75% NP + 100 K + *Azotobacter* + *Azospirillum* + VAM emerged as one of the best treatments and effected the saving of fertilizers to the extent of 25%. Also, an investigation was carried out under Madurai conditions of Tamil Nadu, India to study the influence of nitrogen, application of nitrogen and phosphorus on *Azospirillum* which gave the highest plant height, essential oil yield and harvest index. The changes were directly attributed to positive bacterial effects on mineral uptake by the plant. Enhancement in uptake of NO_3^-, NH_4^-, PO_4^{2-}, K^+ and Fe^{++} by *Azospirillum* (Barton et al., 1986; Murty and Ladha, 1987) was proposed to cause an increase in dry matter and accumulation.

Conclusion

In general, it appears that, as expected, application of azotobacter improved yield and other plant criteria. Therefore, it appears that application of azotobacter and animal manure could be promising in production of black cumin by reduction of chemical fertilizer application. Our finding may give application advice to farmers for management and concern on fertilizer strategy and carefully estimate chemical fertilizer supply by biofertilizers application.

REFERENCES

Barton IL, Johnson GV, Arbock MS (1997).The effect of azosprillum brasilnse on iron absorption and translocation by sorghum. J. Plant Nutr. 9:557- 565.

Bashan Y, Levanony H (1990). Current status ofzospirillum inoculation technology:Azospirillum as a challeng for agriculture. Can J. Microbial. 36:591-608.

Chen J (2006).The combined use of chemical and organic fertilizers and/or biofetilizer for crop growth and soil fertility.International Workshop on Sustained Management of the Soil-Rhizosphere System for Efficient Crop Production and Fertilizer Use.16- 20 October, Thailand.

Deka BC, Bora GC, Shaequel provide initial of author (1992). Effect of Azopirillum growth and yield of chilli (Capsicum annum L) cultivr Pusa Jawala.Haryana. J. Hot. Sci. 38:41-46.

Dixon R, Kahn D (2004). Jenetic iegulation of biological nitrogen fixation. Nat. Rev. Microbial. 2(8):621-631.

Gholami A, Shahsavani S, Nezarat S (2009).The effect of PlantGrowth Rhizobacteria(PGPR) on germination,seedling growth and yield of maize.World Acad. Sci. Eng.Technol. 49:19-24.

Koocheki A, Nadjafi F(2003) .The status of medicinal and aromatic plants in Iran and strategies for sustainable utilization. In: Abstract Book of The 3rd World Congress on Medicinal Aromatic Plants for HumanWelfare, Februrary3-7,2003,Chaing Mai, Thailland, p.283.

Kumar TS, Swaminathan V, Kumar S (2009). Influence of nitrogen, phosphorus and biofertilizers on growth, yield and essential oil constituents in ratoon crop of davana (Artemisia pallens Wall). Electronic J. Environ. Agric. Food Chem. 8(2):86-95.

Mandal A, Patra AK, Singh D, Swarup A, Ebhin Mast R (2007). Effect of long-term application of manure and fertilizer on biological and biochemical activities in soil during crop development stages. Biores. Technol. 98:3585-3592.

Manjunatha R, Farooqi AA, Vasundhara M, Srinivasappa KN (2002).Effect of biofertilizer on growth, yield and essential oil content in patchouli (Pogostemon cablin Pellet.). Indian Perfumer. 46 (2):97-104.

Migahed HA, Ahmed AE, Abd El-Ghany BF(2004). Effect of different bacterial strains as biofertilizer agents on growth, production and oil of Apium graveolense under Calcareous soil. J. Agric. Sci. 12:511-525.

Murty MG, Iadha JK (1987). Differential colonization of azospirillum lipoferum on roots of two varieties of rice (oryza sativa). Biol Fertil. Soil 4:3-7.

Sen N, Kar Y (2012).Pyrolysis of black cumin seed cake in a fixed-bed reactor. J. Biomass Bioenergy 35:4297-4304.

Siddiqui AA, Sharma PKR (1996).Clinical importance of Nigella sativa L. A review. Hamdard Med. 39(2):23-26.

Tilak KVBRM (1992). *Azospirillum brasilense* and *Azotobacter chrooccocum inoculum* effect of maize and sorghum. Soil Bio. Biochem.14;417-418.

Turan M, Ataoglu N, Sahin A (2006). Evaluation of the capacity of phosphate solubilizing bacteria and fungi on different forms of phosphorus in liquid culture. Sus. Agric. 28:99-108.

Vessey JK (2003). Plant growth promoting rhizobacteria as biofertilizers. Plant Soil 255:571-586.

Worthen DR, Ghoshen OA, Crooks PA (1998). The *in vitro* anti-tumor activity of some crude and purified components of black seed, *Nigella sativa* L. Anticancer Res. 18:1527-1532.

Wu SC, Caob ZH, Lib ZG, Cheung KC, Wong MH (2005). Effects of biofertilizer containing N-fixer, P and K solubilizers and AM fungi on maize growth : a greenhouse trial. Geoderma. 125:155-166.

3

Beta glucuronidase activity in early stages of rice seedlings and callus: A comparison with *Escherichia coli* beta glucuronidase expressed in the transgenic rice

Poosakkannu Anbu[1,2] and Loganathan Arul[1]

[1]Department of Plant Molecular Biology and Biotechnology, Centre for Plant Molecular Biology, Tamil Nadu Agricultural University, Coimbatore-641 003, India.
[2]Department of Biological and Environmental Sciences, University of Jyväskylä, P.O. Box, 35, FIN-40014, Finland.

We have chosen rice as a model crop to ascertain endogenous β-glucuronidase (family 79) activity and to differentiate the same from *Escherichia coli* based β-glucuronidase (family-2). The investigation dwells on characterizing endogenous β-glucuronidase (GUS) activity during the early stages of seed germination and from rice callus. Also, similar studies were made from homozygous transgenic rice line expressing *E. coli* GUS under the control of *glyoxalase I* promoter. Endogenous GUS activity was detected in plumules, shoots and calli of rice, nevertheless, showing differential response to pH. Further, endogenous GUS in rice was specifically inhibited by saccharic acid 1,4-lactone (SL) but, the *E. coli* β-glucuronidase remain unaffected, indicating distinct biochemical properties of family-2 and family-79 β-glucuronidase.

Key words: Family 2, family 79, X-gluc, saccharic acid, 1,4-lactone.

INTRODUCTION

Glycosyl hydrolases hydrolyze the glycosidic bond in carbohydrates or between a carbohydrate and a non carbohydrate moiety. β-Glucuronidase (GUS) is classified into three glycosyl hydrolase families 1, 2 and 79. Found in the GH1 family, klotho is a type I membrane protein from mammals that hydrolyzes steroid beta-glucuronides (Tohyama et al., 2004). The family-2 β-glucuronidase is reported in a wide range of organisms. The bacterial gene uidA, encoding the family 2 β-glucuronidase, has been used extensively as a reporter gene in genetic transformation experiments (Jefferson et al., 1987; 1989). Another category of β-glucuronidase belongs to the family-79 of glycosyl hydrolases in the carbohydrate-active enzymes (CAZY) database, which also includes

mammalian heparanases that degrade the carbohydrate moieties of cell surface proteoglycans, flavones specific beta glucuronidase (sGUS) from *Scutellaria baicaleinsis* (Sasaki et al., 2004) and an *Arabidopsis thaliana* beta-D-glucuronidase (AtGUS) was recently shown to hydrolyse glucuronic acids from carbohydrate chains of arabino-galactan protein (Eudes et al., 2008; Konishi et al., 2008).

Biochemical studies of family 79 GUS in plants are limited. Schulz and Weissenbock (1987) reported partial purification and characterization of a specific GUS from rye primary leaves and further, Hu et al. (1990) surveyed 52 plant species for intrinsic GUS like activity using either the quantitative flourimetric GUS assay where the tissues were assayed for 24 h or the histochemical assay which

Table 1. Composition of GUS staining solution.

Ingredient	Volume (μl mL^{-1})
0.1 M EDTA (pH 8.0)	100
100 mM Phosphate buffer[*]	500
1% Triton X-100	100
50 mM potassium ferrocyanide	20
50 mM potassium ferricyanide	20
Methanol	200
100 mM X-Gluc	20
Sterile distilled water	40

*Citrate phosphate and sodium phosphate buffers were used to produce the pH gradient (3.0 - 7.0) in the GUS assay solution.

required an overnight incubation in the staining solution. Under these conditions, they reported that with few exceptions, the GUS activity was detected in certain part(s) of the fruit wall, seed coat, endosperm or the embryos of the tested plants. In addition, *S. baicalensis* has long been known to possess a GUS, called baicalinase (Levvy, 1954). The GUS enzyme from *S. baicalensis* has been purified and was found to provide protection to *Scutellaria* cells against oxidative stress (Matsuda et al., 1995; Morimoto et al., 1995, 1998). Muhitch (1998) reported endogenous GUS activity in the pedicel of developing maize kernels which had an estimated Mw of ca. 32 kDa, stimulated by assay at 60°C and showed inhibition of activity at high ionic strength or in the presence of EDTA. Sudan et al. (2006) used a pharmacological inhibitor of β-GUS, saccharic acid 1,4-lactone (SL) and demonstrated that its application to seedlings of model plant species, such as *Nicotiana tabacum*, resulted in the arrest of growth and the inhibition of root-hair development. Further, Schoenbeck et al. (2007) studied the beta-glucuronidase activity in seedlings of the parasitic angiosperm *Cusctua pentagona* and developmental impact of the beta-glucuronidase inhibitor saccharic acid 1,4-lactone. Also, *Coffea arabica* and *Coffea canephora* embryogenic calli and somatic embryos (Sreenath and Naveen, 2004), *Capsicum chinense* zygotic embryo (Solís-Ramos et al., 2010) and rapeseed microspores and microspore-derived embryos (Abdollahi et al., 2011) were found to have endogenous GUS activity which interferes with the expression of bacterial β-glucuronidase that was transiently expressed in these tissues.

While undertaking the molecular characterization of transgenic Pusa Basmati 1 carrying *Escherichia coli* uidA driven by rice *glyoxalase I* promoter, we carried out GUS assay, an intense blue color developed not only in the transformed explants but also in the untransformed control explants. Captivatingly, the present study was undertaken to characterize the endogenous beta glucuronidase in rice and to differentiate the same from *E. coli* beta glucuronidase.

MATERIALS AND METHODS

Plant material

Rice cultivars, Pusa Basmathi 1 and ADT 43 (obtained from Paddy Breeding Station, TNAU, Coimbatore) and transgenic Pusa Basmati 1 carrying *E. coli* uidA driven by rice glyoxalase I promoter (homozygous transgenic lines (T$_4$ generation) were developed by Dr. L. Arul in an independent study meant for isolating abiotic stress inducible promoters in rice, unpublished data) were used in this investigation. Seeds were surface sterilized with 70% ethanol and 0.1% HgCl$_2$, intervened by several washes with sterile double distilled water. Sterilized seeds were placed in jam bottles containing 0.6% agar for germination. All the cultures were maintained at a photoperiod of 16 h light and 8 h dark at 25±1°C for germination. Three days old plumules and five days old shoots were used for assaying GUS activity.

Callus induction

Calli were induced from ADT 43 and transgenic Pusa Basmati 1 (transgenic and non-transgenic) as per Sudhakar et al. (1998). Dehusked and surface sterilized seeds were placed in a Petri dish containing MS medium supplemented with 2.5 mg L^{-1} of 2,4-D and 3% sucrose. The seeds were incubated in dark at 25 ± 1°C. Fifteen days old calli were used for analysing GUS activity.

Histochemical assay

GUS assay was performed as suggested by Jefferson (1987) and, the assay was carried out at different pH conditions. The GUS assay solutions (composition shown in Table 1) buffered with different pH was prepared using citrate phosphate buffer (pH 3.0, 4.0 and 5.0) and sodium phosphate buffer (pH 6.0 and 7.0). Plant materials were kept in 1.5 mL Eppendorf tubes by completely immersing in GUS staining solution and, incubated overnight at 37°C. For removal of chlorophyll from the GUS stained tissues, the plant materials were immersed in 70% ethanol and incubated for 6 h at 37°C. The ethanol solution was changed twice at 2 to 3 h intervals.

Saccharic acid 1, 4-lactone (SL) treatment

Three days old plumules and five days old shoots of ADT 43 and transgenic Pusa Basmati 1 were soaked in 40 mM SL and incubated for 3 h at room temperature. SL solutions at pH 4.0 and 7.0 were prepared using citrate phosphate buffer and sodium phosphate buffer, respectively. Simultaneously, a set of plumules and shoots were maintained as controls at pH 4.0 and 7.0 without SL. The treated and control seeds were washed with sterile distilled water 3 to 4 times and GUS assay was performed at pH 4.0 and 7.0.

Microtome sectioning

GUS assayed tissues were preserved in 70% ethanol. Transverse section of plumules and shoots were taken without any additional staining and mounted on slides for long time preservation.

RESULTS

Histochemical assay shows GUS activity in rice Non-transgenic, and transgenic rice carrying GUS reporter

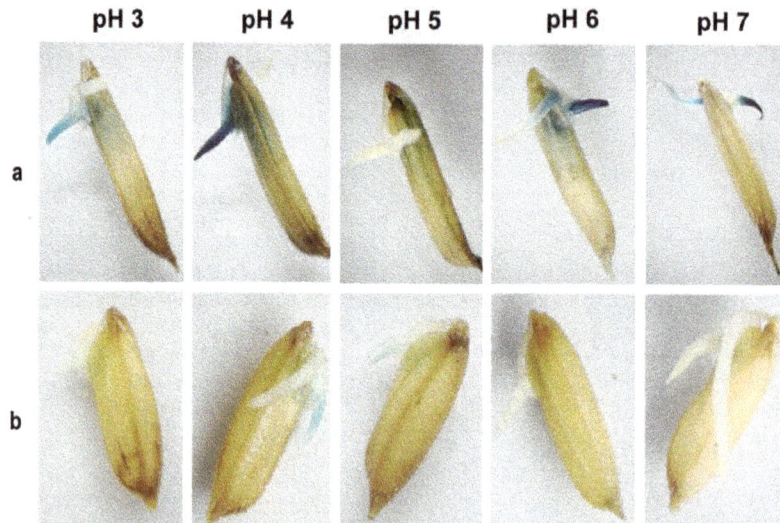

Figure 1. Plumules of transgenic rice (a) and non-transgenic rice (b) showing differential GUS activity between pH 3 and 7.

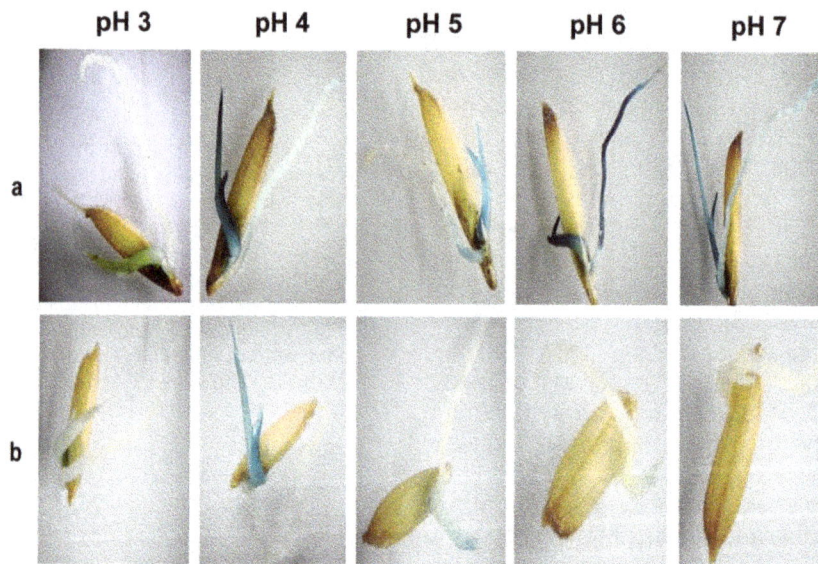

Figure 2. Shoots of transgenic rice (a) and non-transgenic rice (b) showing differential GUS activity between pH 3 and 7.

under the control of rice *glyoxalase I* promoter, showed differential GUS staining when assayed for β-glucuronidase activity with X-gluc at varying pH conditions. Three days old plumules, five days old shoots and fifteen days old scutellar derived calli were used for assaying GUS activity. Transgenic rice harbouring *E. coli* borne uidA showed continuous β-glucuronidase activity between pH 3.0 and 7.0, the maximal colour development was observed at pH 4.0 and 7.0, respectively (Figures 1, 2, 3 and 4). In the case of non-transgenic rice, plumules, shoots and calli showed blue colour but restricted to lower pH 3.0, 4.0 and 5.0, respectively (Figures 1, 2, 3 and 4). In the latter, maximum histochemical staining was

observed at pH 4.0.

Saccharic acid 1,4-lactone (SL), an inhibitor of GUS activity

Non-transgenic and transgenic plumules and shoots were treated with 40 mM saccharolactone prior to GUS assay. The results of the study revealed the complete absence of histochemical staining at pH 4.0 and 7.0, in non-transgenic rice (Figures 5 and 6). In contrast, plumules and shoots of transgenic rice treated with SL gave rise to blue colour only at pH 7.0, but lacked histochemical staining at pH 4.0 (Figures 5 and 6).

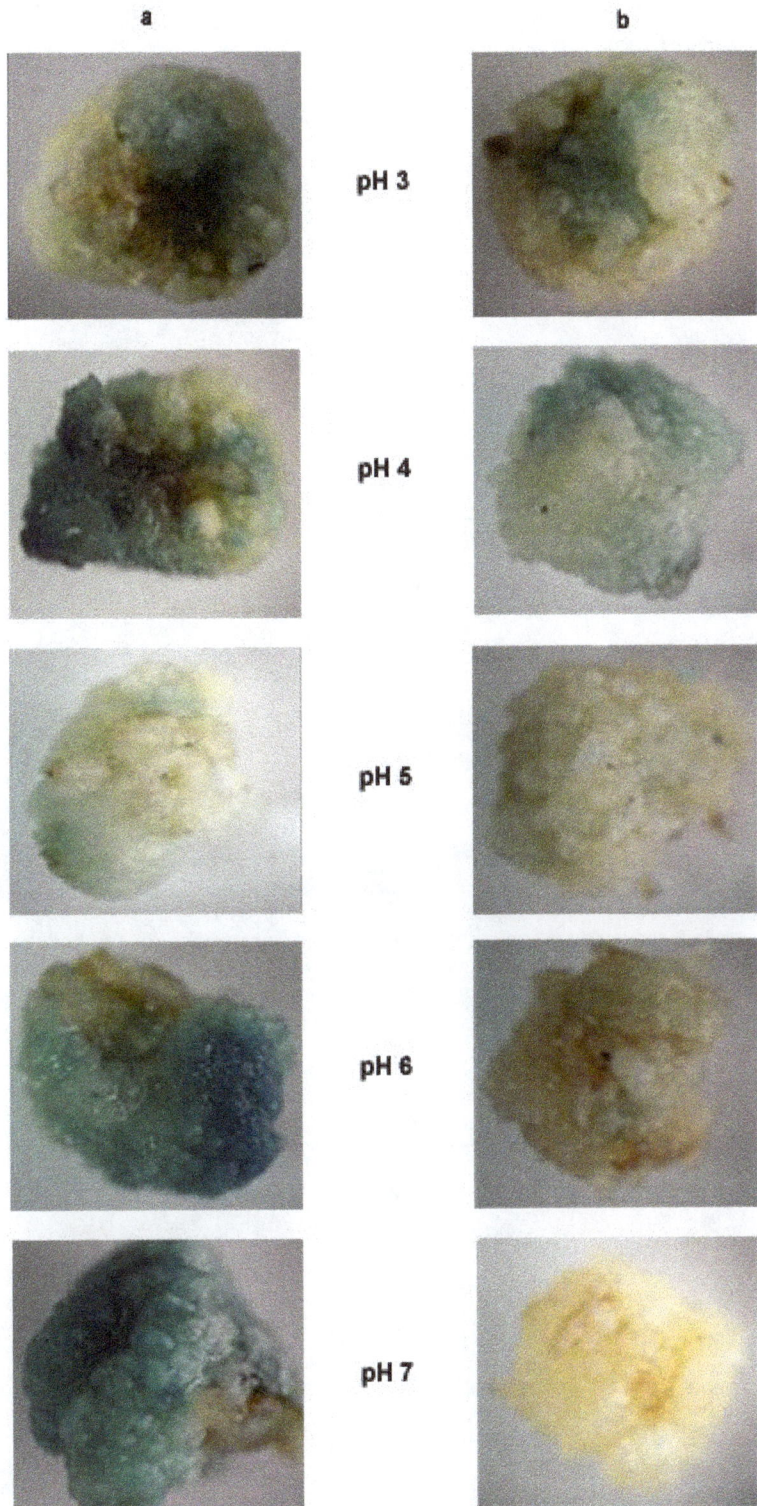

Figure 3. Transgenic rice (a) and non-transgenic rice (b) calli showing differential GUS activity between pH 3 and 7.

DISCUSSION

β-Glucuronidase (GUS) is a glycosyl hydrolase and well known to the plant biologists because of the use of uidA from *E. coli* for gene expression studies (Jefferson et al., 1987). Most β-glucuronidases characterized so far have been classified under glycosyl hydrolase family-2. However, a small number of β-glucuronidases are categorized

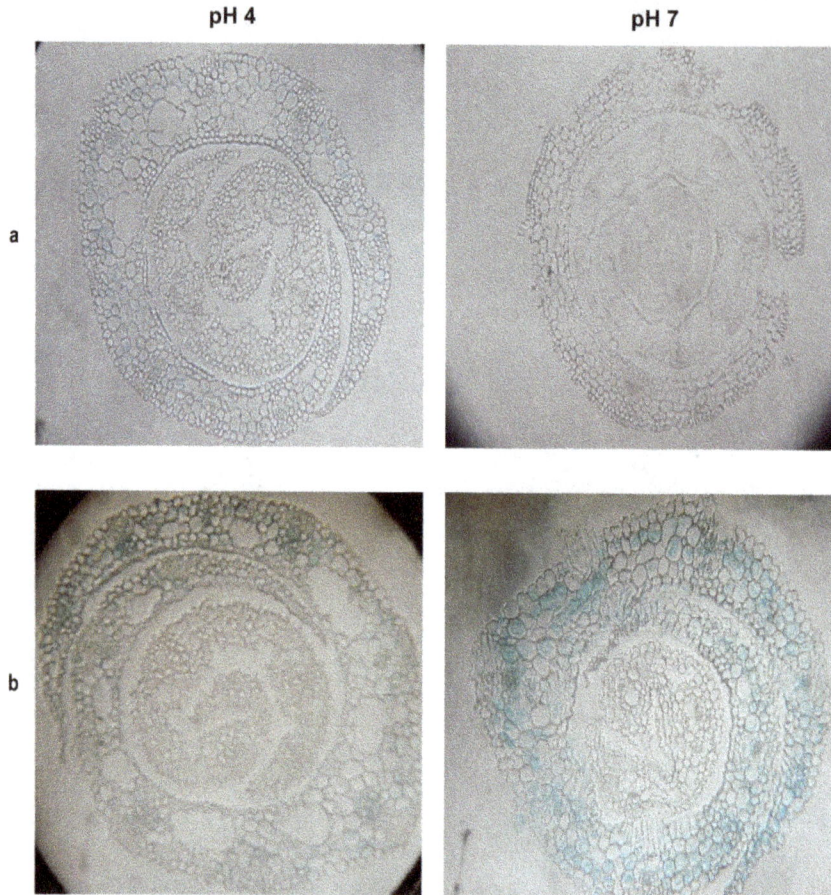

Figure 4. Transverse section of the roots of non-transgenic rice (a) and transgenic rice (b) showing differential GUS activity staining at pH 3 to 7, respectively. Lack of blue colour was observed in the shoots of non-transgenic rice at pH 7.

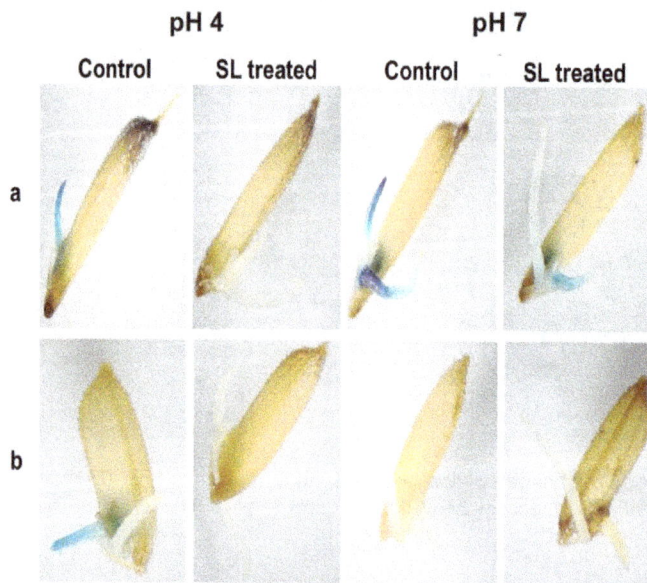

Figure 5. Saccharic acid 1,4-lactone (SL) treated and untreated (control) transgenic rice (a) and non-transgenic rice (b) plumules showing differential GUS activity at pH 4 to 7, respectively.

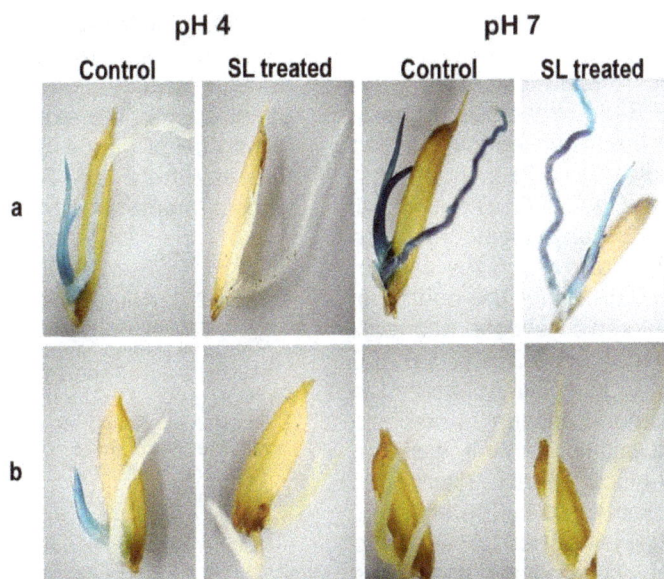

Figure 6. Saccharic acid 1,4-lactone (SL) treated and untreated (control) transgenic rice (a) and non-transgenic rice (b) shoots showing differential GUS activity staining at pH 4 to 7, respectively.

under family-1 and 79 glycosyl hydrolases, but their properties and biological functions have not yet been extensively investigated.

The family-79 β-glucuronidase is also referred to as heparanase, in human, it catalyzes the hydrolysis of heparan sulfate by cleaving the β-1,4-glycosidic bond between D-glucuronate and D-glucosamine in heparan sulfate (a sulfated polysaccharide that is found on the surface of most mammalian cells as part of proteoglycans). Besides vertebrates, heparanase orthologous genes have been reported in a few microorganisms (*Bradyrhizobium japonicum*, *Burkholderia mallei*, *Burkholderia pseudomallei*, *Marinomonas* sp., *Novosphingobium aromaticivorans*, *Saccharophagus degradans*, *Solibacter usitatus*) and in plants as well (*Scutellaria baicalensis*, *Arabidopsis thaliana*, *Oryza sativa*, *Hordeum vulgare*, *Zea mays* and *Medicago truncatula*). The occurrence of endogenous GUS (family-79) activity in plants was reported more than half a century ago by Levvy (1954). The only plant β-glucuronidase which has been thoroughly characterized till date is sGUS from *S. baicalensis* Georgi (Sasaki et al., 2000). Three *AtGUS* genes showing high similarity with *sGUS* were cloned from *A. thaliana*, the *AtGUS1/2* encoded proteins were predicted to be family-79 β-glucuronidase and showed appreciable similarity to heparanase of human, mouse and rat (Woo et al., 2007). In our study, we have chosen rice, a model crop to ascertain endogenous β-glucuronidase (family-79) activity and to differentiate the same from *E. coli* based β-glucuronidase (family-2). Histochemical assay with X-gluc was done along with/without a specific competitive inhibitor saccharic acid 1,4-lactone (SL) which interfered with the

GUS activity. The investigation dwells on characterizing endogenous GUS activity during the early stages of seed germination and also from rice callus. Also, similar studies were made from homozygous transgenic rice line (T_4-generation) expressing *E. coli* GUS under the control of glyoxalase I promoter. Histochemical assay was carried out in rice plumule, shoots and calli. The assay was done between pH 3.0 and pH 7.0 for transgenic and non-transgenic rice, concurrently. The pH of the assay buffer turned out to be very critical for the detection of GUS activity in plants. Non-transgenic rice was found to display differential GUS staining when assayed at varying pH conditions. The plumule, shoots and calli of the non-transgenic rice showed blue stain only between pH 3.0 and 5.0 demonstrating the presence of endogenous β-glucuronidase activity at a lower pH range. Earlier, Sasaki et al. (2000) had reported that family-79 β-glucuronidase (sGUS) from *Scutellaria* catalyzed the cleavage of glucuronic acid from baicalein 7-O-β-D-glucuronide in an H_2O_2 induced acidic cellular environment. Further, Woo et al. (2007) reported the presence of endogenous GUS activity in vegetative and floral organs of *A. thaliana* at pH 5.0. Alwen et al. (1992) also reported endogenous GUS activity at pH 5.0 in a wide variety of plant species. It has also been reported that endogenous GUS activity in rye, potato, apple and almonds is optimal between pH 4.0 and 5.0 (Hodal et al., 1992). Besides, heparanase in animals (vertebrates and invertebrates) are known to have an acidic pH optimum for its activity. The human heparanase has a pH optimum between 3.5 and 5.0 (Levvy and Marsh, 1959; Dutton, 1980). In *Caenorhabditis elegans*, the GUS has its optimum activity at pH 5.0 (Sebastiano et al., 1986) and between pH 3.0 and 5.5 in

Drosophila (Langley et al., 1983). In contrast, *E. coli* β-glucuronidase belonging to family-2 glycosyl hydrolase has an optimal activity at pH of 7.0 (Jefferson, 1987). It is understandable that, family-79 β-glucuronidase (heparanase) is largely responsible for the histochemical staining that we observed at acidic pH (3.0 - 5.0) in non-transgenic rice. On the other hand, the lack of GUS staining at pH 7.0 indicates the absence of any β-glucuronidase activity on the physiological pH. However, in the case of transgenic rice carrying *E. coli* uidA under the control of rice glyoxalase I promoter, plumule, shoots and calli developed blue colour in almost all pH 3.0, 4.0, 5.0, 6.0 and 7.0. The wide spectrum of GUS activity observed in transgenic rice as compared to non-transgenic rice could be traced back to two different origins, partly it is due to the action of endogenous β-glucuronidase (family-79) between pH 3.0 and 5.0, complemented by the action of *E. coil* β-glucuronidase (family-2) between pH 6.0 and 7.0. These results are consistent with findings of previous researchers in which they used transiently expressed plant tissues (Sreenath and Naveen, 2004; Solís-Ramos et al., 2010; Abdollahi et al., 2011).

Further in this direction, we carried out GUS assay in the presence of saccharic acid 1,4-lactone (SL), a well known inhibitor of endogenous β-glucuronidase. There was a complete absence of blue staining at pH 4.0 and pH 7.0 in non-transgenic rice where as the control (untreated with SL) showed histochemical reaction at pH 4.0 but not at pH 7.0, indicating specific inhibition of endogenous GUS activity only at pH 4.0. Alwen et al. (1992) reported 50% inhibition with 5 mM SL and up to 75% inhibition of GUS activity with 25 mM of SL in plant species belonging to different families. In our study, we have observed 100% inhibition with 40 mM SL. In contrast, shoots of transgenic rice treated with SL gave rise to blue colour at pH 7.0, but showed no GUS staining at pH 4.0 indicating the suppression of only the endogenous GUS activity. This is suggestive of the fact that β-glucuronidase activity at pH 7.0 which is due to *E. coli* GUS (family-2) remains unaffected. On expected lines, transgenic shoots untreated for the inhibitor (SL) showed histochemical staining at pH 4.0 and 7.0 as well. Our study presents a comparative account on family-79 and family-2 β-glucuronidase in a stably transformed plant (T_4 generation) model system such as rice. We have demonstrated the occurrence of endogenous GUS activity in the early developmental stages of rice. The use of a specific inhibitor, saccharic acid 1,4-lactone, clearly demonstrates that family-2 and 79 β-glucuronidases are biochemically different from each other however, are involved in a common function, that is, cleavage of the glucuronide moiety from their respective substrates. Although this property is shared by the endogenous and *E. coli* β-glucuronidases, the two activities can be distinguished by: (i) their different pH optima (4.0) for the endogenous activity and close to neutral (7.0) for the *E. coli* beta glucuronidase and (ii) their different sensitivity to the

specific inhibitor saccharic acid-1,4-lactone. The present study suggested that care should be taken to analyse the transgenic plants with GUS reporter system. Therefore, under appropriate experimental conditions such as maintaining pH of the GUS assay buffer to pH 7, it is possible to assay the *E. coli* β-glucuronidase in transgenic plants without interference from the endogenous plant activity.

REFERENCES

Abdollahi MR, Rajabi Memari H, van Wijnen AJ (2011). Factor affecting the endogenous β-glucuronidase activity in rapeseed haploid cells: How to avoid interference with the Gus transgene in transformation studies. Gene 487:96-102.

Alwen A, Benito Moreno RM, Vicente O, Heberle-Bors E (1992). Plant endogenous beta-glucuronidase activity: how to avoid interference with the use of the *E. coli* betaglucuronidase as a reporter gene in transgenic plants. Trans. Res.1:63-70.

Arul L, Benita G, Sudhakar D, Thayumanavan B, Balasubramanian P (2008). Beta-glucuronidase of family-2 glycosyl hydrolase: A missing member in plants. Bioinform. 3:194-197.

Dutton CJ (1980). Glucuronidation of drugs and other compounds. CRC Press, Boca Raton.

Eudes A, Mouille G, Thévenin J, Minic Z, Jouanin L (2008). Purification, cloning and functional characterization of an endogenous beta-glucuronidase in *Arabidopsis thaliana*. Plant Cell Physiol. 49:1331-1341.

Hodal L, Bochardt A, Nielsen JE, Mattsson O, Okkels FT (1992). Detection, expression and specific elimination of endogenous β-glucuronidase activity in transgenic and non-transgenic plants. Plant Sci. 87:115-122.

Hu CY, Chee PP, Chesney RH, Zhou JH, Miller PD, O'Brien WT (1990). Intrinsic GUS-like activities in seed plants. Plant Cell Rep. 9:1-5.

Jefferson RA (1987). Assaying chimeric genes in plants: The β-glucuronidase gene fusion system. Plant Mol. Biol. Rep. 5:387-405.

Jefferson RA (1989). The GUS reporter gene system. Nat. 342:837-838.

Jefferson RA, Kavanagh TA, Bevan MW (1987). GUS fusions:β-glucuronidase as a sensitive and versatile gene fusion marker in plants. EMBO. J. 6:3901-3907.

Konishi T, Kotake T, Soraya D, Matsuoka K, Koyama T, Kaneko S, Igarashi K, Samejima M, Tsumuraya Y (2008). Properties of family 79 beta-glucuronidases that hydrolyze beta-glucuronosyl and 4-O-methyl-beta-glucuronosyl residues of arabinogalactan-protein. Carbohydr. Res. 343:1191-1201.

Langley SD, Wilson SD, Gros AS, Warner CK, Finnerty V (1983). A genetic variant of β-glucuronidase in *Drosophila melanogaster*. J. Biol. Chem. 258:7416-7424.

Levvy GA (1954). Baicalinase, a plant β-glucuronidase. Biochem. J. 56:462-469.

Levvy GA, Marsh CA (1959). Preparation and properties of β-glucuronidase. Adv. Carbohydr. Chem.14:381-428.

Matsuda T, Hatano K, Harioka T, Taura F, Tanaka H, Tateishi N, Shan S, Morimoto S, Shoyama Y (1995). Histochemical investigation of β-glucuronidase in culture cells and regenerated plants of *Scutellaria baicalensis* Georgi. Physiol. Plant. 19:390-394.

Morimoto S, Harioka T, Shoyama Y (1995). Purification and characterization of flavone-specific β-glucuronidase from callus cultures of *Scutellaria baicalensis* Georgi. Planta 195:535-540.

Morimoto S, Tateishi N, Matsuda T, Tanaka H, Taura F, Furuya N, Matsuyama N, Shoyama Y (1998). Novel hydrogen peroxide metabolism in suspension cells of *Scutellaria baicalensis* Georgi. J.Biol. Chem. 273:12606-12611.

Muhitch MJ (1998). Characterization of pedicel β-glucuronidase activity in developing maize (*Zea mays*) kernels. Physiol. Plant. 104:423-430.

Sasaki K, Taura F, Shoyama Y, Morimoto S (2000). Molecular characterization of a novel beta-glucuronidase from *Scutellaria baicalensis* Georgi. J. Biol. Chem. 275:27466-27472.

Sasaki N, Higashi N, Taka T, Nakajima M, Irimura T (2004). Cell surface localization of heparanase on macrophages regulates degradation of extracellular matrix heparin sulfate. J. Immunol. 172:3830-3835.

Schoenbeck MA, Swanson GA, Brommer SJ (2007). β-Glucuronidase activity in seedlings of the parasitic angiosperm *Cusctua pentagona*: developmental impact of the β–glucuronidase inhibitor saccharic acid 1,4-lactone. Funct. Plant Biol. 34:81-821.

Schulz M, Weissenbock G (1987). Partial purification and characterization of a luteolintriglucuronide-specific β-glucuronidase from rye primary leaves (*Secale cereale*). Phytochem. 26:933-937.

Sebastiano M, D'Alessio M, and Bazzicalupo P (1986). β-glucuronidase mutants of the nematode *Caernohabditis elegans*. Genet. 112:459-468.

Solís-Ramos LY, González-Estrada T, Andrade-Torres A, Godoy-Hernández G, de la Serna EC (2009). Endogenous GUS-like activity in *Capsicum chinense* Jacq. Electronic J. Biotech. 13:1-7

Sreenath HL, Naveen KS (2004). Survey of endogenous β-glucuronidase (GUS) activity in coffee tissues and development of an assay for specific elimination of this activity in transgenic coffee tissues. 20th International Conference on Coffee Science, Bangalore, India, 11–15 October.

Sudan C, Prakash S, Bhomkar P, Jain S, Bhalla-Sarin N (2006). Ubiquitous presence of beta-glucuronidase (GUS) in plants and its regulation in some model plants. Planta 224:853-854.

Sudhakar D, Duc LT, Bong BB, Tinjuangjun P, Maqbool SB, Valdez M, Jefferson R, Christou P (1998). An Efficient Rice Transformation System Utilizing Mature Seed-derived Explants and a Portable, Inexpensive Particle Bombardment Device. Transgenic Res. 7:289-294.

Tohyama O, Imura A, Iwano A, Freund JN, Henrissat B, Fujimori T, Nabeshima Y (2004). Klotho is a novel beta-glucuronidase capable of hydrolyzing steroid betaglucuronides. J. Biol. Chem. 279:9777-9784.

Woo HH, Jeong BR, Hirsch AM, Hawes MC (2007). Characterization of *Arabidopsis* AtUGT85A and AtGUS gene families and their expression in rapidly dividing tissues. Genom. 90:143-153.

4

Development of cost-effective media for the culture of *Chilo partellus* larvicide in Kenya

Daniel Anyika[1]*, Hamadi Boga[2] and Romano Mwirichia[1]

[1]Institute for Biotechnology Research, Jomo Kenyatta University of Agriculture and Technology (JKUAT),
P.O. Box 62000, Nairobi, 00200, Kenya.
[2]Department of Botany, Faculty of Science, Jomo Kenyatta University of Agriculture and Technology (JKUAT),
P.O. Box 62000, Nairobi, 00200, Kenya.

Stem borers (*Chilo partellus*) are important field insect pests of maize (*Zea mays* L.) and sorghum (*Sorghum bicolor* L.) in Africa. They account for more than 30% yield losses depending on the composition of the pest community. *C. partellus* larvicide like *Bacillus thuringiensis* have been widely and effectively used in *C. partellus* control programs, but the industrial production of theses bacilli is expensive. Here we have attempted to develop three cost-effective media, based on legumes, potato, and whey. Growth and production of the insecticidal proteins from these bacteria were satisfactory; protein concentration yields of 27.60 mg/ml, spore counts of 5.60×10^8 CFU/ ml and first-instar *Chilo partellus* larvicidal activity (LC_{50}) of 78 µg/l were obtained with a 72 h culture of this bacterium. Therefore, this investigation suggests that legume, potato and whey-based culture media are more economical and effective for the industrial production of *B. thuringiensis* insecticidal crystal proteins.

Key words: *Bacillus thuringiensis*, larvicidal, *Chilo partellus*, insecticidal crystal proteins, LC_{50}, optical density, sulphate polyacrylamide gel electrophoresis (SDS-PAGE), spore counts.

INTRODUCTION

In Kenya, the spotted stem borers (*Chilo partellus*) destroy an estimated 400,000 metric tons or 13.5% of farmers annual harvest of maize costing about >US$72 million (De Groote, 2002). The management of *C. partellus* has largely been based on chemicals, which are rarely effective particularly due to misuse and resistance development by the pest (Camilla, 2000). In addition, small scale farmers, who form the bulk of the maize producers in Kenya, cannot afford those (Bonhof et al., 2001). Technologies that can reduce yield losses from *C. partellus* damage are necessary to increase maize production to cope with increasing demand for maize in Kenya. Berliner (*Bt*) was thus considered as a possible component in such a pest management system and a series of investigations was undertaken to elucidate its potential for inclusion in such a program (Mugo et al., 2007). In the recent past, it has been the most successful commercial biopesticide with its worldwide application (Pena et al., 2007). When compared with the chemical pesticides, *Bt* has the advantages of being biologically degradable, selectively active on pests and less likely to cause resistance (Lambert and Peferoen, 1992). *Bt* synthesizes an insecticidal cytoplasmic protein inclusion during the stationary phase of its growth cycle (Pena et al., 2007). These crystalline inclusions comprise relatively high quantities of one or more glycoproteins known as delta-endotoxins or cryotoxins (Schnepf et al., 1998). The

*Corresponding authors. E-mail: dankwalimwa@gmail.com.

insecticidal activity of *Bt* was attributed largely or completely (depending on the insect) to these parasporal crystals (Bravo et al., 2007). The crystal proteins accumulate in the mother cell and are released upon completion of sporulation (Aronson et al., 1995). Usually *Bt* strains isolated locally are more effective than imported strains due to higher specificity on target host, greater field persistence due to higher adaptation to the natural environment and toxicity at a higher temperature range (Brownbridge, 1991). To derive full benefit from the *Bt* based biopesticides, there is a need for studying influence of carbon-source from cost-effective raw materials on growth, sporulation and crystal protein production by local *Bt* strains that would be used as biopesticides for the indigenous crops.

MATERIALS AND METHODS

Bacteria

Cultures of *B, thuringiensis* subspecies *kenyae (Bt)* were provided by Mr. Richard Rotich, from the Kenya Agricultural Research Insitute (KARI), Nairobi Kenya. Also used in this study were *Bt* strains isolated from soils and termite mounds collected from Kalunya Glade and Lirhanda Hill in Kakamega Forest, Kenya and also from soil samples from Juja, Kenya.

Bacterial culture media

The conventional laboratory culture broth Nutrient Yeast Extract Medium (NYSM), used as reference medium in the present study was prepared by mixing glucose (5 g), peptone (5 g), NaCl (5 g), beef extract (3 g), yeast extract (0.5 g), mineral solutions (10.0 g/l cow blood; 0.02 g/l $MnCl_2.4H_2O$ (s. d. fine-chem ltd); 0.05 g/l $MgSO_4.7H_2O$ (Lab Tech Chemicals); and 1.0 g/l $CaCO_3$ (Sigma-Aldrich, Germany) (10 ml) in an appropriate volume (1 L) of double distilled water (pH 7.5). Legumes, potato and whey-based culture media was collected from farms and brought to the laboratory, washed in tap water, air-dried and stored at room temperature. A known quantity of these dried substrates (10 g/l) was boiled in ordinary tap water for 15 min. After cooling, the extracts were filtered and the pH of the filtrate was adjusted (pH 7.5). 1 L volume of the extract medium was dispensed in each of the three conical flasks (2 L capacities each) for culturing *Bt*. Similarly, flasks were kept for conventional medium (NYSM) also. All the culture media were autoclaved (at 120 °C/20 lb/in^2/20 min).

Bacterial growth

A small amount of *Bt* was inoculated separately in 2 ml each NYSM medium and allowed to grow for 12 h at 37°C as pre-cultures (50 µl each) were inoculated into sterile culture media. The cultures were allowed to grow under constant agitation (120 rev/min) at 37°C in an orbital shaker. Culture samples (2 ml) were drawn from each culture medium at 6 h intervals from 0 to 72 h. The pH and culture turbidity were measured using a digital pH meter and UV-VIS spectrophotometer. These were also examined microscopically for the presence of spore-crystal mixtures (Maniatis et al., 1982).

Total viable cell count and spore count

Total viable cell and spore counts were determined in the final whole culture by the pour plate method. Serial decimal dilutions of the final whole culture were made in sterile 1% peptone water (Oxoid), and 0.5 ml of each dilution in triplicate was added to a Petri dish, followed by the addition of 10 ml of plate count agar (Oxoid) at 45°C. The culture and agar were mixed thoroughly and allowed to set. Plates were incubated at 32°C for 24 to 48 h. Plates with 30 to 300 colonies were counted with a colony counter (Gallenkamp Ltd.). For spore counts, cultures were pasteurized at 65°C for 20 min before serial dilutions were made (Hoben and Somasegaran, 1982).

Spore-crystal toxin recovery from culture media

As soon as the cultures were fully sporulated, the spore-crystal toxin complex was recovered by centrifugation (10,000 *g*/30 min/4°C) using super speed centrifuge and the spore-crystal free supernatants were discarded. The spore-crystal mixtures were thoroughly washed three times each with 0.1 M NaCl and sterile double distilled water (10,000 *g*/30 min/4°C). Finally, these were washed with protease inhibitor, phenyl methyl sulphonyl fluoride (PMSF, 1mM, Sigma), re-suspended in the required volume of double distilled water and stored at -20°C, until further use, for biochemical studies and toxicity bioassays (Wessel and Flugge, 1984).

Protein estimation

A small volume of the stored spore/crystal sample was centrifuged (10,000 *g*/15 min/4°C) and the pellets were solubilized in solubilization buffer (50 mM $NaHCO_3$, 10 mM dithiothreitol, pH 10) and incubated for 2 to 3 h, at 25 to 30°C. After centrifugation and extraction (same rpm as above), the pure solubilized protein (from *Bt*) was quantified for protein estimation (Bradford, 1976) with bovine serum albumin (BSA, Sigma) as standard.

SDS-PAGE

A total of 5 µg protein equivalent samples from *Bt* spores-crystals (NYSM and the test media) was mixed with an equal volume of sample loading buffer and boiled for 5 min and separated on sodium dodecyl sulphate polyacrylamide gel electrophoresis (SDS-PAGE) unit, according to Laemmli (1970). The protein bands were stained with Coommasie Brilliant Blue R-250 and visualized.

Toxicity studies

Powders of *Bt* produced from the three cost-effective media and control were assayed against laboratory-reared first instar larvae of *C. partellus*. A standard primary powder of *Bt* subspecies *kurstaki* (Btk) was included in the assay for comparison. 100 mg of NYSM, potato, legumes, and whey powder was suspended respectively in 1,000 ml of distilled water containing 1% (vol/vol) Tween 80. Serial dilutions of this suspension were made in distilled water. 15 larvae were added to 150 ml of each dilution in 250 ml white plastic cups. Three cups were used per dilution. Controls consisted of three cups each containing 150 ml of distilled water and 15 larvae for each powder assayed. Larval food was provided by adding a small

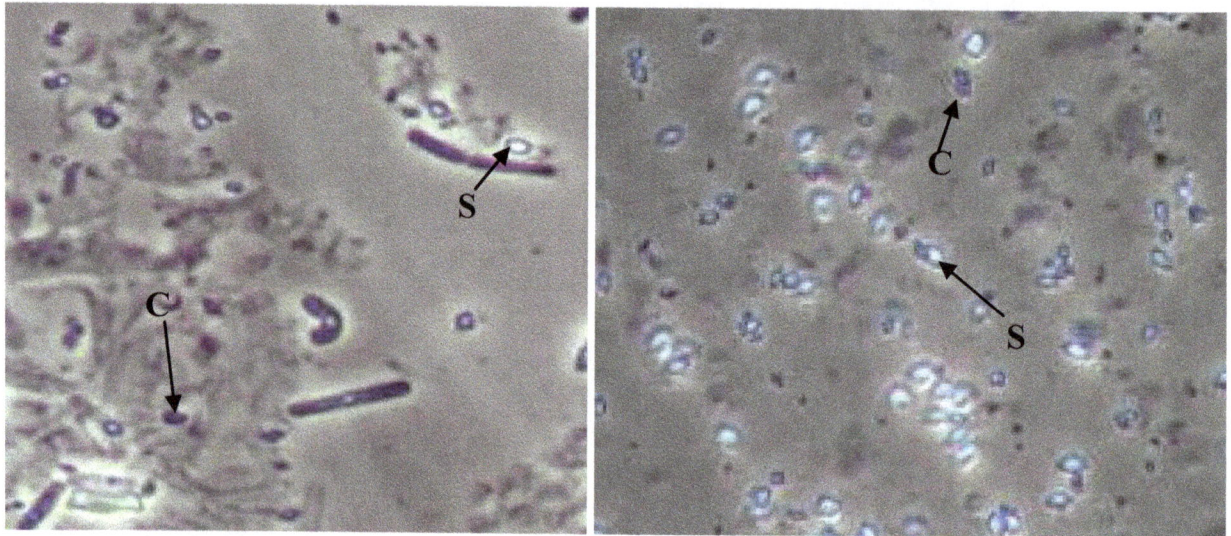

Figure 1. Photomicrograph of *Bt* spore-crystal mixture produced from potato, legume and whey formulated media. S, spores; C, Crystal (×1000).

portion of finely ground oaf flakes (Quaker) mixed with dried yeast powder. Each experiment was incubated at 20 ± 5°C for 48 h, and each assay repeated three times. Observations were made at 6 h for paralysis and knockdown effects. Mortality counts were made at 24 h and 48 h. A larva was presumed dead if it did not move when touched with a blunt needle.

Statistical studies

A one-way ANOVA test was used to compare mean maximum spore count among media and pairwise comparison of the media was done using the Duncan's multiple comparison test based on least significance difference. Probit analysis for calculation of LC_{50} values was carried out using the statistical software SPSS 18.0 for windows.

RESULTS

During activation and multiplication of the isolates, the growth of the local *Bt* and *Btk* isolates occurred between 24 to 72 h producing smooth creamish-white colonies which were rough edged and slightly raised from the nutrient agar. Under the culture conditions described, lysis of the *Bt* cells was complete after 72 h and most of the released protein crystals settled at the bottom of the flask. Almost complete separation of the endotoxin protein crystals from the spores and cell debris was achieved by decantation of the frothy spent culture and high speed centrifugation at 10,000 rpm where the crystals formed a white pellet at the bottom of the tube leaving the spores and cell debris in the supernatant fraction. Serial washing, decanting and centrifugation rid the crystals of spent culture components, spores and cell debris. Microscopy revealed a high concentration of the crystalline inclusions in the pellets obtained (Figure 1).

The highest optical densities were obtained at 37°C from isolates: 62LBG37°C, *Bt* 20, 63KAG37°C, 1SKAG37°C, *Bt* 47, *Bt* 12 and *Bt* 54 respectively. The results of optical density show that pH 7 was the most suitable pH for the maximum growth of 62LBG37C, *Bt* 21, *Bt* 47, and *Bt* 52 while pH 7.5 was suitable for 14SLA30°C and pH 5.5 was suitable for *Bt* 20.

The mass of the resulting pellets ranged from 0.460 g for *Bt* 30 to 0.225 g for *Bt* 20 (mean = 0.314 g ±0.084 g) (Table 1). The protein mass of the pellets was significantly different among the isolates ($t_{16.616, 19, 0.000}$). Spore counts in the pellets ranged from 4.89×10^8 to 5.60×10^8 (mean = 5.23 ±1.53) (Table 1). There was significant difference ($t_{16.014, 19, 0.000}$) on the percent protein content in the pellets. Isolates *Bt* 30 and *Bt* 47 recorded higher contents while 24LBN30°C, 63KAG37°C, and *Bt* 20 had low protein content. The protein yield in the nutrient broth ranged from 2.22 to 4.60 mg/ml of broth (mean = 3.112 mg ± 0.938 mg) and was significantly different ($t_{23.328, 19, 0.000}$) across the different *Bt* isolates.

When compared to high molecular weight standards in SDS-PAGE analysis, the solution and pellet of the dissolved spore-crystal product from each treatment had proteins with molecular weights of approximately 110 to 120 and 60 to 70 kDa (Figures 2 and 3). The major polypeptides present in the spore-crystal complex of *Bt* produced from Legume medium (1SKAG37°C and 24LBN30°C), NYSM medium (58SLA25°C and *Bt* 20), potato medium (58SLA25°C and *Bt* 30) and whey medium

Table 1. Masses of pellets of *Bt* isolates and their protein quantities.

Bt isolate number	Media	Mean absorbance (OD 600)	Spore count (CFU/ml)	Protein in pellet (mg/ml)
46	Legume	1.47	3.80×10^8	4.18
	Potato	1.80	5.10×10^8	2.22
	Whey	1.00	2.50×10^8	3.25
37	Legume	1.48	3.80×10^8	4.01
	Potato	1.92	5.00×10^8	3.22
	Whey	1.07	2.90×10^8	3.68
62LBG37C	Legume	1.45	2.60×10^8	4.51
	Potato	1.82	4.10×10^8	3.09
	Whey	1.21	2.40×10^8	3.78
30	Legume	1.40	3.40×10^8	3.87
	Potato	1.92	5.30×10^8	3.02
	Whey	1.33	1.40×10^8	4.15
20	Legume	1.44	3.40×10^8	4.12
	Potato	1.84	4.10×10^8	3.00
	Whey	0.71	2.00×10^8	3.45
21	Legume	1.35	3.50×10^8	3.69
	Potato	1.91	3.30×10^8	3.07
	Whey	1.30	1.30×10^8	2.68
47	Legume	1.33	4.00×10^8	4.60
	Potato	1.95	3.70×10^8	2.71
	Whey	0.51	1.00×10^7	3.72
63KAG37C	Legume	1.29	2.40×10^8	4.12
	Potato	1.90	3.70×10^8	3.04
	Whey	1.09	2.60×10^8	4.02
14SLA30C	Legume	1.33	3.80×10^8	3.92
	Potato	1.99	4.40×10^8	3.14
	Whey	0.99	1.00×10^7	3.91
53	Legume	1.14	3.50×10^8	4.04
	Potato	1.64	4.90×10^8	3.02
	Whey	1.21	3.00×10^8	3.34
24LBN30C	Legume	1.04	2.70×10^8	4.12
	Potato	2.39	4.70×10^8	3.08
	Whey	0.94	2.20×10^8	3.85
1SKAG37C	Legume	1.05	3.00×10^8	4.43
	Potato	1.66	4.70×10^8	3.32
	Whey	0.72	2.00×10^8	3.00
58SLA25C	Legume	1.38	3.00×10^8	4.63
	Potato	1.93	4.80×10^8	3.11
	Whey	1.27	2.50×10^8	4.45
54	Legume	1.35	3.40×10^8	4.52
	Potato	1.79	5.40×10^8	3.05
	Whey	0.61	2.20×10^8	3.73
12	Legume	1.45	3.30×10^8	4.17
	Potato	1.90	5.30×10^8	3.09
	Whey	1.13	1.90×10^7	3.71
14	Legume	1.44	3.20×10^8	4.08
	Potato	1.92	5.60×10^8	3.12
	Whey	0.52	2.70×10^8	3.09

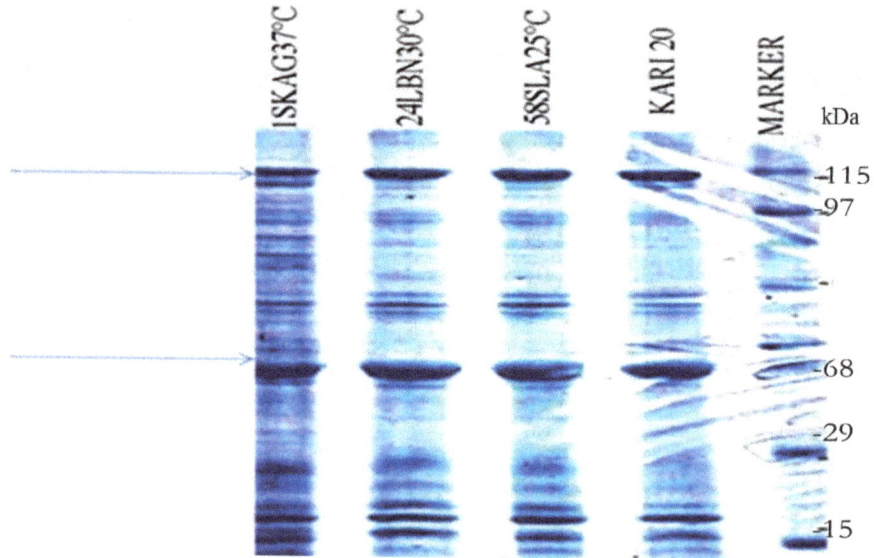

Figure 2. The protein bands (arrows) of delta-endotoxin and spore mixture of *Bt* isolates during its fermentation from Legume medium (1SKAG37°C and 24LBN30°C) and NYSM medium (58SLA25°C and *Bt* 20) as determined by SDS-PAGE.

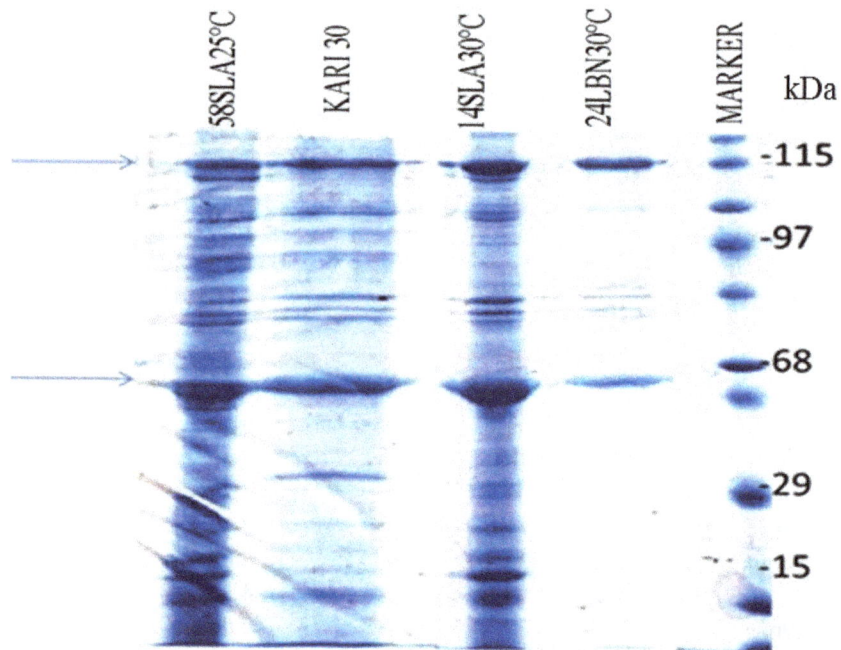

Figure 3. The protein bands (arrows) of delta-endotoxin and spore mixture of *Bt* isolates during its fermentation

(14SLA30°C and 24LBN30°C) were clear and conspicuous. The protein profiles as indicator of *Bt*.

Crystal toxins were correspondingly related to their larvicidal activity.

The neonate larvae started feeding immediately after introduction into the Petri dish and preferred the underside of the leaf. Their feeding intensity slowed down with time and some larvae moved away from the meal

Table 2. Percent mortality of neonate *C. partellus* larvae on treatment with five toxin concentrations of, the standard, *Bacillus thuringiensis* subspecies *kurstaki* (*Btk*).

Concentration (mg/ ml)	Mean larval mortality at 48 (%)	Intercept	Slope (±SE)	LC$_{50}$ (mg/ml)	x^2 (df)
0	10	1.2	0.8 ±0.33	0.001	5.462
0.015	78	2	1.1 ±0.25	0.011	
0.15	72	1.8	1.2 ±0.19	0.008	
1.5	49	1.7	1 ±0.21	0.006	
15	20	1.4	0.9 ±0.27	0.003	

after 24 h. Most larvae in the treatment especially with higher delta-endotoxin concentrations stopped feeding after 48 h, appeared weak and stunted in growth compared to the control upon when death was also observed. For instance, with the 0.015 mg/ml endotoxin treatment, 78% of the larvae were found to be dead from the diet after 48 h. After 48 h, only 10% of larvae were dead with the 0 mg/ml endotoxin treatment, 72% were dead with the 0.15 mg/ml endotoxin treatment, 49% dead with the 1.5 mg/ml endotoxin treatment and 20% of the larvae were dead with the 15 mg/ml endotoxin treatment. Leaf damage was observed to be less on inoculated leaf disks compared to that in the control. Upon death, the larvae appeared dark and shrunk compared to the control. A dead larva was washed, ground and aseptically inoculated onto nutrient agar plate, creamish growth was observed around the larvae which confirmed that the larval mortality was due to ingestion of *Bt* endotoxins. In the set of starved larvae, mortality was 100% in 144 h (Table 2).

A 10% larval mortality on the control treatment was observed after 48 h while 30% recorded after 48 h (Table 2). The cause of this mortality was probably due to drastic changed of weather and laboratory conditions from source of larvae to bioassay laboratory resulting in weak neonates, dehydration or infection; in the subsequent bioassays, eggs were sourced in the yellow state and allowed to acclimatize to the bioassay lab conditions before hatching and maize leaves were also thoroughly washed with distilled water, the filter paper in the Petri dish wetted daily with distilled water and the larvae placed back on the leaf if they had moved far away and got trapped under the filter paper which greatly reduced control larvae mortality. The LC$_{50}$ value estimate for reference isolate *Btk* was 0.011 mg/ml after 48 h (regression coefficient = 0.031005, 95% confidence limit, SE = 0.13747).

Among the different *Bt* treatments, only isolates 24LBN30°C, 63KAG37°C and *Bt* 20 recorded mortality of 10% at 48 h of observation (Table 3). However, while *Btk* increased mortality towards the end of the observation, *Bt* 30, *Bt* 47 and *Bt* 54 stabilized at 60% from 48 h.

Although, isolate 58SLA25°C recorded the first mortality of 40% at 24 h, it is the only isolate that recorded 73% mortality in the observation period, at 48 h. The *Btk* recorded 83% mortality at 48 h. No mortality was observed with 14SLA30°C, ISKAG37°C, *Bt* 21, *Bt* 12 and the control throughout the experiment period. Calculations of LT$_{50}$ shows that *Btk* was the most toxic, causing 50% mortality after only 24 h, followed by 58SLA25°C at 48 h and *Bt* 30 at 48 h. One way ANOVA (repeated measures) revealed that the difference in percent larval mortalities of the standard isolate *Btk* and the *Bt* isolates was statistically significant (p<0.05) except the isolates with less than 20% mortality; *Bt* 37 ($F_{(1.0,5.0)}$ = 6.4, p>0.05) and *Bt* 20 ($F_{(1.0,5.0)}$ = 0.122, p>0.05).

DISCUSSION

The growth of the Kenyan isolates on nutrient agar and nutrient broth was similar to that reported by Wamaitha (2006) which shows the viability of local (Kenyan) *Bt* isolates. The protein purity values recorded by this study were highly variable probably due to the large diversity of isolates that may have differences in optimum growth conditions and a variety of insecticidal crystal protein produced (Aronson et al., 1995) which suggests that the culturing and extraction method may need to be optimized for each isolate in order to obtain equally high delta-endotoxin yields of high purity. The procedure used by this study has been reported to be well suited for large scale production of endotoxin extracts for pesticidal application (Osir and Vundla, 1999). The mean protein yield from the pellets varied from 20 to 30% similar to what is reported by Lereclus et al. (1993) although using different protocol. Higher protein values may have resulted from using lower centrifugation speeds and prior decantation of froth containing cell debris and spores effectively resulting in a lighter pellet.

Two commonly used *Bt* strains in commercial formulations for control of lepidopterans are *Bt kurstaki* and *Bt aizawai*, with the letter strains showing better larval control in situations where *Bt kurstaki* is becoming

Table 3. Percent cumulative mortality of *C. partellus* first-instar larvae exposed to 0.015 mg/ ml endotoxins from *Bt* isolates.

Bt isolate	Mean larval mortality at 48 h (%)	Intercept	Slope (±SE)	LC$_{50}$ (mg/ml)	x^2 (df)
Bt kurstaki	83	1.9	1.1 ±0.33	0.011	11.425 (2)
58SLA25°C	73	1.8	1.1 ±0.33	0.009	
30	60	1.8	1 ±0.25	0.008	
47	60	1.8	1 ±0.25	0.008	
54	30	1.5	0.8 ±0.19	0.005	
62LBG37°C	30	1.5	0.8 ±0.19	0.005	
46	30	1.5	0.8 ±0.19	0.005	
14	30	1.5	0.8 ±0.19	0.005	
53	30	1.5	0.8 ±0.19	0.005	
37	20	1.3	0.6 ±0.21	0.003	
24LBN30°C	10	1.1	0.5 ±0.27	0.0001	
63KAG37°C	10	1.1	0.5 ±0.27	0.0001	
20	10	1.1	0.5 ±0.27	0.0001	
14SLA30°C	0				
ISKAG37°C	0				
21	0				
12	0				

less effective due to resistance development of the pests like the diamond black moth (Schnepf et al., 1998; Polanczyk et al., 2000). The findings of this study closely resemble those of Wang'ondu (2001) with the more toxic isolates (*Bt* 44 and *Bt* 48) being obtained from the lowest LT$_{50}$ values. Significant correlations between endotoxin yield and toxicity among the different isolates illustrates that different *Bt* isolates produce different delta-endotoxins which may differ in toxicity against different target pests (Uribe et al., 2003).

RECOMMENDATIONS

These results form a basis for further investigation of the local *Bt* isolates showing efficacy against *C. partellus* such as determination of the Cry proteins therein and how temperature and pH would affect their toxicity. It is also recommended that the toxicity of these isolates be investigated against other local lepidopteran pests in order to determine their target range.

ACKNOWLEDGEMENTS

I would like to appreciate the cooperation of Dr. Dan Masiga, International Center for Insect Physiology and Ecology (ICIPE) Nairobi, Kenya. He tirelessly worked to ensure the success of this work and his cooperation in providing the available facilities.

REFERENCES

Aronson AI, Wu D, Zhang C (1995). Mutagenesis of specificity and toxicity regions of a *Bacillus thuringiensis* protoxin gene. J. Bacteriol. 177:4059-4065.

Bonhof MJ, Van Huis A, Kiros FG, Dibogo N (2001). Farmers' perceptions of importance, control methods and natural enemies of maize stem borers at the Kenyan coast. Insect Sci. Appl. 21:33-42.

Bradford MM (1976). A rapid and sensitive method for the quantification of microgram quantities of protein utilizing the principle of protein-dye binding. Anal. Biochem. 74:248-254.

Bravo A, Gill SS, Soberon M (2007). Mode of action of *Bacillus thuringiensis* Cry and Cyt toxins and their potential for insect control. Toxicon. 49:423-435.

Brownbridge M (1991). Native *Bacillus thuringiensis* isolates for the management of Leptidopteran cereal pests. Insect Sci. Appl. 12:57-61.

Camilla CN (2000). Managing resistance to *Bacillus thuringiensis* toxins. University of Chicago, B.A. Thesis. p. 70.

De Groote H (2002). Maize Yield Losses from Stem borers in Kenya. Insect Sci. Appl. 22:89-96.

Hoben HJ, Somasegaran P (1982). Comparison of the pour, spread, and drop plate methods for enumeration of Rhizobium spp. In inoculants made form presterilized peat. Appl. Environ. Microbiol. 44:1246-1247.

Laemmli UK (1970) Cleavage of structural proteins during the assembly of the head of bacteriophage T4. Nature 227:680-685.

Lambert B, Hofte H, Annys K, Jansens S, Soetaert P, Peferoen M (1992). Novel *Bacillus thuringiensis* insecticidal crystal protein with a silent activity against coleopteran larvae. Appl. Environ. Microbiol. 58:2536-2542.

Lereclus D, Delecluse A, Lecadet MM (1993). Diversity of *Bacillus thuringiensis* toxins and genes. In: Entwistle PF, Cory JS, Bailey MJ and Higgs S. Chichester (Eds) *Bacillus thuringiensis*, an Environmental biopesticide: Theory and practice. John Wiley and Sons Ltd. pp. 37-69.

Maniatis T, Fritsch EF, Sambrook J (1982). Molecular cloning. pp. 61-

62, 68, 442, 444.

Mugo S, Gethi M, Okuro J, Bergvinson D, Groote HD, Songa J (2007). Evaluation of insect resistant maize open pollinated varieties and hybrids on-station and on-farm in the moist mid-altitude maize ecologies of Kenya. Afr. Crop Sci. Conf. pp. 959-964.

Osir EO, Vundla WRM (1999). Characterisation of the δ-endotoxin of a Bacillus thuringiensis isolate active against tsetse, Glossina morsitans, and a stem borer, Chilo partellus. Biocontr. Sci. Technol. 9:247-258.

Polanczyk RA, Silva RFP, Fiuza LM (2000). Effectiveness of Bacillus thuringiensis strains against Spodoptera frugiperda (lepidoptera: noctuidae). Brazilian J. Microbiol. 31:165-167.

Schnepf E, Crickmore N, Van Rie J, Lereclus D, Baum J, Feitelson J, Zeigler DR, Dean DH (1998). Bacillus thuringiensis and its pesticidal crystal proteins. Microbiol. Mol. Biol. Rev. 62:775-806.

Uribe D, Martinez W, Cerón . (2003). Distribution and diversity of cry genes in native strains of Bacillus thuringiensis obtained from different ecosystems from Columbia. J. Invertebrate Pathol. 82:119-127.

Wamaitha JM (2006). Isolation, evaluation and molecular characterisation of Bacillus thuringiensis isolates against Prostephanus truncatus, a major storage pest in maize. Kenyatta University M.Sc. Thesis. pp. 47-51.

Wang'ondu VW (2001). Isolation and partial characterization of Bacillus thuringiensis from Kakamega and Machakos districts in Kenya. University of Nairobi M.Sc. Thesis. pp. 96-105.

Wessel D, Flugge UI (1984). Acetone Precipitation Protocol. Analyt. Biochem.138:141-143.

5

Green energy from chemicals and bio-wastes

Abdeen Mustafa Omer

Energy Research Institute, Khartoum, Sudan. E-mail: abdeenomer2@yahoo.co.uk.

This paper discusses a comprehensive review of biomass energy sources, environment and sustainable development. This includes the biomass energy technologies, energy efficiency systems, energy conservation scenarios, energy savings and other measures necessary to reduce climate change. Energy use reductions can be achieved by minimising the energy demand, by rational energy use, and by recovering heat. The increased availability of reliable and efficient energy services stimulates the use of more green energies. The adoption of green or sustainable approaches to the way in which society is run is seen as an important strategy in finding a solution to the energy problem. The key factors to reducing and controlling CO_2 emissions to the atmospheric sink, which is the major contributor to global warming, are the use of alternative approaches to energy generation and the exploration of how these alternatives are used today and may be used in the future as green energy sources.

Key words: Biomass, wastes, bi-wastes, bioenergy, bioheat, biogas.

INTRODUCTION

Energy is an essential factor in development since it stimulates, and supports economic growth and development. Fossil fuels, especially oil and natural gas, are finite in extent, and should be regarded as depleting assets, and efforts are oriented to search for new sources of energy. The clamour all over the world for the need to conserve energy and the environment has intensified as traditional energy resources continue to dwindle whilst the environment becomes increasingly degraded. Alternative energy sources can potentially help fulfil the acute energy demand and sustain economic growth in many regions of the world (Haripriye, G., 2000; WB, 2003b; DEFRA, 2002; and EUO; 2000). Energy security, economic growth and environment protection are the national energy policy drivers of any country of the world. As world populations grow, many faster than the average 2%, the need for more and more energy is exacerbated (Anne and Michael, 2005). Enhanced lifestyle and energy demand rise together and the wealthy industrialised economics, which contain 25% of the world's population, consume 75% of the world's energy supply (REN21, 2001; and UN, 2001).

The world's energy consumption today is estimated to be 22 billion kWh per year (UNECA, 2002; UNECA, 2003a; and UNECA; 2003b). About 6.6 billion metric tones carbon equivalent of greenhouse gas (GHG)

emission are released in the atmosphere to meet this energy demand (UNECE, 2004; UNEP, 2000; WB, 2003a; WB, 2006; and WB, 2007). Approximately 80% is due to carbon emissions from the combustion of energy fuels (WB, 2003b; and WB, 2004). At the current rate of usage, taking into consideration population increases and higher consumption of energy by developing countries, oil resources, natural gas and uranium will be depleted within a few decades. Bioenergy is beginning to gain importance in the global fight to prevent climate change (Omer, 2008a, 2008b; IEA, 2008; Paul, 2001). The scope for exploiting organic waste as a source of energy is not limited to direct incineration or burning refuse-derived fuels. Biogas, biofuels and woody biomass are other forms of energy sources that can be derived from organic waste materials. These biomass energy sources have significant potential in the fight against climate change. Technological progress has dramatically changed the world in a variety of ways. It has, however, also led to developments, e.g., environmental problems, which threaten man and nature. Build-up of carbon dioxide and other GHGs is leading to global warming with unpredictable but potentially catastrophic consequences. When fossil fuels burn, they emit toxic pollutants that damage the environment and people's health with over 700,000 deaths resulting each year, according to the

World Bank review of 2000 (Huttrer, 2001; Reddy et al., 2007; Lam, 2000; Mortal, 2002). At the current rate of usage, taking into consideration population increases and higher consumption of energy by developing countries, oil resources, natural gas and uranium will be depleted within a few decades (Shao et al., 2002; Roriz, 2001; Witte and Gelder, 2002; CEC, 2000). The sources to alleviate the energy situation in the world are sufficient to supply all foreseeable needs (Trevor, 2007; IEA, 2007; Brain and Mark, 2007; Omer, 2009, 2005; Pernille, 2004).

Conservation of energy and rationing in some form will however have to be practised by most countries, to reduce oil imports and redress balance of payments positions. Meanwhile development and application of nuclear power and some of the traditional solar, wind, biomass and water energy alternatives must be set in hand to supplement what remains of the fossil fuels.

The encouragement of greater energy use is an essential component of development. In the short-term, it requires mechanisms to enable the rapid increase in energy/capita, and in the long-term we should be working towards a way of life, which makes use of energy efficiency and clean environment without causing safety problems (IPCC, 2001; Lazzarin et al., 2002; David, 2003). Such a programme should as far as possible be based on renewable energy resources. Large-scale, conventional, power plant such as hydropower has an important part to play in development. It does not, however, provide a complete solution. There is an important complementary role for the greater use of small- scale, rural based-power plants. Such plant can be used to assist development since it can be made locally using local resources, enabling a rapid built-up in total equipment to be made without a corresponding and unacceptably large demand on central funds. Renewable resources are particularly suitable for providing the energy for such equipment and its use is also compatible with the long-term aims. In compiling energy consumption data one can categorise usage according to a number of different schemes:

1. Traditional sector- industrial, transportation, etc.
2. End-use- space heating, process steam, etc.
3. Final demand- total energy consumption related to automobiles, to food, etc.
4. Energy source- oil, coal, etc.
5. Energy form at point of use- electric drive, low temperature heat, etc.

The scope for exploiting organic waste as a source of energy is not limited to direct incineration or burning refuse-derived fuels. Biogas, biofuels and woody biomass are other forms of energy sources that can be derived from organic waste materials. These biomass energy sources have significant potential in the fight against climate change. Energy is a vital prime mover to the

development whether in urban or rural areas. The rural energy needs are modest compared to urban. A shift to renewables would therefore help to solve some of these problems while also providing the population with higher quality energy, which will in turn, improve living standards and help reduce poverty. For proper rural development the following must be considered:

1. Analyse the key potentials and constraints of development of rural energy. Assess the socio-technical information needs for decision-makers and planners in rural development.
2. Utilise number of techniques and models supporting planning rural energy.
3. Design, import and interpret different types of surveys to collect relevant information and analyse them to be an input to planners.

MATERIALS AND METHODS

Bio-wastes development

Waste is defined as an unwanted material that is being discarded. Waste includes items being taken for further use, recycling or reclamation. Waste produced at household, commercial and industrial premises are control waste and come under the waste regulations. Waste Incineration Directive (WID) emissions limit values will favour efficient, inherently cleaner technologies that do not rely heavily on abatement (Abdeen, 2004, 2000, 2005, 2006). For existing plant, the requirements are likely to lead to improved control of:

1. NOx emissions, by the adoption of infurnace combustion control and abatement techniques.
2. Acid gases, by the adoption of abatement techniques and optimisation of their control.
3. Particulate control techniques, and their optimisation, e.g., of bag filters and electrostatic precipitators.

Bioenergy[1] is energy from the sun stored in materials of biological origin (Aroyeun et al., 2009; Dragana, 2008; UN, 2002a). This includes plant matter and animal waste, known as biomass. Plants store solar energy through photosynthesis in cellulose and lignin, whereas animals store energy as fats. When burned, these sugars break down and release energy exothermically, releasing carbon dioxide, heat and steam. The by-products of this reaction can be captured and manipulated to create power, commonly called bioenergy (UN, 2002b; UN, 2002c; UNECA, 2002). Biomass is considered renewable because the carbon is taken out of the atmosphere and replenished more quickly than the millions of years required for fossil fuels to form. The use of biofuels to replace fossil fuels contributes to a reduction in the overall release of carbon dioxide into the atmosphere and hence helps to tackle global

---

[1] Bioenergy is biomass energy made available from agricultural materials (crops, trees, etc.) and animal residues/wastes (dung) derived from biological sources. In its most narrow sense it is a synonym to biofuel, which is fuel derived from biological sources. It is usually meant as fuel produced from organic crops, most of which are grown specifically to be used as fuel. Energy produced from renewable biomass (plant derived organic matter) resources, can yield electricity, liquid, solid, and gaseous fuels, heat, chemicals, and other materials.

Table 1. Sources of energy for poor people (Abdeen, 2008a).

Energy source	Energy carrier	Energy end-use
Vegetation	Fuel-wood	Cooking Water heating Building materials Animal fodder preparation
Oil	Kerosene	Lighting Ignition fires
Dry cells	Dry cell batteries	Lighting Small appliances
Muscle power	Animal power	Transport Land preparation for farming Food preparation (threshing)
Muscle power	Human power	Transport Land preparation for farming Food preparation (threshing)

Table 2. Energy applications (Abdeen, 2007a).

Systems	Applications
Water supply	Rain collection, purification, storage and recycling
Wastes disposal	Anaerobic digestion (CH4)
Cooking	Methane
Food	Cultivate the 1 hectare plot and greenhouse for four people
Electrical demands	Wind generator
Space heating	Solar collectors
Water heating	Solar collectors and excess wind energy
Control system	Ultimately hardware
Building fabric	Integration of subsystems to cut costs

warming (FEC, 2000; Brain and Mark, 2007; ASHRAE, 1993; McKennan, Crisp and Cooper, 1988; Dieng and Wang, 2001; UNEP, 2003; Abdeen, 2007b, and 2008d; and Jeremy, 2005). The range of waste treatment technologies that are tailored to produce bioenergy is growing. There are a number of key areas of bioenergy from wastes including (but not limited to) biogas, biofuels and bioheat. When considering using bioenergy, it is important to take into account the overall emission of carbon in the process of electricity production (Zuatori, 2005; Abdeen, 2004, 2000).

The biomass energy resources are particularly suited for the provision of rural power supplies and a major advantage is that equipment such as flat plate solar driers, wind machines, etc., can be constructed using local resources and without the high capital cost of more conventional equipment. Further advantage results from the feasibility of local maintenance and the general encouragement such local manufacture gives to the build up of small-scale rural based industry. Table 1 lists the energy sources available for poor people. Currently the 'non-commercial' fuels

wood, crop residues and animal dung are used in large amounts in the rural areas of developing countries, principally for heating and cooking; the method of use is highly inefficient. Table 2 presented some renewable applications (Omer, 2006, 2007b; ASHRAE, 1993) for household. Considerations when selecting power plant include the following:

1. Power level- whether continuous or discontinuous.
2. Cost- initial cost, total running cost including fuel, maintenance and capital amortised over life.
3. Complexity of operation.
4. Maintenance and availability of spares.
5. Life.
6. Suitability for local manufacture.

The internal combustion engine is a major contributor to rising CO_2 emissions worldwide and some pretty dramatic new thinking is needed if our planet is to counter the effects. With its use increasing

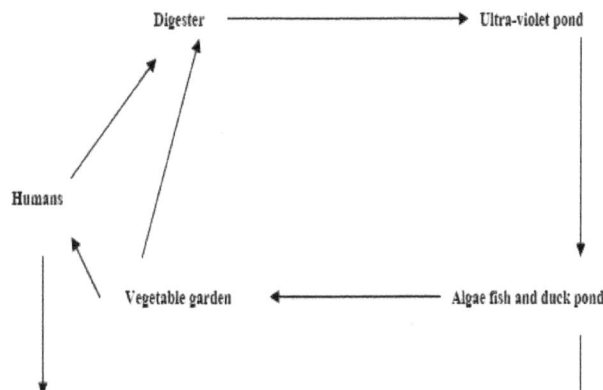

Figure 1. Biomass utilisation concept

in developing world economies, there is something to be said for the argument that the vehicles we use to help keep our inner-city environments free from waste, litter and grime should be at the forefront of developments in low-emissions technology (Abdeen, 2008b, 2008c). Materials handled by waste management companies are becoming increasingly valuable. Those responsible for the security of facilities that treat waste or manage scrap will testify to the precautions needed to fight an ongoing battle against unauthorised access by criminals and crucially, to prevent the damage they can cause through theft, vandalism or even arson. Of particular concern is the escalating level of metal theft, driven by various factors including the demand for metal in rapidly developing economies such as India and China.

There is a need for greater attention to be devoted to this field in the development of new designs, the dissemination of information and the encouragement of its use. International and government bodies and independent organisations all have a role to play in biomass energy technologies.

Environment has no precise limits because it is in fact a part of everything. Indeed, environment is, as anyone probably already knows, not only flowers blossoming or birds singing in the spring, or a lake surrounded by beautiful mountains. It is also human settlements, the places where people live, work, rest, the quality of the food they eat, the noise or silence of the street they live in. Environment is not only the fact that our cars consume a good deal of energy and pollute the air, but also, that we often need them to go to work and for holidays. Obviously man uses energy just as plants, bacteria, mushrooms, bees, fish and rats do (Figure 1). Man largely uses solar energy- food, hydropower, wood- and thus participates harmoniously in the natural flow of energy through the environment. But man also uses oil, gas, coal and nuclear power. By using such sources of energy, man is thus modifying his environment. Economic importance of environmental issue is increasing, and new technologies are expected to reduce pollution derived both from productive processes and products, with costs that are still unknown. This is due to market uncertainty, weak appropriability regime, lack of a dominant design, and difficulties in reconfiguring organisational routines. The degradation of the global environment is one of the most serious energy issues. Various options are proposed and investigated to mitigate climate change, acid rain or other environmental problems.

Energy use and the environment

Energy use is one of several essential components for developing

countries:

1. The overall situation and the implications of increased energy use in the future.
2. The problem of the provision of power in rural areas, including the consideration of energy resources and energy conversion.

In addition to the drain on resources, such an increase in consumption consequences, together with the increased hazards of pollution and the safety problems associated with a large nuclear fission programmes. This is a disturbing prospect. It would be equally unacceptable to suggest that the difference in energy between the developed and developing countries and prudent for the developed countries to move towards a way of life which, whilst maintaining or even increasing quality of life, reduce significantly the energy consumption per capita. Such savings can be achieved in a number of ways:

1. Improved efficiency of energy use, for example better thermal insulation, energy recovery, and total energy.
2. Conservation of energy resources by design for long life and recycling rather than the short life throwaway product and systematic replanning of our way of life, for example in the field of transport. The aim of any modern biomass energy systems must be:

1. To maximise yields with minimum inputs.
2. Utilisation and selection of adequate plant materials and processes.
3. Optimum use of land, water, and fertiliser.
4. Create an adequate infrastructure and strong R and D base.

Furthermore, investigating the potential to make use of more and more of its waste. Household waste, vegetable market waste, and waste from the cotton stalks, leather, and pulp; and paper industries can be used to produce useful energy either by direct incineration, gasification, digestion (biogas production), fermentation, or cogeneration. Therefore, effort has to be made to reduce fossil energy use and to promote green energies, particularly in the building sector. Energy use reductions can be achieved by minimising the energy demand, by rational energy use, by recovering heat and the use of more green energies.
Energy ratio is defined as the ratio of:

Energy content of the food product/Energy input to produce the

Table 3. Annual GHG emissions from different sources of power plants (Abdeen, 2008e).

Primary source of energy	Emissions		Waste (x 10^3 metric tons)	Area (km^2)
	Atmosphere	Water		
Coal	380	7-41	60-3000	120
Oil	70-160	3-6	Negligible	70-84
Gas	24	1	-	84
Nuclear	6	21	2600	77

Table 4. Energy consumption per population (Abdeen, 2008f).

Region	Population (millions)	Energy (Watt/m^2)
Africa	820	0.54
Asia	3780	2.74
Central America	180	1.44
North America	335	0.34
South America	475	0.52
Western Europe	445	2.24
Eastern Europe	130	2.57
Oceania	35	0.08
Russia	330	0.29

food (1).

Combined heat and power (CHP)

The atmospheric emissions of fossil fuelled installations are mostly aldehydes, carbon monoxide, nitrogen oxides, sulphur oxides and particles (that is, ash) as well as carbon dioxide. Table 3 shows estimates include not only the releases occurring at the power plant itself but also cover fuel extraction and treatment, as well as the storage of wastes and the area of land required for operation (Table 4). A review of the potential range of recyclables is presented in Table 5. Combined heat and power (CHP) installations are quite common in greenhouses, which grow high-energy, input crops (e.g., salad vegetables, pot plants, etc.).

Scientific assumptions for a short-term energy strategy suggest that the most economically efficient way to replace the thermal plants is to modernise existing power plants to increase their energy efficiency and to improve their environmental performance. However, utilisation of wind power and the conversion of gas-fired CHP plants to biomass would significantly reduce the dependence on imported fossil fuels. Although a lack of generating capacity is forecasted in the long-term, utilisation of the existing renewable energy potential and the huge possibilities for increasing energy efficiency are sufficient to meet future energy demands in the short-term. A total shift towards a sustainable energy system is a complex and long process, but is one that can be achieved within a period of about 20 years. Implementation will require initial investment, long-term national strategies and action plans. However, the changes will have a number of benefits including: a more stable energy supply than at present and major improvement in the environmental performance of the energy sector, and certain social benefits (Figure 2). A vision used a methodology and calculations based on computer modelling that utilised:

1. Data from existing governmental programmes.

2. Potential renewable energy sources and energy efficiency improvements.
4. Assumptions for future economy growth.
5. Information from studies and surveys on the recent situation in the energy sector.

The main advantages are related to energy, agriculture and environment problems, are foreseeable both at national level and at worldwide level and can be summarised as follows:
1. Reduction of dependence on import of energy and related products.
2. Reduction of environmental impact of energy production (greenhouse effect, air pollution, and waste degradation).
3. Substitution of food crops and reduction of food surpluses and of related economic burdens.
4. Utilisation of marginal lands and of set aside lands and reduction of related socio-economic and environmental problems (soil erosion, urbanisation, landscape deterioration, etc.).
5. Development of new know-how and production of technological innovation.

In some countries, a wide range of economic incentives and other measures are already helping to protect the environment. These include:

1. Taxes and user charges that reflect the costs of using the environment, e.g., pollution taxes and waste disposal charges.
2. Subsidies, credits and grants that encourage environmental protection.
3. Deposit-refund systems that prevent pollution on resource misuse and promote product reuse or recycling.
3. Financial enforcement incentives, e.g., fines for non-compliance with environmental regulations.
4. Tradable permits for activities that harm the environment.

District Heating (DH), also known as community heating can be a

Table 5. Summary of material recycling practices in the construction sector (Robinson, 2007)

Construction and demolition material	Recycling technology options	Recycling product
Asphalt	Cold recycling: heat generation; Minnesota process; parallel drum process; elongated drum; microwave asphalt recycling system; finfalt; surface regeneration	Recycling asphalt; asphalt aggregate
Brick	Burn to ash, crush into aggregate	Slime burn ash; filling material; hardcore
Concrete	Crush into aggregate	Recycling aggregate; cement replacement; protection of levee; backfilling; filter
Ferrous metal	Melt; reuse directly	Recycled steel scrap
Glass	Reuse directly; grind to powder; polishing; crush into aggregate; burn to ash	Recycled window unit; glass fibre; filling material; tile; paving block; asphalt; recycled aggregate; cement replacement; manmade soil
Masonry	Crush into aggregate; heat to 900oC to ash	Thermal insulating concrete; traditional clay
Non-ferrous metal	Melt	Recycled metal
Paper and cardboard	Purification	Recycled paper
Plastic	Convert to powder by cryogenic milling; clopping; crush into aggregate; burn to ash	Panel; recycled plastic; plastic lumber; recycled aggregate; landfill drainage; asphalt; manmade soil
Timber	Reuse directly; cut into aggregate; blast furnace deoxidisation; gasification or pyrolysis; chipping; moulding by pressurising timber chip under steam and water	Whole timber; furniture and kitchen utensils; lightweight recycled aggregate; source of energy; chemical production; wood-based panel; plastic lumber; geofibre; insulation board

key factor to achieve energy savings, reduce CO_2 emissions and at the same time provide consumers with a high quality heat supply at a competitive price. DH should generally only be considered for areas where the heat density is sufficiently high to make DH economical. In countries like Denmark DH may today be economical even to new developments with lower density areas due to the high level of taxation on oil and gas fuels combined with the efficient production of DH (Sims, 2007). To improve the opportunity for DH local councils can adapt the following plan:

1. Analyse the options for heat supply during local planning stage.
2. In areas where DH is the least cost solution it should be made part of the infrastructure just like for instance water and sewage connecting all existing and new buildings.
3. Where possible all public buildings should be connected to DH.
4. The government provides low interest loans or funding to minimise conversion costs for its citizens.
5. Use other powers, for instance national legislation to ensure the most economical development of the heat supply and enable an obligation to connect buildings to a DH scheme.

Denmark has broadly seen three scales of CHP which were largely implemented in the following chronological order (Omer and Yemen, 2003):

1. Large scale CHP in cities (>50 MWe).

2. Small (5 kWe - 5 MWe) and medium scale (5-50 MWe).
3. Industrial and small scale CHP.

Most of the heat is produced by large CHP plants (gas-fired combined cycle plants using natural gas, biomass, waste or biogas). DH is energy efficient because of the way the heat is produced and the required temperature level is an important factor. Buildings can be heated to temperature of 21 °C and domestic hot water (DHW) can be supplied with a temperature of 55 °C using energy sources that are most efficient when producing low temperature levels (<95 °C) for the DH water. Most of these heat sources are CO_2 neutral or emit low levels. Only a few of these sources are available to small individual systems at a reasonably cost, whereas DH schemes because of the plant's size and location can have access to most of the heat sources and at a low cost. Low temperature DH, with return temperatures of around 30-40 °C can utilise the following heat sources:

1. Efficient use of CHP by extracting heat at low calorific value (CV).
2. Efficient use of biomass or gas boilers by condensing heat in economisers (Table 6).
3. Efficient utilisation of geothermal energy.
4. Direct utilisation of excess low temperature heat from industrial processes.
5. Efficient use of large-scale solar heating plants.

Methane → Methanol

Reforming — Synthesis gas → Synthesis — Crude → Purification — Chemical

Natural gas (methane)

Recycle   Purge

Synthesis gas

Reforming

(CO_2, H_2, CO)

Synthesis

$CH_3OH + H_2O$
Methanol + Water

Crude

Purification

Chemical

(CH_3OH)
Methanol

Steam

Overall reaction: $CH_4 + H_2O = CH_3OH + H_2$

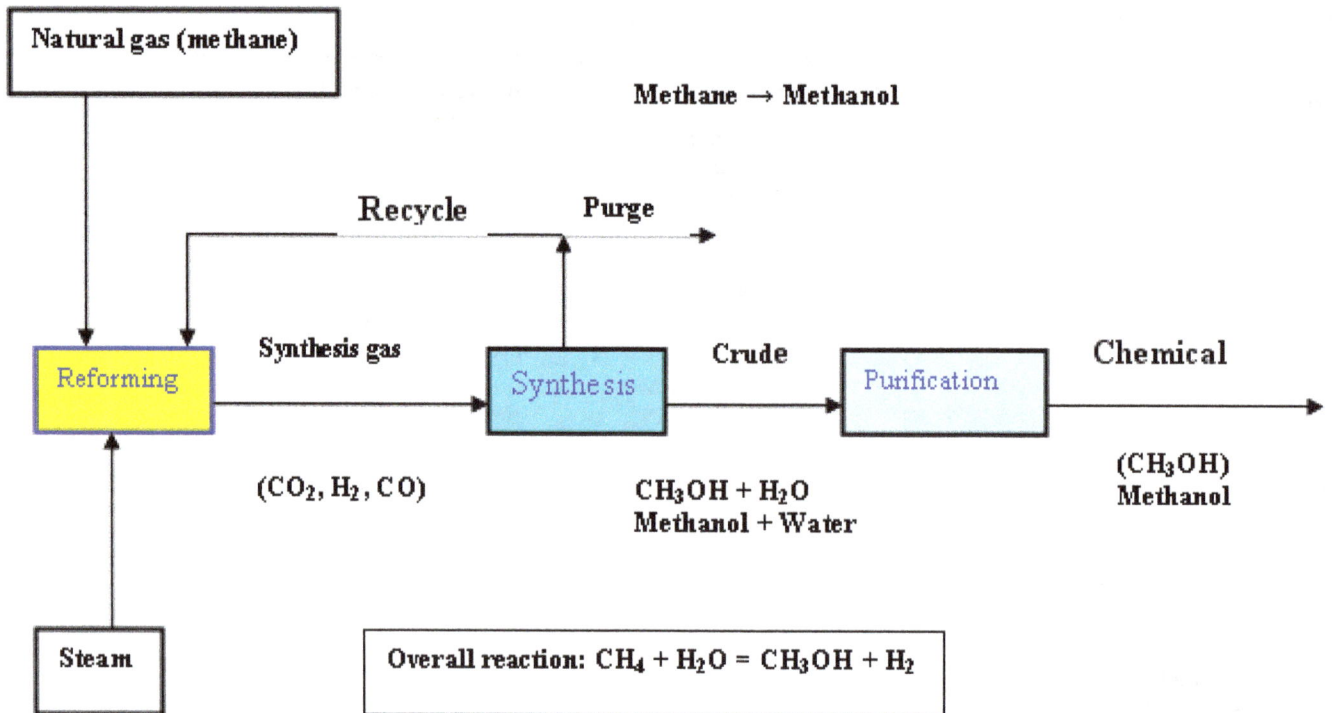

Figure 2. Schematic process flow sheet.

Table 6. Final energy projections including biomass (Mtoe) (Omer, 2007a).

Region	1995			
	Biomass	**Conventional** energy	**Total**	**Share of biomass (%)**
Africa	205	136	341	60
China	206	649	855	24
East Asia	106	316	422	25
Latin America	73	342	415	18
South Asia	235	188	423	56
Total developing countries	825	1632	2457	34
Other non-OECD countries	24	1037	1061	2
Total non-OECD countries	849	2669	3518	24
OECD countries	81	3044	3125	3
World	930	5713	6643	14

Region	2020			
	Biomass	**Conventional** energy	**Total**	**Share of biomass (%)**
Africa	371	266	637	59
China	224	1524	1748	13
East Asia	118	813	931	13
Latin America	81	706	787	10
South Asia	276	523	799	35
Total developing countries	1071	3825	4896	22
Other non-OECD countries	26	1669	1695	2
Total non-OECD countries	1097	5494	6591	17
OECD countries	96	3872	3968	2
World	1193	9365	10558	11

Table 7. Classifications of data requirements.

	Plant data	System data
Existing data	Size	Peak load
	Life	Load shape
	Cost (fixed and var. O and M)	Capital costs
	Forced outage	Fuel costs
	Maintenance	Depreciation
	Efficiency	Rate of return
	Fuel	Taxes
	Emissions	
Future data	All of above, plus	System lead growth
	Capital costs	Fuel price growth
	Construction trajectory	Fuel import limits
	Date in service	Inflation

Heat tariffs may include a number of components such as: a connection charge, a fixed charge and a variable energy charge. Also, consumers may be incentivised to lower the return temperature. Hence, it is difficult to generalise but the heat practice for any DH company no matter what the ownership structure can be highlighted as follows:

1. To develop and maintain a development plan for the connection of new consumers.
2. To evaluate the options for least cost production of heat.
3. To implement the most competitive solutions by signing agreements with other companies or by implementing own investment projects.
4. To monitor all internal costs and with the help of benchmarking, improve the efficiency of the company.
5. To maintain a good relationship with the consumer and deliver heat supply services at a sufficient quality.

Installing DH should be pursued to meet the objectives for improving the environment through the improvement of energy efficiency in the heating sector. At the same time DH can serve the consumer with a reasonable quality of heat at the lowest possible cost. The variety of possible solutions combined with the collaboration between individual companies, the district heating association, the suppliers and consultants can, as it has been in Denmark, be the way forward for developing DH in the United Kingdom (Abdeen, 2007b).

Biomass utilisation and development of conversion technologies

Sustainable energy is energy that, in its production or consumption, has minimal negative impacts on human health and the healthy functioning of vital ecological systems, including the global environment. It is an accepted fact that renewable energy is a sustainable form of energy, which has attracted more attention during recent years. A great amount of renewable energy potential, environmental interest, as well as economic consideration of fossil fuel consumption and high emphasis of sustainable development for the future will be needed. Explanations for the use of inefficient

agricultural-environmental polices include: the high cost of information required to measure benefits on a site-specific basis, information asymmetries between government agencies and farm decision makers that result in high implementation costs, distribution effects and political considerations (Abdeen, 2007c). Achieving the aim of agric-environment schemes through:

1. Sustain the beauty and diversity of the landscape.
2. Improve and extend wildlife habitats.
3. Conserve archaeological sites and historic features.
4. Improve opportunities for countryside enjoyment.
5. Restore neglected land or features, and
6. Create new habitats and landscapes.

Efficient bio-energy use and improvement

The data required to perform the trade-off analysis simulation can be classified according to the divisions given in Table 7, the overall system or individual plants, and the existing situation or future development. The effective economic utilisations of these resources are shown in Table 8, but their use is hindered by many problems such as those related to harvesting, collection, and transportation, besides the photo-sanitary control regulations. Biomass energy is experiencing a surge in interest stemming from a combination of factors, e.g., greater recognition of its current role and future potential contribution as a modern fuel, global environmental benefits, its development and entrepreneurial opportunities, etc. Possible routes of biomass energy development are shown in Table 9. The key to successful future appears to lie with successful marketing of the treatment by products. There is also potential for using solid residue in the construction industry as a filling agent for concrete. Research suggests that the composition of the residue locks metals within the material, thus preventing their escape and any subsequent negative effect on the environment (Abdeen, 2009e).

The use of biomass through direct combustion has long been, and still is, the most common mode of biomass utilisation as shown in Tables 7 to 9. Examples for dry (thermo-chemical) conversion processes are charcoal making from wood (slow pyrolysis), gasification of forest and agricultural residues (fast pyrolysis- this is

Table 8. Effective biomass resource utilisation (Omer, 2009a).

Subject	Tools	Constraints
Utilisation and land clearance for agriculture expansion	Stumpage fees Control Extension Conversion Technology	Policy Fuel-wood planning Lack of extension Institutional
Utilisation of agricultural residues	Briquetting Carbonisation Carbonisation and briquetting Fermentation Gasification	Capital Pricing Policy and legislation Social acceptability

Table 9. Agricultural residues routes for development.

Source	Process	Product	End use
Agricultural residues	Direct	Combustion	Rural poor, Urban household, Industrial use
	Processing	Briquettes	Industrial use Limited household use
	Processing	Carbonisation (Small scale)	Rural household (self sufficiency)
	Carbonisation	Briquettes Carbonised	Urban fuel
	Fermentation	Biogas	Energy services Household Industry
Agricultural and animal residues	Direct	Combustion	(Save or less efficiency as wood)
	Briquettes	Direct combustion	(Similar end use devices or improved)
	Carbonisation	Carbonised	Use
	Carbonisation	Briquettes	Briquettes use
	Fermentation	Biogas	Use

still in demonstration phase), and of course, direct combustion in stoves, furnaces, etc. Wet processes require substantial amount of water to be mixed with the biomass. Biomass technologies include:

1. Briquetting.
2. Improved stoves.
3. Biogas.
4. Improved charcoal.
5. Carbonisation.
6. Gasification.

The increased demand for gas and petroleum, food crops, fish and large sources of vegetative matter mean that the global harvesting of carbon has in turn intensified. It could be said that mankind is mining nearly everything except its waste piles. It is simply a matter of time until the significant carbon stream present in municipal solid waste is fully captured. In the meantime, the waste industry needs to continue on the pathway to increased awareness and better-optimised biowaste resources. Optimisation of waste carbon may require widespread regulatory drivers (including strict limits on the Landfilling of organic materials), public acceptance of the benefits of waste carbon products for soil improvements/crop enhancements and more investment in capital facilities. In short, a significant effort will be required in order to capture a greater portion of the carbon stream and put it to beneficial use. From the standpoint of waste practitioners, further research and pilot programmes are necessary before the available carbon in the waste stream can be extracted in sufficient quality and quantities to create the desired end products.

Table 10. Anaerobic degradation of organic matter (Bacaoui et al., 1998).

Level	Substance	Molecule	Bacteria
Initial	Manure, vegetable, wastes	Cellulose, proteins	Cellulolytic, proteolytic
Intermediate	Acids, gases, oxidized, inorganic salts	CH_3COOH, $CHOOH$, SO_4, CO_2, H_2, NO_3	Acidogenic, hydrogenic, sulfate reducing
Final	Biogas, reduced inorganic compounds	$CH4$, $CO2$, H_2S, NH_3, NH_4	Methane formers

Other details need to be ironed out too, including measurement methods, diversion calculations, sequestration values and determination of acceptance contamination thresholds.

Briquette

Charcoal stoves are very familiar to African society. As for the stove technology, the present charcoal stove can be used, and can be improved upon for better efficiency. This energy term will be of particular interest to both urban and rural households and all the income groups due to the simplicity, convenience, and lower air polluting characteristics. However, the market price of the fuel together with that of its end-use technology may not enhance its early high market penetration especially in the urban low income and rural households.

Briquetting is the formation of a char (an energy-dense solid fuel source) from otherwise wasted agricultural and forestry residues. One of the disadvantages of wood fuel is that it is bulky with a low energy density and is therefore enquire to transport. Briquette formation allows for a more energy-dense fuel to be delivered, thus reducing the transportation cost and making the resource more competitive. It also adds some uniformity, which makes the fuel more compatible with systems that are sensitive to the specific fuel input.

Improved cook stoves

Traditional wood stoves can be classified into four types: three stone, metal cylindrical shaped, metal tripod and clay type. Another area in which rural energy availability could be secured where woody fuels have become scarce, are the improvements of traditional cookers and ovens to raise the efficiency of fuel saving. Also, by planting fast growing trees to provide a constant fuel supply. The rural development is essential and economically important since it will eventually lead to better standards of living, people's settlement, and self sufficient in the following:

1. Food and water supplies.
2. Better services in education and health care.
3. Good communication modes.

Biogas

Biogas technology can not only provide fuel, but is also important for comprehensive utilisation of biomass forestry, animal husbandry, fishery, agricultural economy, protecting the environment, realising agricultural recycling, as well as improving the sanitary conditions, in rural areas. The introduction of biogas

technology on wide scale has implications for macro planning such as the allocation of government investment and effects on the balance of payments. Factors that determine the rate of acceptance of biogas plants, such as credit facilities and technical backup services, are likely to have to be planned as part of general macro-policy, as do the allocation of research and development funds (Omer, 2008c). Bacteria form biogas during anaerobic fermentation of organic matters. The degradation is very complex process and requires certain environmental conditions as well as different bacteria population. The complete anaerobic fermentation process is briefly described as shown in Table 10, and Figure 3. Biogas is a relatively high-value fuel that is formed during anaerobic degradation of organic matter. The process has been known, and put to work in a number of different applications during the past 30 years, for rural needs such as in (Pernille, 2004): food security, water supply, health cares, education and communications.

Biogas is a generic term for gases generated from the decomposition of organic material. As the material breaks down, methane (CH_4) is produced as shown in Figure 3. Sources that generate biogas are numerous and varied. These include landfill sites, wastewater treatment plants and anaerobic digesters. Landfills and wastewater treatment plants emit biogas from decaying waste. To date, the waste industry has focused on controlling these emissions to our environment and in some cases, tapping this potential source of fuel to power gas turbines, thus generating electricity. The primary components of landfill gas are methane (CH_4), carbon dioxide (CO_2), and nitrogen (N_2). The average concentration of methane is ~45%, CO_2 is ~36% and nitrogen is ~18%. Other components in the gas are oxygen (O_2), water vapour and trace amounts of a wide range of non-methane organic compounds (NMOCs). For hot water and heating, renewables contributions come from biomass power and heat, geothermal direct heat, ground source heat pumps, and rooftop solar hot water and space heating systems. Solar assisted cooling makes a very small but growing contribution. When it comes to the installation of large amounts of PV, the cities have several important factors in common. These factors include:

1. A strong local political commitment to the environment and sustainability.
2. The presence of municipal departments or offices dedicated to the environment, sustainability or renewable energy.
3. Information provision about the possibilities of renewables.
4. Obligations that some or all building include renewable energy.

During the last decades thousands of biogas units were built all over the world in different areas, producing methane CH_4 for cooking, water pumping and electricity generation. In order not to repeat successes in depth on local conditions and conscientious planning urged (D'Apote, 1998). The goals should be achieved through:

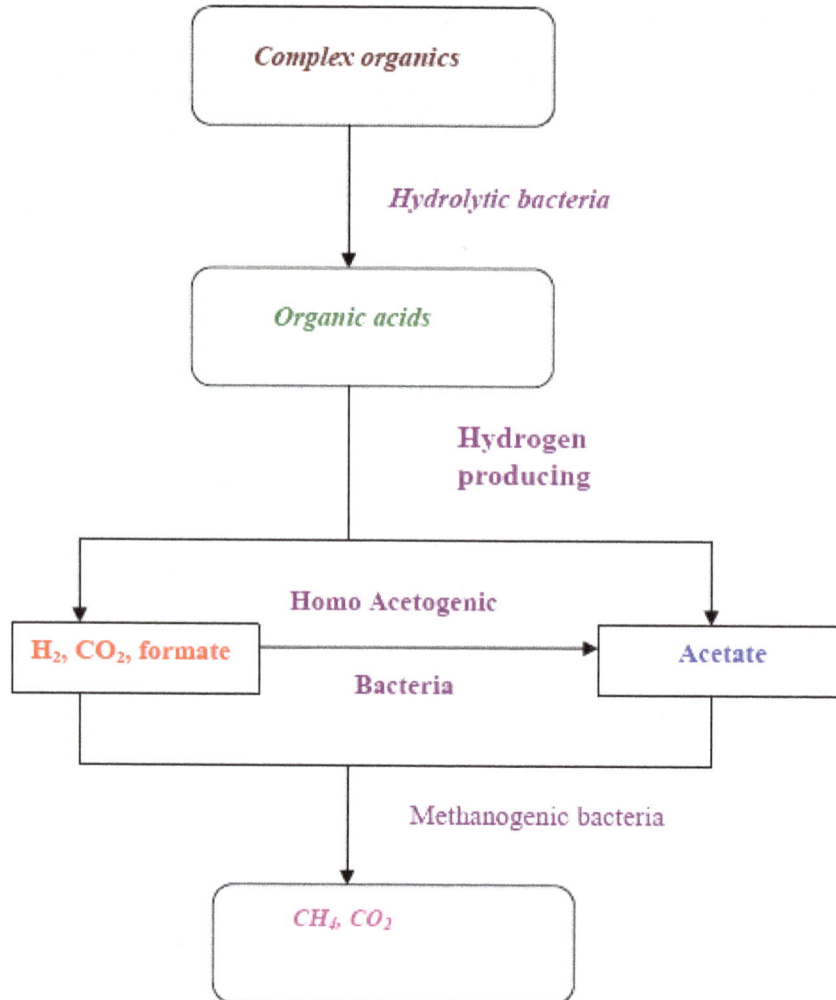

Figure 3. Biogas production process.

1. Review and exchange of information on computer models and manuals useful for economic evaluation of biogas from biomass energy.

2. Exchange and compile information on methodologies for economic analysis and results from type causes.

3. Investigation of the constraints on the implementation of the commercial supply of biogas energy.

4. Investigation of the relations between supplies and demand for the feedstock from different industries.

5. Documentation of the methods and principles for evaluation of indirect consequences as effects on growth, silvicultural treatment, and employment.

Biogas is a mixture containing predominantly methane (50-65% by volume) and carbon dioxide and in a natural setting it is formed in swamps and anaerobic sediments, etc., due to its high methane concentration, biogas is a valuable fuel. Wet (40-95%) organic materials with low lignin and cellulose content are generally suitable for anaerobic digestion. A key concern is that treatment of sludge tends to concentrate heavy metals, poorly biodegradable trace organic compounds and potentially pathogenic organisms (viruses, bacteria and the like) present in wastewaters. These materials can pose a serious threat to the environment. When deposited in soils, heavy metals are passed through the food chain, first entering crops, and then animals that feed on the crops and eventually human beings, to whom they appear to be highly toxic. In addition they also leach from soils, getting into groundwater and further spreading contamination in an uncontrolled manner. European and American markets aiming to transform various organic wastes (animal farm wastes, industrial and municipal wastes) into two main by-products:

1. A solution of humic substances (a liquid oxidant).
2. A solid residue.

In the past two decades the world has become increasingly aware of the depletion of fossil fuel reserves and the indications of climatic changes based on carbon dioxide emissions. Therefore extending the use of renewable resources, efficient energy production and the reduction of energy consumption are the main goals to reach a sustainable energy supply. Renewable energy sources include water and wind power, solar and geothermal energy, as well as energy from biomass. The technical achievability and the actual usage of these energy sources are different around Europe, but

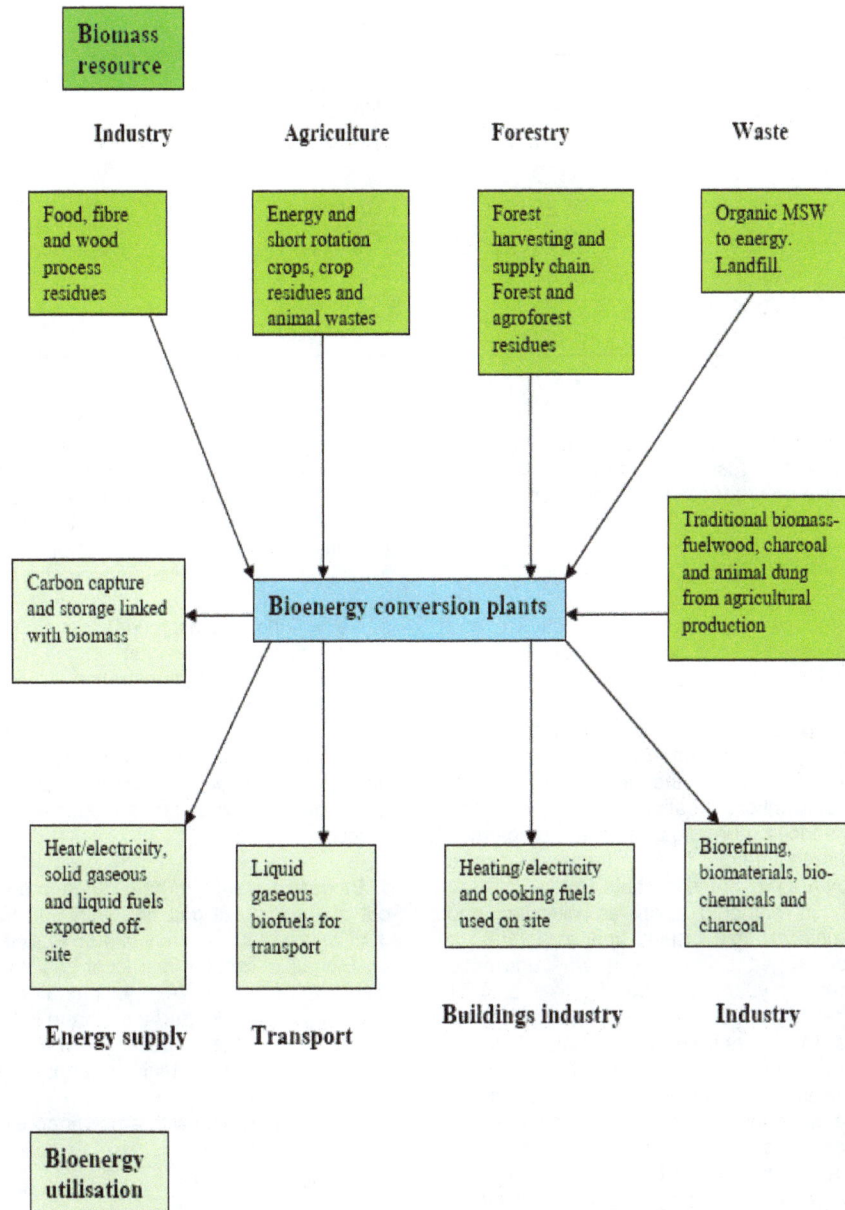

Figure 4. Biomass resources from several sources are converted into a range of products for use by transport, industry and building sectors (Pernille, 2004).

biomass is seen to have a great potential in many of them. An efficient method for the conversion of biomass to energy is the production of biogas by microbial degradation of organic matter under the absence of oxygen (anaerobic digestion). It is now possible to produce biogas at rural installation, upgrade it to bio-methane, feed it into the gas grid, use it in a heat demand-controlled CHP and to receive revenues (UNEP, 2000).

Improved forest and tree management

Dry cell batteries are a practical but expensive form of mobile fuel that is used by rural people when moving around at night and for powering radios and other small appliances. The high cost of dry cell batteries is financially constraining for rural households, but their popularity gives a good indication of how valuable a versatile fuel like electricity is in rural area. Dry cell batteries can constitute an environmental hazard unless they are recycled in a proper fashion. Direct burning of fuel-wood and crop residues constitute the main usage of biomass, as is the case with many developing countries. However, the direct burning of biomass in an inefficient manner causes economic loss and adversely affects human health. In order to address the problem of inefficiency, research centres around the world have investigated the viability of converting the resource to a more useful form, namely solid briquettes and fuel gas (Figure 4). Biomass resources play a significant role in energy

Table 11. Comparison of various fuels (Bacaoui et al., 1998).

Fuel	Calorific value (kcal)	Burning mode	Thermal efficiency (%)
Electricity, kWh	880	Hot plate	70
Coal gas, kg	4004	Standard burner	60
Biogas, m^3	5373	" "	60
Kerosene, l	9122	Pressure stove	50
Charcoal, kg	6930	Open stove	28
Soft coke, kg	6292	" "	28
Firewood, kg	3821	" "	17
Cow dung, kg	2092	" "	11

supply in all developing countries. Biomass resources should be divided into residues or dedicated resources, the latter including firewood and charcoal can also be produced from forest residues.

Gasification

Gasification is based on the formation of a fuel gas (mostly CO and H_2) by partially oxidising raw solid fuel at high temperatures in the presence of steam or air. The technology can use wood chips, groundnut shells, sugar cane bagasse, and other similar fuels to generate capacities from 3 kW to 100 kW. Three types of gasifier designs have been developed to make use of the diversity of fuel inputs and to meet the requirements of the product gas output (degree of cleanliness, composition, heating value, etc.). The requirements of gas for various purposes, and a comparison between biogas and various commercial fuels in terms of calorific value, and thermal efficiency are presented in Table 11.

Sewage sludge is rich in nutrients such as nitrogen and phosphorous. It also contains valuable organic matter, useful for remediation of depleted or eroded soils. This is why untreated sludge has been used for many years as a soil fertiliser and for enhancing the organic matter of soil. A key concern is that treatment of sludge tends to concentrate heavy metals, poorly biodegradable trace organic compounds and potentially pathogenic organisms (viruses, bacteria and the like) present in wastewaters. These materials can pose a serious threat to the environment. When deposited in soils, heavy metals are passed through the food chain, first entering crops, and then animals that feed on the crops and eventually human beings, to whom they appear to be highly toxic. In addition they also leach from soils, getting into groundwater and further spreading contamination in an uncontrolled manner (UNECA, 2003b). Biomass is a raw material that has been utilised for a wide variety of tasks since the dawn of civilisation. Important as a supply of fuel in the third world, biomass was also the first raw material in the production of textiles. The gasification of the carbon char with steam can make a large difference to the surface area of the carbon. The corresponding stream gasification reactions are endothermic and demonstrate how the steam reacts with the carbon char (D'Apote, 1998):

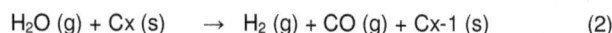

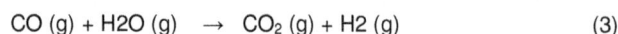

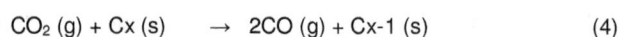

$$H_2O\ (g) + Cx\ (s) \rightarrow H_2\ (g) + CO\ (g) + Cx\text{-}1\ (s) \qquad (2)$$

$$CO\ (g) + H2O\ (g) \rightarrow CO_2\ (g) + H2\ (g) \qquad (3)$$

$$CO_2\ (g) + Cx\ (s) \rightarrow 2CO\ (g) + Cx\text{-}1\ (s) \qquad (4)$$

Agricultural wastes are abundantly available globally and can be converted to energy and useful chemicals by a number of microorganisms. The organic matter was biodegradable to produce biogas and the variation show a normal methanogene bacteria activity and good working biological process as shown in Figures 5 to 6. The success of promoting any technology depends on careful planning, management, implementation, training and monitoring. Main features of gasification project are:

1. Networking and institutional development/strengthening.
2. Promotion and extension.
3. Construction of demonstration projects.
4. Research and development, and training and monitoring.

An easier situation can be found when looking at the ecological effects of different biogas utilisation pathways. The key assumptions for the comparison of different biogas utilisation processes are:

1. Biogas utilisation in heat demand controlled gas engine supplied out of the natural gas grid with 500 kWe - electrical efficiency of 37.5%, thermal efficiency of 42.5%, and a methane loss of 0.01.
2. Biogas utilisation in a local gas engine, installed at the biogas plant wqith 500 kWe - electrical efficiency of 37.5%, thermal efficiency of 42.5%, and a methane loss of 0.5.
3. Biogas production based on maize silage using a biogas plant with covered storage tank - methane losses were 1% of the biogas produced.
4. Biogas upgrading with a power consumption 0.3 $kWhe/m^3$ biogas - methane losses of 0.5.

RESULTS AND DISCUSSIONS

Energy and environmental problems

Technological progress has dramatically changed the world in a variety of ways. It has, however, also led to developments of environmental problems, which threaten man and nature. During the past two decades the risk and reality of environmental degradation have become more apparent. Growing evidence of environmental problems is due to a combination of several factors since the environmental impact of human activities has grown dramatically because of the sheer increase of world population, consumption, industrial activity, etc. throughout the 1970s most environmental analysis and legal control instruments concentrated on conventional

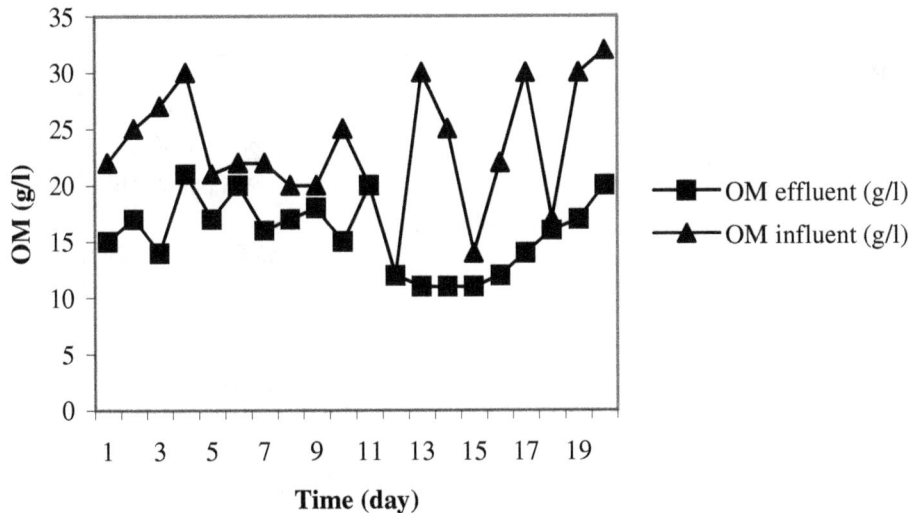

Figure 5. Organic matters before and after treatment in digester.

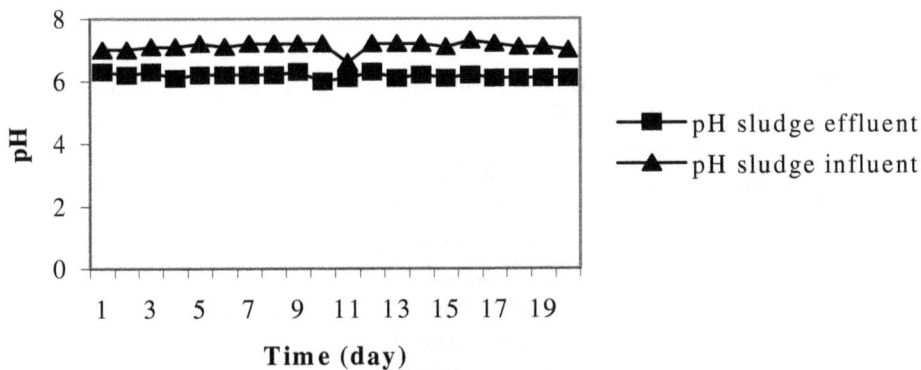

Figure 6. pH sludge before and after treatment in the digester.

effluent gas pollutants such as SO_2, NOx, CO_2, particulates, and CO (Table 12). Recently, environmental concerns has extended to the control of micro or hazardous air pollutants, which are usually toxic chemical substances and harmful in small doses, as well to that of globally significant pollutants such as CO_2. Aside from advances in environmental science, developments in industrial processes and structures have led to new environmental problems. For example, in the energy sector, major shifts to the road transport of industrial goods and to individual travel by cars has led to an increase in road traffic and hence a shift in attention paid to the effects a nd sources of NO_x and volatile organic compound (VOC) emissions.

Environmental problems span a continuously growing range of pollutants, hazards and ecosystem degradation over wider areas. The main areas of environmental problems are: major environmental accidents, water pollution, maritime pollution, land use and sitting impact, radiation and radioactivity, solid waste disposal, hazardous air pollutants, ambient air quality, acid rain, stratospheric ozone depletion and global warming (greenhouse effect, global climatic change) (Table 13). The four more important types of harm from man's activities are global warming gases, ozone destroying gases, gaseous pollutants and microbiological hazards (Table 14). The earth is some 30°C warmer due to the presence of gases but the global temperature is rising.

This could lead to the sea level rising at the rate of 60 mm each decade with the growing risk of flooding in low-lying areas (Figure 7). At the United Nations Earth Summit at Rio in June 1992 some 153 countries agreed to pursue sustainable development (D'Apote, 1998). A main aim was to reduce emission of carbon dioxide and other GHGs. Reduction of energy use in buildings is a major role in achieving this. Carbon dioxide targets are

Table 12. EU criteria pollutant standards in the ambient air environment (Abdeen, 2009a).

Pollutant	EU limit
CO	30 mg/m^2; 1h
NO$_2$	200 µg/m^2; 1h
O$_3$	235 µg/m^2; 1h
SO$_2$	250-350 µg/m^2; 24 h
	80-120 µg/m2; annual
PM10	250 µg/m^2; 24 h
	80 µg/m2; annual
SO2 + PM10	100-150 µg/m^2; 24 h
	40-60 µg/m^2; annual
Pb	2 µg/m^2; annual
Total suspended particulate (TSP)	260 µg/m^2; 24 h
HC	160 µg/m^2; 3 h

Table 13. Significant EU environmental directives in water, air and land environments (Abdeen, 2009b).

Environment	Directive name
Water	Surface water for drinking
	Sampling surface water for drinking
	Drinking water quality
	Quality of freshwater supporting fish
	Shellfish waters
	Bathing waters
	Dangerous substances in water
	Groundwater
	Urban wastewater
	Nitrates from agricultural sources
Air	Smokes in air
	Sulphur dioxide in air
	Lead in air
	Large combustion plants
	Existing municipal incineration plants
	New municipal incineration plants
	Asbestos in air
	Sulphur content of gas oil
	Emissions from petrol engines
	Air quality standards for NO$_2$
	Emissions from diesel engines
Land	Protection of soil when sludge is applied

Table 14. The external environment (Abdeen, 2009c).

Damage	Manifestation	Design
NO_x, SO_x	Irritant	Low NO_x burners
	Acid rain land damage	Low sulphur fuel
	Acid rain fish damage	Sulphur removal
CO_2	Global warming	Thermal insulation
	Rising sea level	Heat recovery
	Drought, storms	Heat pumps
O_3 destruction	Increased ultra violet	No CFC's or HCFC's
	Skin cancer	Minimum air conditioning
		Refrigerant collection
Legionnellosis	Crop damage	Careful maintenance
	Pontiac fever	Dry cooling towers
	Legionnaires	

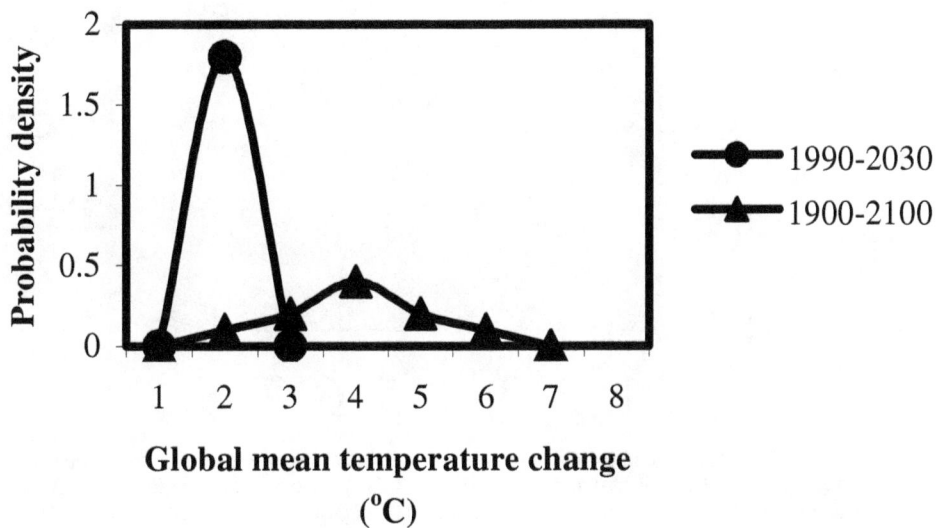

Figure 7. Global mean temperature changes over the period of 1990-2100 and 1990-2030.

proposed to encourage designers to look at low energy designs and energy sources (World Bank, 2001).

Problems with energy supply and use are related not only to global warming that is taking place, due to effluent gas emission mainly CO_2, but also to such environmental concerns as air pollution, acid precipitation, ozone depletion, forest destruction and emission of radioactive substances. These issues must be taken into consideration simultaneously if humanity is to achieve a bright energy future with minimal environmental impacts. Much evidence exists, which suggests that the future will be negatively impacted if humans keep degrading the environment (Table15). During the past century, global surface temperatures have increased at a rate near 0.6oC/century and the average temperature of the Atlantic, Pacific and Indian oceans (covering 72% of the earth surface) have risen by 0.06oC since 1995. Global temperatures in 2001 were 0.52°C above the long-term 1880-2000 average (the 1880-2000 annually averaged combined land and ocean temperature is 13.9°C). Also, according to the USA Department of Energy, world emissions of carbon are expected to increase by 54% above 1990 levels by 2015 making the earth likely to warm 1.7 - 4.9°C over the period 1990-2100, as shown in

Table 15. Global emissions of the top twelve nations by total CO_2 volume (billion of tones).

Rank	Nation	CO_2	Rank	Nation	CO_2
1	USA	1.36	7	Canada	0.11
2	Russia	0.98	8	Italy	0.11
3	China	0.69	9	Mexico	0.09
4	Japan	0.30	10	Poland	0.08
5	India	0.19	11	S. Africa	0.08
6	UK	0.16	12	S. Korea	0.07

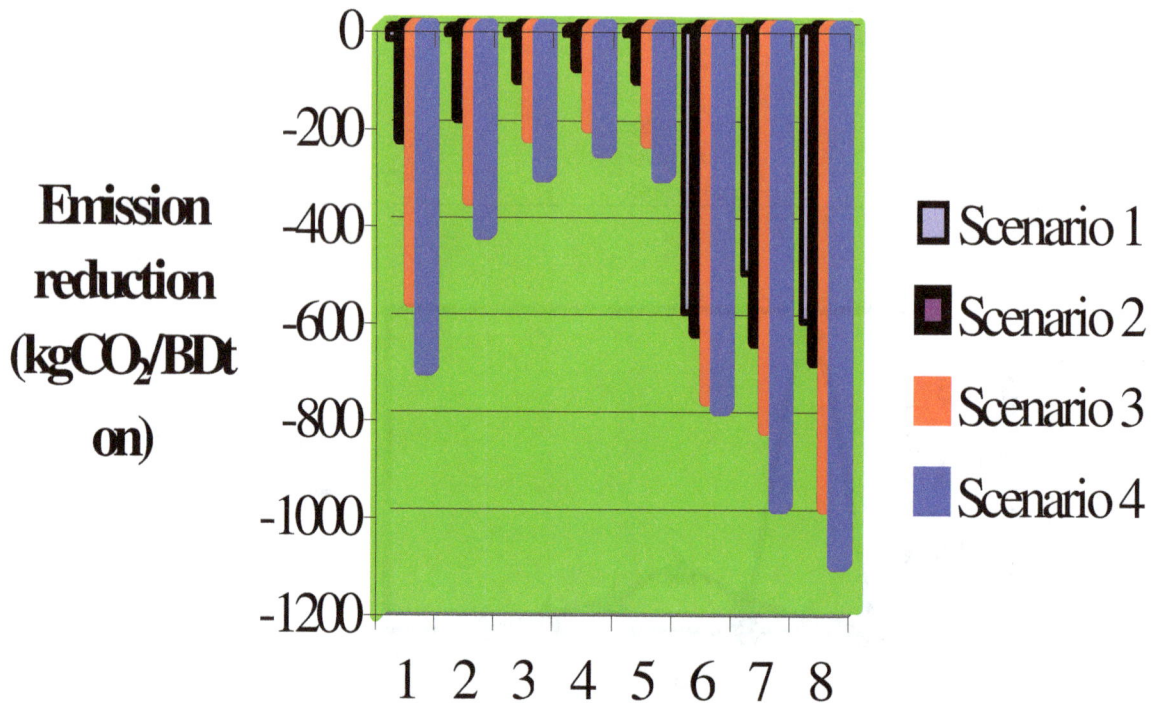

Figure 8. Comparison of thermal biomass usage options, CHP displacing natural gas as a heat source.
*1 Large steam power (LSP); *2 Small steam power (SSP); *3 Brayton cycle power (BCP); *4 Bio-oil conversion power (B-CP); *5 Gasification power (GP); *6 Small steam CHP (SSCHP); *7 Turboden cycle CHP (TCCHP); *8 Entropic cycle CHP (ECCHP).

Figure 8. Such observation and others demonstrate that interests will likely increase regarding energy related environment concerns and that energy is one of the main factors that must be considered in discussions of sustainable development (CEC, 2000).

Lifecycle analysis of several ethanol feedstocks shows the emission displacement per ton of feedstock is highest for corn stover and switch grass (about 0.65 tons of CO_2 per ton of feedstock) and lowest for corn (about 0.5 tone). Emissions due to cultivation and harvesting of corn and wheat are higher than those for lignocellulosics, and although the latter have a far higher process energy requirement (Figure 8). GHG emissions are lower because this energy is produced from biomass residue, which is carbon neutral.

Sulphur in fuels and its environmental consequences

Coal is formed from the deposition of plant material according to the peat to anthracite series:

Vegetation → Peat
          → Lignite (brown coal)
          → Sub-bituminous coal
          → Bituminous coal   →   Anthracite

Table 16. Representative sulphur contents of coals (Abdeen, 2009d).

Source	Rank	Sulphur content (%)
Ayrshire, Scotland	Bituminous	0.6
Lancs. /Cheshire, UK	Bituminous	Up to 2.4
S. Wales, UK	Anthracite	Up to 1.5
Victoria, Australia	Lignite	Typically 0.5
Pennsylvania, USA	Anthracite	0.7
Natal, S. Africa	Bituminous	Up to 4.2
Bulgaria	Lignite	2.5

Table 17. Examples of SO_2 control procedures (Abdeen, 2009d).

Type of control	Fuel	Details
Pre-combustion	Fuels from crude oil	Alkali treatment of crude oil to convert thiols RSSR, disulphides; solvent removal of the disulphides
Post-combustion	Coal or fuel oil	Alkali scrubbing of the flue gases with $CaCO_3/CaO$
Combustion	Coal	Limestone, $MgCO_3$ and/or other metallic compounds used to fix the sulphur as sulphates

Organic sulphur is bonded within the organic structure of the coal in the same way that sulphur is bonded in simple thio-organics, e.g., thiols. Sulphur contents of coals vary widely, and Table 16 gives some examples.

Control of SO_2 emissions

Emissions will also, of course, occur from petroleum-based or shale-based fuels, and in heavy consumption, such as in steam rising. There will frequently be a need to control SO_2 emissions. There are, broadly speaking, three ways of achieving such control:

1. Pre-combustion control: involves carrying out a degree of desulphurisation of the fuel.
Combustion control: incorporating into the combustion system something capable of trapping SO_2.
2. Post-combustion control: removing SO_2 from the fuel gases before they are discharged into the atmosphere.

Table 17 gives brief details of an example of each.

The control of NO_x release by combustion processes

Emission of nitrogen oxides is a major topic in fuel technology. It has to be considered even in the total absence of fuel nitrogen if the temperature is high enough for thermal NO_x, as it is in very many industrial applications. The burnt gas from the flame is recirculated in two ways:

1. Internally, by baffling and restricting flow of the burnt gas away from the burner, resulting in flame re-entry of part of it.
2. Externally, by diverting up to 10% of the flue gas back into the flame.

Several definitions of sustainable development have been put forth, including the following common one: development that meets the needs of the present without compromising the ability of future generations to meet their own needs. A recent World Energy Council (WEC) study found that without any change in our current practice, the world energy demand in 2020 would be 50-80% higher than 1990 levels. According to a recent USA Department of Energy (DoE) report, annual energy demand will increase from a current capacity of 363 million kilowatts to 750 million kilowatts by 2020. The world's energy consumption today is estimated at 22 billion kWh per year, 53 billion kWh by 2020. Such ever-increasing demand could place significant strain on the current energy infrastructure and potentially damage world environmental health by CO, CO_2, SO_2, NO_x effluent gas emissions and global warming. Achieving solutions to environmental problems that we face today requires long-term potential actions for sustainable development. In this regards, renewable energy resources appear to be the one of the most efficient and effective solutions since the intimate relationship between renewable energy and sustainable development. More rational use of energy is an important bridge to help transition from today's fossil fuel dominated world to a world powered by non-polluting fuels and advanced

Table 18. Particle control techniques.

Technique	Principle	Application
Gravity settlement	Natural deposition by gravity of particles from a horizontally flowing gas, collection in hoppers	Removal of coarse particles (>50 µm) from a gas stream, smaller particles removable in principle but require excessive flow distances
Cyclone separator	Tangential entry of a particle-laden gas into a cylindrical or conical enclosure, movement of the particles to the enclosure wall and from there to a receiver	Numerous applications, wide range of particles sizes removable, from = 5 µm to = 200 µm, poorer efficiencies of collection for the smaller particles
Fabric filters	Retention of solids by a filter, filter materials include woven cloth, felt and porous membranes	Used in dust removal for over a century
Electrostatic precipitation	Passage of particle-laden gas between electrodes, application of an electric field to the gas, resulting in acquisition of charge by the particles and attraction to an electrode where coalescence occurs, electrical resistivity of the dust an important factor in performance	Particles down to 0.01 µm removable, extensive application to the removal of flyash from pulverised fuel (pf) combustion

technologies such as photovoltaic (PV) and fuel cells (FC).

Growing concerns about social and environmental sustainability have led to increased interest in planning for the energy utility sector because of its large resource requirements and production of emissions. A number of conflicting trends combine to make the energy sector a major concern, even though a clear definition of how to measure progress toward sustainability is lacking. These trends include imminent competition in the electricity industry, global climate change, expected long-term growth in population and pressure to balance living standards (including per capital energy consumption). Designing and implementing a sustainable energy sector will be a key element of defining and creating a sustainable society. In the electricity industry, the question of strategic planning for sustainability seems to conflict with the shorter time horizons associated with market forces as deregulation replaces vertical integration. Sustainable low-carbon energy scenarios for the new century emphasise the untapped potential of renewable resources. Rural areas can benefit from this transition. The increased availability of reliable and efficient energy services stimulates new development alternatives. It is concluded that renewable environmentally friendly energy must be encouraged, promoted, implemented, and demonstrated by full-scale plant especially for use in remote rural areas (Omer, 1996; Lund et al., 2005)). Some of the available control procedures for particles are summarised in Table 18. This is the step in a long journey to encourage a progressive economy, which continues to provide us with high living standards, but at the same time helps reduce pollution, waste mountains, other environmental degradation, and environmental rationale for future policy-making and intervention to improve market mechanisms. This vision will be accomplished by:

1. 'Decoupling' economic growth and environmental degradation. The basket of indicators illustrated shows the progress being made. Decoupling air and water pollution from growth, making good headway with CO_2 emissions from energy, and transport. The environmental impact of our own individual behaviour is more closely linked to consumption expenditure than the economy as a whole.
2. Focusing policy on the most important environmental impacts associated with the use of particular resources, rather than on the total level of all resource use.
3. Increasing the productivity of material and energy use that are economically efficient by encouraging patterns of supply and demand, which are more efficient in the use of natural resources. The aim is to promote innovation and competitiveness. Investment in areas like energy efficiency, water efficiency and waste minimisation.
4. Encouraging and enabling active and informed individual and corporate consumers.

Wastes

Waste is defined as an unwanted material that is being discarded. Waste includes items being taken for further use, recycling or reclamation. Waste produced at household, commercial and industrial premises are control waste and come under the waste regulations. Waste Incineration Directive (WID) emissions limit values will favour efficient, inherently cleaner technologies that do not rely heavily on abatement. For existing plant, the requirements are likely to lead to improved control of:

1. NO_x emissions, by the adoption of infurnace combustion control and abatement techniques.
2. Acid gases, by the adoption of abatement techniques and optimisation of their control.
3. Particulate control techniques, and their optimisation, e.g., of bag filters and electrostatic precipitators.

The waste and resources action programme has been working hard to reduce demand for virgin aggregates and market uptake of recycled and secondary alternatives. The programme targets are:

1. To deliver training and information on the role of recycling and secondary aggregates in sustainable construction for influences in the supply chain, and
2. To develop a promotional programme to highlight the new information on websites.

Conclusions

The adoption of green or sustainable approaches to the way in which society is run is seen as an important strategy in finding a solution to the energy problem. The key factors to reducing and controlling CO_2, which is the major contributor to global warming, are the use of alternative approaches to energy generation and the exploration of how these alternatives are used today and may be used in the future as green energy sources. Even with modest assumptions about the availability of land, comprehensive fuel-wood farming programmes offer significant energy, economic and environmental benefits. These benefits would be dispersed in rural areas where they are greatly needed and can serve as linkages for further rural economic development. The nations as a whole would benefit from savings in foreign exchange, improved energy security, and socio-economic improvements. With a nine-fold increase in forest - plantation cover, a nation's resource base would be greatly improved. The international community would benefit from pollution reduction, climate mitigation, and the increased trading opportunities that arise from new income sources. The non-technical issues, which have recently gained attention, include: (1) Environmental and ecological factors, e.g., carbon sequestration, reforestation and revegetation. (2) Renewables as a CO_2 neutral replacement for fossil fuels. (3) Greater recognition of the importance of renewable energy, particularly modern biomass energy carriers, at the policy and planning levels. (4) Greater recognition of the difficulties of gathering good and reliable renewable energy data, and efforts to improve it. (5) Studies on the detrimental health efforts of biomass energy particularly from traditional energy users:

1) Biogas technology can not only provide fuel, but also

important for comprehensive utilisation of biomass forestry, animal husbandry, fishery, evoluting the agricultural economy, protecting the environment, realising agricultural recycling, as well as improving the sanitary conditions, in rural areas.
(2) The biomass energy, one of the important options, which might gradually replace the oil in facing the increased demand for oil and may be an advanced period in this century. Any county can depend on the biomass energy to satisfy part of local consumption.
(3) Development of biogas technology is a vital component of alternative rural energy programme, whose potential is yet to be exploited. A concerted effect is required by all if this has to realise. The technology will find ready use in domestic, farming, and small-scale industrial applications.
(4) Support biomass research and exchange experiences with countries that are advanced in this field. In the meantime, the biomass energy can help to save exhausting the oil wealth.

Biomass is a renewable energy source, which can be converted into liquid fuels and/or gas fuels with different technologies available today. Ethanol production via fermentation, extraction and extractive-distillation is one such method and has been practiced for long time in most developing countries with agricultural surplus. However, the intensive research and development activities still needed. Furthermore, investigating the potential to make use of more and more of its waste. Household waste, vegetable market waste, and waste from the cotton stalks, leather, and pulp; and paper industries can be used to produce useful energy either by direct incineration, gasification, digestion (biogas production), fermentation, or cogeneration. Therefore, effort has to be made to reduce fossil energy use and to promote green energies, particularly in the building sector.

ACKNOWLEDGEMENTS

The financial support for this research work from the Energy Research Institute is gratefully acknowledged. It is a pleasure to acknowledge, with gratitude, all those who, at different times and in different ways, have supported the development and evaluation of biomass energy technologies. A special thanks to my spouse Kawthar Abdelhai Ali for her support and her unwavering faith in me. Her intelligence, humour, spontaneity, curiosity and wisdom added to this article.

REFERENCES

Abdeen MO (2000). Biomass energy potential and applications, Agriculture Development in Arab World, Khartoum, Sudan, 19(4): 1-15.

Abdeen MO (2004). Water resources development and management in the Republic of the Sudan. Water Energy Int. J. New Delhi, India, October-December, 61(4): 27-39.

Abdeen MO (2005). Agricultural biomass production is an energy option for the future, In: Proceedings of the Dubrovnik Conference on Sustainable Development of Energy, Water and Environment systems, ES2 Energy Evaluation, Dubrovnik, Croatia, p.17.

Abdeen MO (2006). The puzzle of consumption, development and sustainability, In: Proceedings of the National Conference for development and Environment, Khartoum, Sudan, Sudan Eng. Soc. J., 52(47): 35-43.

Abdeen MO (2007a). Green energy saving mechanisms, In: Proceedings of the First Plan-Arab Conference on environmental Science & Technology, Renewable Energy Sources- Solar and Geothermal Energy, Sharjah, UAE, p. 6.

Abdeen MO (2007b). Green energy saving mechanisms, In: Proceedings of the 6th Jordanian International Mechanical Engineering Conference (JIMEC'6), Amman, Jordan, 22-24 October 2007.

Abdeen MO (2007c). Chapter 6: Energy, water and sustainable development, In: Focus on Sustainable Development Research Advances, Editor: Barton A. Larson, 2007 NOVA Science Publishers, Inc., New York, USA, pp. 189-205.

Abdeen MO (2008a). Renewable building energy systems and passive human comfort solutions. Renewable Sustainable Energy Review, United Kingdom, 12(6): 1562-1587.

Abdeen MO (2008b). People, power and pollution, Renewable and Sustainable Energy Reviews, United Kingdom, 12(7): 1864-1889.

Abdeen MO (2008c). Energy, environment and sustainable development, Renewable Sustain. Energy Rev., United Kingdom, 12(9): 2265-2300.

Abdeen MO (2008d). Focus on low carbon technologies: the positive solution, Renewable Sustain. Energy Rev., United Kingdom, 12(9): 2331-2357.

Abdeen MO (2008e). Chapter 10: Development of integrated bioenergy for improvement of quality of life of poor people in developing countries, In: Energy in Europe: Economics, Policy and Strategy- IB, Editors: Flip L. Magnusson and Oscar W. Bengtsson, 2008 NOVA Science Publishers, Inc., New York, USA, pp. 341-373.

Abdeen MO (2008f). The environmental and economical advantages of agricultural wastes for sustainable development, In: Proceedings of the 16th European Biomass Conference & Exhibition from Research to Industry and Markets, Biomass for Energy, Industry and Climate Protection, Feria Valencia, Spain, pp. 35-40.

Abdeen MO (2009a). Environmental and socio-economic aspect of possible development in renewable energy use, In: Proceedings of the 5th International Congress for South-East Europe on Energy Efficiency and Renewable Energy Sources, Sofia, Bulgaria.

Abdeen MO (2009b). Environmental and socio-economic aspect of possible development in renewable energy use, In: Proceedings of the 4th International Symposium on Environment, Athens, Greece.

Abdeen MO (2009c). Energy use, environment and sustainable development, In: Proceedings of the 3rd International Conference on Sustainable Energy and Environmental Protection (SEEP 2009), Dublin, Republic of Ireland, p. 1011.

Abdeen MO (2009d). Energy use and environmental: impacts: A general review, J. Renewable Sustain. Energy, United State of America, 1(053101): 1-29.

Abdeen MO (2009e). Chapter 3: Energy use, environment and sustainable development, In: Environmental Cost Management, Editors: Randi Taylor Mancuso, 2009 NOVA Science Publishers, Inc., New York, USA, 2009, pp. 129-166.

Anne G, Michael S (2005). Building and land management. 5th Edition. Oxford: UK. 2005, pp. 10-20.

Aroyeun SO, Adegoke GO, Varga J, Teren J (2009). Reduction of aflatoxin B1 and Ochratoxin A in cocoa beans infected with Aspergillus via Ergosterol Value. World Rev. Sci. Technol. Sustain. Dev., 6(1): 75-90.

ASHRAE. (1993). Energy efficient design of new building except new low-rise residential buildings. BSRIASHRAE proposed standards 90-

2P-1993, alternative GA. American Society of Heating, Refrigerating, and Air Conditioning Engineers Inc., USA, 1993.

Bacaoui A, Yaacoubi A, Dahbi C, Bennouna J, Mazet A (1998). Activated carbon production from Moroccan olive wastes-influence of some factors. Environ. Technol., 19: 1203-1212.

Brain G, Mark S (2007). Garbage in, energy out: landfill gas opportunities for CHP projects. Cogeneration and On-Site Power, 8 (5): 37-45.

Commission of the European Communities (CEC). (2000). Towards a European strategy for the security of energy supply. Green Paper, Brussels, 29 November 2000 COM (2000) 769. www.cec.org.

McKennan G, Crisp V, Cooper I (1988). Daylighting as a passive solar energy option: an assessment of its potential in non-domestic buildings.Garston. UK. p.129.

D'Apote SL (1998). IEA biomass energy analysis and projections. In: Proceedings of Biomass Energy Conference: Data, analysis and Trends, Paris: OECD.

David E (2003). Sustainable energy: choices, problems and opportunities. R. Soc. Chem., 19: 19-47.

DEFRA. (2002). Energy Resources. Sustainable Development and Environment. Doncaster, UK.

Dieng A, Wang R (2001). Literature review on solar absorption technologies for ice making and air conditioning purposes and recent development in solar technology. Renewable Sustain. Energy Rev., 5 (4): 313-42.

Dragana V (2008). Plant medicines: A herbalist's perspective. World Rev. Sci. Technol. Sustain. Dev., 5(2): 140-151.

Energy Use in Offices (EUO) (2000). Energy Consumption Guide 19 (ECG019). Energy efficiency best practice programme. UK Government. London.

Farm Energy Centre (FEC). (2000). Helping agriculture and horticulture through technology, energy efficiency and environmental protection. Warwickshire, 2000.

Haripriye G (2000). Estimation of biomass in India forests. Biomass and Bioenergy, 19: 245-58.

Huttrer G (2001). The status of world geothermal power generation 1995-2000. Geothermics, 30: 1-27.

International Energy Agency (IEA). (2007). Indicators for industrial Energy Efficiency and CO2 Emissions: A Technology Perspective, pp. 5-16.

IEA (2008). Combined heat and power: evaluating the benefits of greater global investment, pp. 7-21.

IPCC (2001). Climate change,United Nations International Panel on Climate Change. Cambridge University Press. UK (3 volumes).

Jeremy L (2005). The energy crisis, global warming and the role of renewables. Renewable Energy World, 8(2).

Lam JC (2000). Shading effects due to nearby buildings and energy implications. Energy Conversion Manage, 47(7): 47-59.

Lazzarin R, D'Ascanio A, Gaspaella A (2002). Utilisation of a green roof in reducing the cooling load of a new industrial building. In: Proceedings of the 1st International Conference on Sustainable Energy Technologies (SET), Porto: Portugal, pp. 32-37.

Lund JW, Freeston DH, Boyd TL (2005). Direct application of geothermal energy: 2005 Worldwide Review. Geothermics, 34: 691-727.

Mortal A (2002). Study of solar powered heat pump for small spaces. Portugal, pp. 6-13.

Omer AM (1996) Biogas technology and the environment, Regional Energy News, 2(4): 2-5.

Omer AM, Yemen F (2003). Biogas energy technology in Sudan. Renewable Energy, 28(3): 499-507.

Omer AM (2005). Biomass energy potential and future prospect in Sudan. Renewable Sustain. Energy Rev., 9: 1-27.

Omer AM (2007a). Review: Organic waste treatment for power production and energy supply. Cells Anim. Biol., 1(2): 34-47.

Omer AM (2007b). Renewable energy resources for electricity generation. Renewable Sustain. Energy Rev. UK, 11(7): 1481-1497.

Omer AM (2008a). Green energies and the environment. Renewable Sustainable Energy Rev., 12: 1789-1821.

Omer AM (2008b). Energy demands for heating and cooling equipment systems and technology advancements. In: Natural Resources: Economics, Management and Policy, pp. 131-165.

Omer AM (2008c). Ground-source heat pumps systems and applications. Renewable Sustain. Energy Rev., 12: 344-371.

Omer AM (2009). The environmental and economical advantages of agricultural wastes for sustainability development in Sudan. In Proceedings of the 1st Diaspora Conference. Brighton, UK, pp. 173-182.

Paul F (2001). Indoor hydroponics: A guide to understanding and maintaining hydroponics' nutrient solution. UK.

Pernille M (2004). Feature: Danish lessons on district heating. Energy Res. Sustain. Manage. Environ., pp. 16-17.

Reddy A, Williams R, Johansson T (2007). Energy after Rio: prospects and challenges. United Nations Development Programme (UNDP). http://www.undp.org/seed/energy/-exec-en.html.

REN21 (2001). Renewables (2007) global status report. www.ren21.net.

Robinson G (2007). Changes in construction waste management. Waste Manage. World, 3: 43-492.

Roriz L (2001). Determining the potential energy and environmental effects reduction of air conditioning systems. Commission of the European Communities DG TREN.

Shao S, Lin RS, Zhejiang DX (2002). Thermodynamic analysis on heat pumps with economiser for cold regions, China, pp. 23-28.

Sims RH (2007). Not too late: IPCC identifies renewable energy as a key measure to limit climate change. Renewable Energy World, 10(4) 31-39.

The World Bank WB (2001). 'World development Report 2000/2001', Oxford University Press. UK, pp. 16-34

Trevor T (2007). Fridge recycling: bringing agents in from the cold. Waste Manag. World, 5: 43-47.

United Nations UN (2001). World Urbanisation Prospect: The 1999 Revision. New York. The United Nations Population Division, 2001.

United Nations (2002a). 'Implementation of the United Nations millennium declaration', Report of the Secretary-General, United Nations General Assembly, http://www.un.org.

United Nations (2002b). Science and Technology as a Foundation for SD. Summary by the Scientific and Technological Community for the Multi-Stakeholder Dialogue Segment of the fourth session of the Commission on SD acting as the preparatory committee for the World Summit on SD. Note by the Secretary-General. Commission on SD acting as the preparatory committee for the World Summit on SD Fourth Preparatory Session.

United Nations (2002c) . 'Global challenge global opportunity: trends in sustainable development', Department of Economics and Social, World Summit on Sustainable Development, Johannesburg, SA.

United Nations Economic Commission for Africa (UNECA) (2002). 'Address by Josué Dioné: science and technology policies for sustainable development and Africa's global inclusion', Sustainable Development Division ATPS Conference, 11 November, Abuja, Nigeria.

United Nations Economic Commission for Africa (UNECA) (2003a). Making Science and Technology Work for the Poor and for SD in Africa, Paper prepared by the SD Division with the assistance of a senior international consultant, Akin Adubifa, January.

United Nations Economic Commission for Africa (UNECA) (2003b) 'The state of food security in Africa', Progress Report of the 3rd Meeting of the Committee on Sustainable Development, Addis Ababa, Ethiopia.

United Nations Economic Commission for Europe (UNECE) (2004). 'Note by the ECE Secretariat, Steering Group on Sustainable Development. Second Meeting of the 2003/2004 Bureau', Conference of European Statisticians, Statistical Commission, Geneva, Switzerland.

UNEP (2003). Handbook for the International Treaties for the Protection of the Ozone Layer. United Nations Environment Programme. Nairobi: Kenya.

United Nations Under-Secretary General and the United Nations Environment Programme (UNEP) (2000) 'Overview: Outlook and recommendations', Global Environment Outlook, http://grid.cr.usgs.gov/geo2000/ov-e/0012.htm, Earthscan, 1999, London.

Witte H, Gelder A (2002). Comparison of design and operation of a commercial UK ground source heat pump project. Groenholland BV, pp. 5-9.

World Bank (WB) (2003a) 'Global economic prospects: realizing the development promise of the Doha agenda', The International Bank for Reconstruction and Development. The World Bank, World Bank: Washington, DC.

World Bank (WB) (2003b) World Development Report, Oxford University Press, New York, pp. 12-17.

World Bank (2004). World Development Report 2004: Making Services Work for Poor People, World Bank: Washington, DC.

World Bank (WB) (2006). Sustainable Development in the 21st Century. http://Inweb18.worldbank.org/ESSD/sdvext.nsf/43ByDocName/Sustai nableDevelopmentint

World Bank (WB) (2007). World Bank Sustainable Development Reference Guide,htttp://www.WorldBankSustainableDevelopmentReferenceGui de.

Zuatori A (2005). An overview on the national strategy for improving the efficiency of energy use. Jordanian Energy Abstracts, 9(1): 31-32.

6

Elaboration of mycotoxins by seed-borne fungi of finger millet (*Eleusine coracana* L.)

Shilpa Penugonda*, S. Girisham and S. M. Reddy

Department of Microbiology, Kakatiya University, Warangal-506009, Andhra Pradesh, India.

Mycotoxin producing potential of fungi associated with finger millet was investigated. Many species of *Aspergillus* elaborated aflatoxins, patulin, terreic acid and sterigmocystin, while species of *Fusarium* elaborated zearalenone, fusarinone-X, deoxynivalenol, nivalenol, diacetoxyscripenol, neosolanil and HT-2 toxins. *Penicillium griseofulvum* elaborated cyclopiazonic acid. The toxigenic potential of individual fungus varied.

Key words: Mycotoxins, seed-borne fungi, finger millet.

INTRODUCTION

Deoxynivalenol (DON) and nivalenol (NIV) are a group of closely related secondary fungal metabolites, that are produced predominantly, although not exclusively, by several species of the genus *Fusarium*, especially *F. graminearum*. Finger millet , known as 'ragi' in India is an important staple food for people belonging to the low socio-economic group, several reports have shown that millet (Pathak et al., 2000) are inexpensive and nutritionally comparable or even superior to major cereals. Regular consumption is known to reduce the risk of diabetes mellitus (Gopalan, 1981) and gastro intestinal tract disorders (Tovey, 1994). These seeds are vulnerable to the huge diversity of opportunistic microbes especially the *Fusarial* species, further, it is anticipated seeds that are more vulnerable to mycotoxin contamination.

Though, there are several recent reports of infestation of finger millet by mycotoxin, producing fungi from different parts of the World (Nikema et al., 2004; Ana et al., 2009). There are only limited studies in India (Rajan et al., 2006; Vinod kumar et al., 2008). Further, very limited information is available from this region. Moulds, besides depleting the nutrients, may also produce toxic substances that are potential health hazards to animals and, in turn to humans (Fazekas et al., 1996; Trucksess, 2001). These mycotoxins can be very stable to food processing (Molini'e et al., 2005) and be present in final products. Hence, an attempt has been made to study the toxigenic potentials of different fungi associated with finger millet in different parts of the state. Majority of the *Fusarium* species produce trichothecene mycotoxins. Trichothecenes are esters of sesquiterpenoid alcohols containing the trichothecene tricyclic ring system (Pestka and Smolinski, 2005).

MATERIALS AND METHODS

A total of 110 pre-packaged samples were selected from local retail commerce in Andhra Pradesh of India. No particular preference was used in selecting samples or locations. The sample size was 250 gm were analyzed. The mycoflora of seed as well as the mycotoxins were assayed.

Fusarial mycotoxins were analyzed using thin layer chromatography (TLC). For this purpose, fusarial culture filtrates were extracted twice with ethylacetate (2 × 50). The combined extracts were passed through an anhydrous Na_2SO_4 bed to remove moisture and then evaporated to dryness before dissolving in 1 ml of methanol and spotting onto the TLC plates. The toxins were identified by spraying the plates with different spray reagents (Table 1) as suggested by Kamimura et al. (1981); Ramakrishna et al. (1985), and the compounds thus separated were identified based on the color of the fluorescence of the spot and by the R_f values, as compared with standards. The R_f was calculated by using the formula:

$$R_f = \frac{\text{Distance travelled by the compound}}{\text{Distance travelled by the solvent}}$$

RESULTS AND DISCUSSION

From Table 1, it is evident that, most of the fungal strains

---

*Corresponding author. E-mail: shilpa.penugonda1@gmail.com

Table 1. Incidence of mycotoxin producing fungi associated with finger millet.

Name of the fungus	Number of strains	Number of strains producing toxin	Solvent system	Fluorescence under UV		Rf value	Chemical conformation	Mycotoxin
				Before spray	After spray			
Aspergillus flavus	120	79	C:A (90:10)	Blue green	-	B1-0.42 B2-0.40 G1-0.32	-	Aflatoxins
Aspergillus nidulans i.e solvent	28	22	C:M:A (1:01:01)	Dull brick	Yellow	0.91	AlCl₃ (Ramakrishna et.al., 1985)	Sterigmocystin
Aspergillus terreus	36	21	T:Ea:F (50:40:10)	Dark brown	Yellow	0.45	2% Phenylhydrazene hydrochloride	Patulin or Terreic acid
Fusarium spp. *Fusarium oxysporum,* *F. moniliforme,* *F. graminearum,* *F. culmorum,* *F. sporotrichoides*	48	24	Ea:T:F (50:40:10)	Green	Blue	0.63 0.35 0.21 0.78 0.42	-	Zearalenone Fusarinone-X Deoxynivalenol Nivalenol Neosolaniol,HT-2
Trichothecium roseum	5	3	C:M (98:2)	Blue Blue-green	Pink	0.97 0.65	Phloroglucinol	Trichothecin
Trichoderma viride	2	2	C:M (98:2)	Blue	Pink	0.97	Pholroglucinol Resorcinol	Trichodermin Gliotoxin
Penicillium griseofulvum	8	4	C:Ea:F:T (50:40:10:2)	Dark brown	Purple	-	FeCl₃	Cyclopiazonic acid

C = chloroform; A = acetone; M = methanol; T= toluene; Ea = ethylacetate; F = formic acid.

isolated from finger millet produced one or the other mycotoxin. However, aflatoxins producing fungi were dominant. The incidence of toxigenic strains of *A. nidulans* and *A. terreus* come next. Species of *Fusarium* also elaborated variety of toxins of which Zearalenone was most common. On the other hand, Vesonder et al. (1978) reported that most of the food samples were contaminated with deoxynivalenol. Other trichothecene producing fungi not only formed minor production of spermosphere but also their toxigenic potentials were limited. Doohan et al. (2003) commented that production of trichothecenes by *F. culmorum* and *F. graminearum* is favoured by warm and humid conditions. The trichothecenes including DON, NIV and fusarenone-X, are common fungal contaminants of millets (Magan and Olsen, 2004; Jennings et al. (2000). Most of the species of *Penicillium* were non-toxigenic and hence less hazardous. Present observations are similar to those of Bilgrami et al. (1981) , Reddy and Reddy (1983), Girisham et al. (1985) who also observed the association of fungi with seeds of maize, sesamum and Pearl millet respectively with varied mycotoxigenic potentials and pose a threat to the health to man.

From the present investigations it can be concluded that variety of fungi harboring finger millet seeds are potentially toxigenic and not only hazardous directly to man but also may be responsible for diseases of poultry and livestock. Consumption of these toxins is a potential problem for humans and farm animals (Erisken et al., 1998; Rotter et al., 1996). Thus these fungi may be responsible for primary and secondary mycotoxicoses in man. Hence, more detailed investigations are desired in order to suggest measures to check the mould infestation of finger millet grains/product.

ACKNOWLEDGEMENTS

The authors thank Prof. M. A. Singara Charya, Head, Department of Microbiology for providing facilities; and financial assistance from Jawaharlal Nehru Memorial Fund, New Delhi is also gratefully acknowledged.

REFERENCES

Ana MP, Emilia CB, Hector HL, Gonzalez EM, White C, Elena JM, Siliva LR (2009). Fungal and fumonisins contamination and Argentine maize (*Zea mays L.*) silico bags. J. Agric. Food Chem., 57: 2778-2781.

Bilgrami KS, Prasad T, Misra RS, Sinha KK (1981). Aflatoxin contamination in maize under field conditions. Indian Phytopath., 34: 67-68.

Doohan FM, Brennan JM, Cooke BM (2003). Influence of climatic factors on *Fusarium* species pathogenic to cereals. Eur. J. Plant Pathol., 109: 755-768.

Fazekas B, Kis M, Haidu ET (1996). Data on the contamination of maize with fumonisins B1 and other fusarial toxins in Hungary. Acta. Vet. Hung, 44, 25-37.

Girisham S, Rao GV, Reddy SM (1985). Mycotoxin producing fungi associated with pearl millet (*Pennisetum typhoides* (Burm. f) stapf & C.E.Hubb.). Nat. Acad. Sci. Lett.,, 8, 333-335.

Gopalan C (1981). Carbohydrates in diabetic diet. India: Bulletin of Nutrition Foundation, P.3

Tovey FI (1994). Diet and duodenal ulcer. J. Gastroenterol. Hepatol. 9: 177-185.

Jennings P, Turner JA, Nicholson P (2000). Overview of Fusarium ear blight in the UK- effect of fungicide treatment on disease control and mycotoxin production. The British crop protection council. Pests Dis., 2: 707-712.

Kamimura H, Nishijima M. Yasuda K, Saito L, Ibe A, Nagayama T, Yoshiyama H, Naoi Y (1981). Simultaneous detection of fusarial toxins. J.Assoc. Off. Anal. Chem., 64: 1067-1073.

Magan N. Olsen M. (2004). Mycotoxins in Food: Detection and control. Wood head Publishing Ltd., Cambridge, UK.

Molini'e A, Faucet V, Castegnaro M, Pfohl-Leszkonicz A (2005). Analysis of some breakfast cereals on the fresh market for their contents of ochratoxin a, citrinin and fumonisins B1: development of method for simultaneous extraction of ochratoxin a and citrinin. Food Chem, 92: 391-400.

Pathak P, Srinivastava S, Grover S (2000). Development of food products based on millet, legumes and fenugreek seeds and their suitability in the diabetic diet. Int. J. Food Sci. Nutr. 51: 409-414.

Pestka JJ, Smolinski AT (2005). Deoxynivaneol: Toxicology and potential effects on humans. J.Toxicol. Environ. Health, part B, 8: 39-69.

Rajan SK, Ashok S (2006). Occurrence of mycotoxigenic fungi and mycotoxins in animal feed from Bihar, India. J. Sci. Food Agric., 56: 39-47.

Ramakrishna Y, Bhat RV (1987). Comparison of different spray reagents for identification of trichothecenes. Curr. Sci., 56, 524-526.

Reddy AS, Reddy SM (1983). Elaboration of mycotoxins by fungi associated with Til (Sesamum *indicum* L.). Curr. Sci., 6(20): 52: 613.

Rotter BA, Prelusky DB, Pestka JJ (1996). Toxicology of deoxynivalenol (vomitoxin). J. Toxicol. Environ. Health, 48: 1-34.

Trucksess W (2001). Joint mycotoxin technical Committee reports. J. AOAC, 83, 2.

Vesonder RF, Ciegler A, Rogers RF, Bumbridege, KA, Bothast RJ, Jensen AB (1978). Natural occurrence of Vomitoxin in Austrian and Canadian Corn. Appl. Microbiol. Biotechnol., 36: 885-888.

Vinod K, Basu MS and Rajendran TP (2008). Mycotoxin research and mycoflora in some commercially important agricultural commodities. Crop Prot., 27, 891-905.

7

Effects of planting dates and compost on mucilage variations in borage (*Borago officinalis* L.) under different chemical fertilization systems

Ahmad Ebrahimi[1], Payam Moaveni[2] and Hossein Aliabadi Farahani[3]*

[1]Islamic Azad University, Iranshahr Branch, Iran.
[2]Islamic Azad University, Shahr-e-Qods Branch, Iran.
[3]Member of Young Researchers Club, Islamic Azad University, Shahr-e Qods Branch, Iran.

The experimental design was a split factorial on the basis of completely randomized block design with three replications at the experimtal field of the Islamic Azad University, Shahr-e-Qods Branch, Iran in 2009. The planting dates (1 March, 15 March and 1 April) were assigned to the main plots and the combination of compost including 5, 10, 15 and 20 ton ha^{-1} and the chemical fertilization systems (N1P1K1 = 160, 128, 160; N2P2K2 = 120, 96, 120; N3P3K3 = 80, 64, 80; N4P4K4 = 40, 32, 40 respectively) were factorially assigned to the subplots. The chemical fertilization systems and compost significantly increased the mucilage percentage, flower yield, grain yield, root dry weight, plant height, flower number per plant and thousand seed weight in borage. Although, the planting date treatment significantly increased the plant features and the highest mucilage percentage (9.4%) was achieved under the treatments of 1 March and N1P1K1. It can be stated that compost is able to enhance the growth of borage under chemical fertilization systems enhancing NPK uptake.

Key words: Planting date, chemical fertilization system, compost, mucilage, borage.

INTRODUCTION

Composts are products containing living cells of different types of microorganisms (Vessey, 2003; Chen, 2006) that have an ability to convert nutritionally important elements from unavailable to available form through biological processes (Vessey, 2003) and are known to help with expansion of the root system and better seed germination. Composts differ from chemical and organic fertilizers in that they do not directly supply any nutrients to crops and are cultures of special bacteria and fungi. They also increase germination and vigor in young plants, leading to improved crop stands (Chen, 2006). Chemical fertilizers are the major nutrient that influences plants yield and protein concentration. When the amount of available soil NPK limits yield potential, additions of NPK fertilizers can substantially increase plants yield. However, plants protein concentration can decrease if the amount of added NPK is not adequate for potential yield

(Olson et al., 1976; Grant et al., 1985). Many researchers have found that late-season top-dress NPK additions as dry fertilizer materials were the most effective in attaining higher plants protein concentration (Fowler and Brydon, 1989; Vaughan et al., 1990; Stark and Tindall, 1992; Wuest and Cassman, 1992; Knowles et al., 1994). Good soil fertility management ensures adequate nutrient availability to plants and increases yields. High aboveground biomass yield is obviously accompanied by an active root system, which releases an array of organic compounds into the rhizosphere (Mandal et al., 2007). It is well known that a considerable number of bacterial and fungal species possess a functional relationship and constitute a holistic system with plants. They are able to exert beneficial effects on plant growth (Vessey, 2003) and also enhance plant resistance to adverse environmental stresses, such as water and nutrient deficiency and heavy metal contamination (Wu et al., 2005). The relationship between essential oil content and planting date has not been established. It has been hypothesized that cultivating medicinal plants for essential oil content could

---

*Corresponding author. E-mail: aliabadi.farahani@yahoo.com.

Table 1. Analysis of variance.

Mean squares							df	Value sources
Plant height	Thousand seed weight	Flower number per plant	Grain yield	Root dry weight	Flower yield	Mucilage percentage		
346.65	4.347	162755.694	4.802	0.036	107.81	107.81	2	Replication
209.167	0.047	360317.291*	136.603**	0.001**	0.001*	31.04	2	PD
37.723	2.701	17703.73	3.792	0.004	0.0001	93.09	4	Error a
31.72	1.97	291690.374**	36.91**	0.003**	0.001**	18921.41**	3	Compost
17.671	2.183	102190.046	8.964	0.003	0.0001	18.93	6	PD × Compost
7874.563**	92.13**	14969087.337**	42.779*	0.694**	0.035**	11.14	3	CFS
5.88	3.05	1736.263	17.977	0.0001	0.0001	5.7	6	PD × CFS
16.459	1.258	142939.147*	2.247	0.002	0.0001	68.11	9	Compost × CFS
4.107	4.421	3072.814	4.204	0.0001	0.0001	1.14	18	PD × Compost × CFS
33.233	2.73	39184.251	6.745	0.009	0.0001	85.17	3	Error bc

CFS = Chemical fertilization systems, PD = Planting date,* and ** : Significant at 5% and 1% levels, respectively.

theoretically be later than medicinal plants for canopy because plants do not have to be harvested at maturity (Zehtab-Salmasi et al., 2001). Early planting increases the total length of time that the plant is in the field and exposed to the environment and also it is associated with increased incidences of several diseases (Bowden, 1997). Thus, early planting increases the probability of adverse consequences relative to essential oil content and planting date may also influence the quality of the essential oil. Several studies have been conducted on the effect of planting date on the essential oil content of cumin (Zehtab-salmasi et al., 2001) and coriander (Carrubba et al., 2002). The objectives of this study were to describe the relationships between planting date and compost on plant features and determine the optimum chemical fertilization systems for the borage mucilage percentage in Iran.

MATERIALS AND METHODS

The experimental design was a split factorial on the basis of completely randomized block design with three replications at the experimtal field of Islamic Azad University, Shahr-e-Qods Branch, Iran in 2009. The planting dates (1 March, 15 March and 1 April) were assigned to the main plots and the combination of compost including 5, 10, 15 and 20 ton ha^{-1} and the chemical fertilization systems (N1P1K1 = 160, 128, 160; N2P2K2 = 120, 96, 120; N3P3K3 = 80, 64, 80; N4P4K4 = 40, 32, 40 respectively) were factorially assigned to the subplots. A total number of 144 plots, each measuring 15 m^2 area (5 × 3 m) and the seedlings were thinned to achieve 40 cm spacing within rows after which the plants were at the 4 leaves stage and also, chemical fertilizers and compost were added in planting time. At the end of flowering stage, we selected 100 g dry matter of flowering shoot from each plot to determine of the mucilage percentage. To determine the flower yield, grain yield, root dry weight, plant height, flower number per plant and thousand seed weight, 10 plants were selected randomly from each plot at maturity. The data were subjected to analysis of variance (ANOVA) using statistical analysis system (SAS Institute, 1988) computer software at P < 0.05.

RESULTS

The final results of plants characters showed that compost significantly increased the mucilage percentage, flower yield, grain yield, root dry weight and flowers number per plant (P ≤ 0.01, Table 1). Also, chemical fertilization systems significantly affected flower yield, root dry weight, plant height, thousand seed weight and flowers number per plant (P ≤ 0.01) and grain yield (P < 0.05, Table 1). Highest thousand seed weight (1.9 g) and plant height (34.2 cm) were achieved by application of 20 ton/ha compost and N2P2K2 and highest root dry weight (0.14 kg/m2) and grain weight (506.8 kg/ha) were performed by N4P4K4 and 5 ton/ha and N2P2K2 and 10 ton/ha respectively, (Table 3). Those findings are in agreement with the observations of Hadj Seyed Hadi et al. (2004) and Hashemi et al. (2008). In addition, planting date had significant effect on grain yield and root dry weight (P ≤ 0.01) and flower yield and flowers number per plant (P < 0.05, Table 1). However, we noted the highest mucilage percentage (9.4%), flower yield (280.91 kg/ha) and flowers number per plant (28.2 flower/plant) were obtained under N1P1K1 and 1 March PD, while other plant characteristics were reduced under this condition (Table 2). Those results were similar with the findings of Hadj Seyed Hadi et al. (2004) and Zehtab-salmasi et al. (2001).

DISCUSSION

The results showed that late-planting decreased quantity and quality features of borage. Selection of borage planting date is one of the most important management decisions to produce mucilage. Planting date affects leaf-spot by avoiding unfavorable weather conditions for disease development. Late planting date was positively associated with more necrosis because of favorable

Table 2. Mean comparison between planting date and chemical fertilization systems.

Plant height (cm)	Thousand seed weight (g)	Flower number per plant (flower/plant)	Grain yield (kg/ha)	Root dry weight (kg/m^2)	Flower yield (kg/ha)	Mucilage percentage (%)	Treatments	
28.4 a	1.9 a	28.2 a	500.12 a	0.13 a	280.91 a	9.4 a	N1P1K1	
27.1 a	0.9 c	28.1 a	491.1 ab	0.12 a	270.1 a	9.3 a	N2P2K2	
20.2 b	0.88 c	27 a	400.1 bc	0.14 a	240.11 b	9 a	N3P3K3	1 March
20.1 b	0.87 c	25.1 a	430.2 b	0.13 a	198.2 c	9.2 a	N4P4K4	
23.2 b	1.57 b	23.1 b	505.2 a	0.11 a	260.45 ab	8.2 ab	N1P1K1	
24.1 b	0.9 c	20.4 b	500.3 a	0.10 a	250.1 ab	8.8 a	N2P2K2	
22.2 b	0.9 c	22.1 b	461.2 b	0.12 a	241.11 b	7.8 ab	N3P3K3	15 March
20.4 bc	0.88 c	19.8 b	400.3 bc	0.10 a	200.3 c	7 b	N4P4K4	
20.1 c	1.84 ab	18.4 c	490.1 ab	0.10 a	190.11 c	7.4 b	N1P1K1	
18.1 cd	0.7 c	18.8 c	470.6 ab	0.11 a	170.2 c	7.1 b	N2P2K2	
18 cd	0.82 c	17.9 c	474.2 ab	0.12 a	177.4 c	7.2 b	N3P3K3	1 April
16.1 d	0.82 c	16.8 c	430.8 b	0.13 a	130.13 d	7 b	N4P4K4	

Table 3. Means comparison between chemical fertilization systems and compost.

Plant height (cm)	Thousand seed weight (g)	Flower number per plant (flower/plant)	Grain yield (kg/ha)	Root dry weight (kg/m^2)	Flower yield (kg/ha)	Mucilage percentage (%)	Treatments (ton/ha)	
25.4 b	1.88 a	11.4 c	495.2 b	0.11 c	140.11 c	4.4 b	5	
27.3 b	1.9 a	14.3 b	497.2 b	0.10 d	145.14 bc	4.7 b	10	
30.2 a	2 a	15.7 b	501.3 a	0.13 b	160.71 b	4.8 b	15	N1P1K1
33.1 a	1.9 a	17.8 a	412.8 bc	0.14 a	210.12 a	8.6 a	20	
20.41 bc	1 ab	12.3 c	491.1 b	0.11 c	134.2 c	4.9 b	5	
27.2 b	1.1 ab	13.8 c	490.6 b	0.10 d	140.1 bc	5.1 b	10	
30.1 a	1.2 ab	16.9 ab	506.8 a	0.13 b	175.1 b	4.7 b	15	N2P2K2
34.2 a	1.9 a	16.8 a	458.1 b	0.14 a	200.3 a	8.3 a	20	
19.8 c	1.1 ab	13.4 c	399.1 c	0.13 b	120.1 c	4.7 b	5	
24.3 bc	1.8 a	13.9 c	380.8 c	0.14 a	118 c	5 b	10	
30.3 a	1.6 ab	15.1 b	390.2 c	0.14 a	168.2 b	3.8 c	15	N3P3K3
30.1 b	1.5 ab	17.4 a	400.1 b	0.13 b	198.4 ab	8.3 a	20	
19.1 c	1 ab	15.1 b	300.41 c	0.14 a	118.1 c	4.6 b	5	
24 bc	1.1 ab	12.1 c	315.1 c	0.13 b	114 c	6.2 ab	10	N4P4K4
29.4 b	1 ab	15 b	301.12 c	0.10 d	160.4 b	4.1 b	15	
26.4 c	1.8 ab	17 a	390.6 bc	0.11 c	180.6 ab	8 a	20	

Means within the same column and factors, followed by the same letter are not significantly difference (P < 0.05).

weather conditions. Early planting increased the forage production potential by extending the vegetative growth period and increased the total length of time that the borage was in the field and exposed to the environment. In areas with limited soil moisture, planting too early can cause excessive fall growth these results in depletion of soil moisture for early spring growth. Early planting of borage also breaks winter dormancy earlier in the spring as temperature increases and, thus, has a greater potential for late spring freeze injury. Borage planted at an intermediate date has mucilage content potential than late-planted borage because of increased lateral stems, leafs and flowering stem. Late-planted borage also develops under different temperature and day-length, has a shortened vegetative growth period and requires greater mucilage rate to compensate partially for reduced flowering stem development. In this study, increases in agronomic criteria were observed following inoculation with compost. This may be due to better utilization of nutrients in the soil through inoculation of efficient microorganisms. A positive effect of compost on yield and yield components has been reported in the literature. In addition, higher dry matter production by the inoculated plant might be because of the augmented uptake of N, P and K which in turn was a consequence of the root proliferation. Also, the increased growth parameters in hyssop might be due to the production of growth hormones by the bacteria. Nitrogen of chemical fertilizer, which is a primary constituent of proteins, is extremely susceptible to loss when considering that average recovery rates fall in the range of 20 to 50% for dry matter production systems in plants. Nitrogenous fertilizers generally cause deficiency of potassium, increased carbohydrate storage and reduced proteins, alteration in amino acid balance and consequently change in the quality of proteins and are a main element in chlorophyll production. Toxic concentrations of nitrogen fertilizers cause characteristic symptoms of nitrite or nitrate toxicity in plants, especially in the leaves. Although, pre plant fertilizer applications decrease the potential for nutrient deficiencies in early stages of growth, presence of residual soil NO_3 - N (plant-available mineral N from the previous season) may pose a risk to the environment. The water of soil be salt by inordinate N application and increase its potential. Finally, the plant use high energy for absorb of salt water that be causes dry matter reduces in this condition. Therefore, dry matter reduced under application of high levels of chemical fertilizer application due to injured roots and reduced the absorption.

Conclusion

In general it appears that, as expected, application of compost improved yield and other plant criteria. Therefore, it appears that application of this compost can be promising in production of borage by reduction of chemical fertilizer application. Our finding may give applicable advice to farmers for management and concern on fertilizer strategy and carefully estimate chemical fertilizer supply by compost application.

ACKNOWLEDGEMENT

The authors are indebted to Dr. Sayed Alireza Valadabadi for providing financial assistance and continuous encouragement to carry out this investigation.

REFERENCES

Bowden RL (1997). Disease management. In: Manhattan, KS [Ed.2, Wheat production handbook. C-529. Kansas State University. Coop. Ext. Serv., pp.18-24.

Carrubba A, la Torre A, Calabrese I (2002). Cultivation trials of coriander (Coriandrum sativum L.) in a semi-arid Mediterranean environment. In medicinal and aromatic plants possibilities and limitations of medicinal and aromatic plant production in the 21st century, Proc. Int. Conf., Budapest. 8–11 July 2001. Acta Hortic. 576: 237-242.

Chen J (2006). The combined use of chemical and organic fertilizers and/or biofetilizer for crop growth and soil fertility. International workshop on sustained management of the Soil-Rhizosphere System for Efficient Crop Production and Fertilizer Use.16 – 20 October, Thailand.

Fowler DB, Brydon J (1989). No-till winter wheat production on the Canadian prairies: Timing of nitrogen fertilizers. Agron. J. 81: 817–825.

Grant CA, Stobbe EH, Racz GJ (1985). The effect of fall-applied N and P fertilizers and timing of N application on yield and protein content of winter wheat grown on zero-tilled land in Manitoba. Can. J. Soil Sci. 65: 621–628.

Knowles TC, Hipp BW, Graff PS, Marshall DS (1994). Timing and rate of top-dress nitrogen for rainfed winter wheat. J. Prod. Agric. 7: 216–220.

Mandal A, Patra AK, Singh D, Swarup A, Ebhin MR (2007). Effect of long-term application of manure fertilizer on biological and biochemical activities in soil during crop development stages. Biores. Technol. 98: 3585–3592.

Olson RV, Swallow CW (1984). Fate of labeled nitrogen fertilizer applied to winter wheat for five years. Soil Sci. Soc. Am. J. 48: 583–586.

SAS Institute (1998). Statistics Analysis System user's guide: Statistics. SAS Inst., Cary, NC.

Stark JC, Tindall TA (1992). Timing split applications of nitrogen for irrigated hard red spring wheat. J. Prod. Agric. 5: 221–226.

Vaughan B, Westfall DG, Barbarick KA (1990). Nitrogen rate and timing effects on winter wheat grain yield, grain protein, and economics. J. Prod. Agric. 3: 324–328.

Vessey JK (2003). Plant growth promoting rhizobacteria as biofertilizers. Plant Soil. 255: 571–586.

Wuest SB, Cassman KG (1992). Fertilizer-nitrogen use efficiency of irrigated wheat: I. Uptake efficiency of pre-plant versus late-season application. Agron. J. 84: 682–688.

Wu SC, Caob ZH, Lib ZG, Cheung KC, Wong MH (2005). Effects of biofertilizer containing N-fixer, P and K solubilizers and AM fungi on maize growth: a greenhouse trial. Geoderma. 125: 155–166.

Zehtab-Salmasi S, Javanshir A, Omidbaigi R, Alyari H, Ghassemi-golezani K (2001). Effects of water supply and planting date on performance and essential oil production of anis (Pimpinella anisum L.). Act. Agro. Hun. 49(1): 75-81.

8

Substrate utilization and inhibition kinetics: Batch degradation of phenol by indigenous monoculture of *Pseudomonas aeruginosa*

S. E. Agarry[1]*, B. O. Solomon[2, 4] and T. O. K. Audu[3]

[1]Biochemical Engineering Research Laboratory, Department of Chemical Engineering, Ladoke Akintola University of Technology, Ogbomoso, Oyo State, Nigeria.
[2]Biochemical Engineering Research Laboratory, Department of Chemical Engineering, Obafemi Awolowo University, Ile-Ife, Osun State, Nigeria.
[3]Department of Chemical Engineering, University of Benin, Benin-City, Edo State, Nigeria.
[4]National Biotechnology Development Agency, Abuja, Nigeria.

The biodegradation potential of an indigenous monoculture of *Pseudomonas aeruginosa* was studied in batch fermentation using synthetic phenol in water in the concentration range of (100 - 500) mg/L as a model limiting substrate. The effect of initial phenol concentration on the degradation process was investigated. Phenol was completely degraded at different cultivation times for various initial phenol concentrations. Increasing the initial phenol concentration from 100 to 500 mg/L, increased the lag phase from 0 to 24 h and correspondingly prolonged the degradation process from 54 to 168 h. This implies that there was decrease in biodegradation rate as initial phenol concentration increased. Four substrate utilization models were examined, and out of these, the adapted Miura model was found to be the best fit for description of kinetics. The $r_{s\,max}$ decreased and K_s increased with higher concentration of phenol. The $r_{s\,max}$ has been found to be a strong function of initial phenol concentration. The bacterial culture followed substrate inhibition kinetics and the specific phenol consumption rates were fitted to five inhibition models. The Haldane and Yano and Koga inhibition models were found to give the best fit. Therefore, the biokinetic constants estimated using these models show good potential of the monoculture of *Pseudomonas aeruginosa* and the possibility of using it in bioremediation of phenolic waste effluents.

Key words: *Pseudomonas aeruginosa*, phenol, biodegradation, kinetic model, batch cultivation, bioreactor, primary culture, secondary culture, bioremediation.

INTRODUCTION

Phenol and its derivatives are the basic structural unit in a wide variety of synthetic organic compounds (Annadurai et al., 2000). It is an organic, aromatic compound that occurs naturally in the environment (Prpich and Daugulis, 2005), but is more commonly produced artificially from industrial activities such as petroleum processing, plastic manufacturing, resin production, pesticide production, steel manufacturing and the production of paints and varnish (Mahadevaswamy et al., 1997; Bandyopadhyay et al., 1998). This aromatic compound is water-soluble and highly mobile (Collins and Daugulis, 1997). Wastewaters generated from these industrial activities contain high concentrations of phenolic compounds (Chang et al., 1998) which eventually may reach down to streams, rivers, lakes and soil, and represent a serious ecological problem (Fava et al., 1995). Phenol is a listed priority pollutant by the U.S. Environmental Protection Agency (EPA, 1979) and is

*Corresponding author. E-mail: sam_agarry@yahoo.com

considered to be a toxic compound by the Agency for Toxic substances and Disease Registry (ATSDR, 2003). The adverse effects of phenol on health are well documented (Calabrese and Kenyon, 1991) and death among adults has been reported with ingestion of phenol ranging from 1 to 32 g (Prpich and Daugulis, 2005). The low volatility of phenol and its affinity for water make oral consumption of contaminated water a greatest risk to humans (Prpich and Daugulis, 2005).

A variety of techniques involving physical, chemical and biological methods have been used for the removal of phenol from industrial effluents and contaminated waters. Bioremediation have received the most attention due to its environmental friendliness, its, ability to completely mineralize toxic organic compounds and its low-cost (Kobayashi and Rittman, 1982; Prpich and Daugulis, 2005). Microbial degradation of phenol with different initial concentrations ranging from 50 – 2000 mg/L have been actively studied using shake flask, fluidized-bed reactor, continuous stirred tank bioreactor, multistage bubble column reactor, air-lift fermenter and two phase partitioning bioreactor methods (Bettmann and Rehm, 1984; Sokol, 1988; Annadurai et al., 2000; Reardon et al., 2000; Ruiz-ordaz et al., 2001; Oborien et al., 2005; Prpich and Daugulis, 2005; Saravanan et al., 2008). These studies have shown that phenol can be aerobically degraded by wide variety of fungi and bacterial cultures such as Candida tropicalis (Ruiz-ordaz et al., 2001; Chang et al., 1998; Ruiz-ordaz et al., 1998), Acinetobacter calcoaceticus (Paller et al., 1995; Hao et al., 2002), Alcaligenes eutrophus (Hughes et al., 1984; Leonard and Lindley, 1998), Pseudomonas putida (Hill and Robinson, 1975; Kotturi et al., 1991; Nikakhtari and Hill, 2006) and Burkholderia cepacia G4 (Folsom et al., 1990; Solomon et al.,1994).

A variety of kinetic substrate utilization and inhibition models have been used to describe the dynamics of microbial growth on phenol. Of these, the Monod and Andrew (Haldane) equations have been extensively used to describe phenol biodegradation and are based on the specific growth rate (Bandyopadhyay et al., 1998; Reardon et al., 2000; Oboirien et al., 2005), but may also be related to the specific substrate consumption rate (Edwards, 1970; Solomon et al., 1994). Other kinetic models have also been propagated. Sokol (1988) has reported a better fit for a modified Monod-Haldane equation, while Schroder et al. (1997) have shown a better fit for Yano and Koga equation amongst the tested inhibition models. In spite of the rather extensive use of phenol biodegradation processes, little work has been published on phenol microbial degradation kinetics based on specific substrate consumption rate ($r_{s\,max}$) using mono or mixed culture systems. The present study investigates the effect of initial phenol (substrate) concentration on the degradation potential of an indigenous monoculture of Pseudomonas aeruginosa isolated from an oil-polluted swampy area of Warri in Niger-Delta region of Nigeria and to determine its kinetics at these different phenol concentrations.

MATERIALS AND METHODS

Microorganism

The microorganism, monoculture of P. aeruginosa being an indigenous bacteria strain isolated from an oil-polluted area in Niger-Delta region of Nigeria was procured from the Department of Microbiology, Obafemi Awolowo University, Ile-Ife, Nigeria. The bacterial culture was maintained on nutrient agar slant and stored at $4 \pm 1\,°C$ for further use.

Culture medium and inoculum preparation

The mineral salt medium used was modified from the one suggested by Bettman and Rehm (1984). The medium had the following composition per litre: 700 ml deionized water, 100 ml buffer solution A, 100 ml trace elements solution B, 50 ml solution C and 50 ml solution D. Compositions of each solution were as follows: Buffer solution A composition: $K_2 HPO_4$ 1.0 g, KH_2PO_4 0.5g, $(NH_4)_2SO_4$ 0.5g, deionized water 100ml. Trace element solution B composition: NaCl 0.5g, $CaCl_2$ 0.02g, $MnSO_4$ 0.02g, $CuSO_4.5H_2O$ 0.02g, $H_3 BO_3$ 0.01g, deionized water 50ml. Solution C composition: $MgSO_4.7H_2O$ 0.5g, deionized water 50 ml, Solution D composition $FeSO_4$ 0.02g, Molybdenum powder 0.02 g, deionized water 50 ml. To prevent the precipitation of $CaSO_4$ and $MgSO_4$ in storage, the water, buffer solution A, trace elements solution B, solution C and solution D were autoclaved at $121\,°C$ for 15 m. After cooling, all the solutions were then mixed together and kept as stock solution from which known quantities were taken for the cultivation of the microorganisms

A primary culture was prepared by transferring two loops full of microorganisms from an agar slant culture into 100 ml of feed medium containing 20 ml of mineral salt medium and 80 ml of 50 mg phenol solution in a 250 ml Erlenmeyer conical flask. This was then incubated in a New Brunswick gyratory shaker (G25-R model, N.J. U.S.A) for 48 h at $30\,°C$ and agitated at 120 rpm. Thereafter, 10 ml of the primary culture was transferred into another 100 ml of feed medium in a 250 ml Erlenmeyer conical flask and the incubation process was repeated. This was the secondary culture that was used as the inoculum for the degradation studies as this ensures that the organisms had fully adapted to growth on phenol as the sole source of carbon and energy.

Experimental design to study the free suspended cell system

The experimental studies were carried out in a New Brunswick Microferm Twin Bioreactor (pH - 22 model, N.J., U.S.A) with 4 l working volume. Autoclaved mineral salt medium (800 ml) and 3 l of phenol solution (100 mg/L) were measured into the bioreactor vessel and 200 ml of the inoculum was introduced aseptically to make up 4 l of working volume. The bioreactor was operated for several hours at $30\,°C$, aeration rate of 3.0 vvm and agitation of 300 rpm. Culture broth was withdrawn every 6 h for biomass and phenol determination.

Estimation of phenol concentration

The undergraded phenol was estimated quantitatively by measuring its   absorbance   at   510 nm   wavelength   using   UV - visible

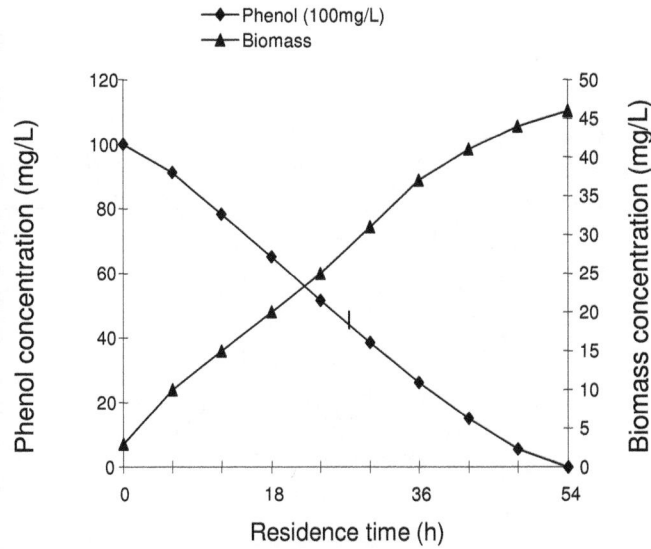

Figure 1. Experimental data obtained from batch degradation of phenol (100 mg/L) by monoculture of *P. aeruginosa*.

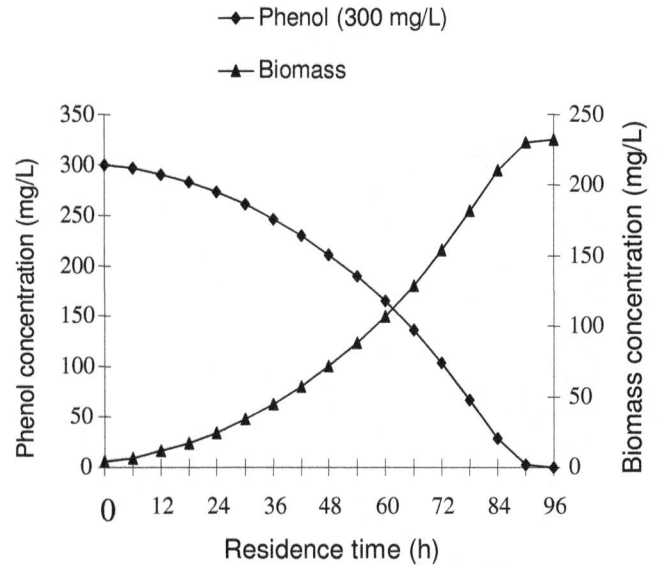

Figure 3. Experimental data obtained from batch degradation of phenol (300 mg/L) by of *P. aeruginosa*.

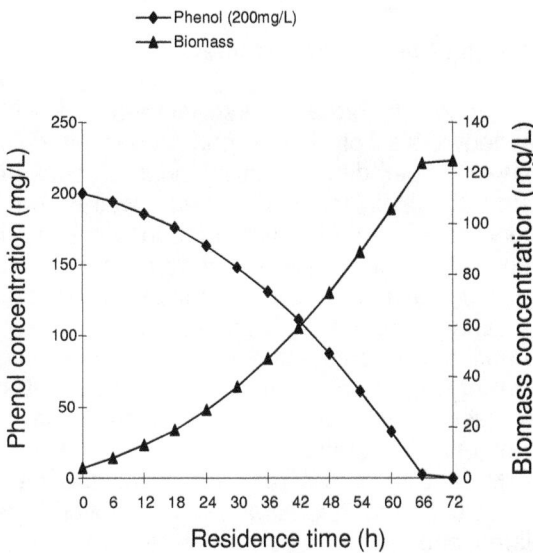

Figure 2. Experimental data obtained from batch degradation of phenol (200 mg/L) by *P. aeruginosa*.

Spectrophotometer (Lambda 35, Perkin-Elmer, USA) and 4 - amino antipyrene as colour indicator (Yang and Humphrey, 1975; Oboirien et al., 2005).

Estimation of biomass concentration

The biomass concentration was estimated using the dry weight method. A sample of culture broth (50 ml) was withdrawn from the bioreactor and centrifuged (Gallenkamp centrifuge) at 4000 rpm for 20 min in plastic centrifuge tubes. The supernatant was decanted into small bottles and stored at 4 °C for subsequent phenol estimation. The pellets was re-suspended in de-ionized water and re-centrifuged. The supernatant was decanted and pellets rinsed off

from the tube into a pre-weighed 1.2 µm pore filter paper (Whatman GF/C). The filter paper was then dried in an oven at 105 °C for 12 - 24 h, cooled in a dessicator at room temperature and re-weighed until a constant dry weight was obtained. The difference between the pre-weighed filter paper and the final constant weight was used to estimate the dry weight of the biomass.

RESULTS AND DISCUSSION

Five batch cultivation experiments were carried out using phenol as single limiting substrate for monoculture of *P. aeruginosa*. The extent of phenol degradation using different initial phenol concentrations (100 – 500 mg/L) was investigated for several batch residence times by intermittent sampling.

Figures 1 – 5 show the biodegradation potential of the indigenous monoculture of *P. aeruginosa* in degrading synthetic phenol waste in the concentration range of 100 to 500 mg/L. Since the degradation proceeds with biomass (cell mass) growth, the Figures also depict a typical cell growth curve with increasing lag phase. Various initial phenol concentrations ranging from 100 – 500 mg/L were completely degraded (consumed) at different residence times of 54, 72, 96, 120 and 168 h, respectively. At these times the biomass correspondingly increased to a maximum of 46, 125, 232, 280 and 385 mg/L, respectively. No lag phase was observed for initial phenol concentrations of 100 and 200 mg/L as shown in (Figures 1 and 2). Similar observations have been reported by Oboirien et al., 2005; Saravanan et al., 2008; Agarry and Solomon, 2008. However, for initial phenol concentrations of 300, 400 and 500 mg/L respectively, corresponding lag phase of 6, 12 and 18 h was observed

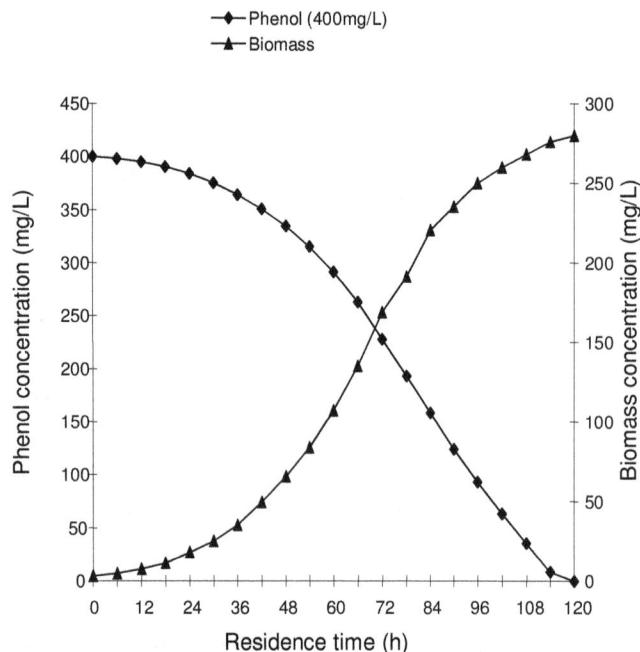

Figure 4. Experimental data obtained from batch degradation of phenol (400 mg/L) by *P. aeruginosa*.

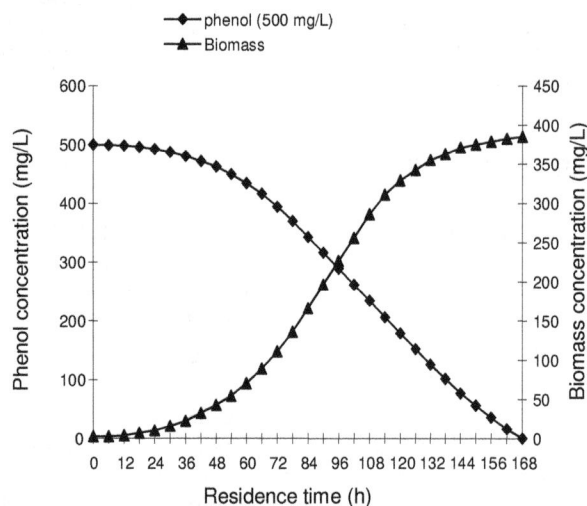

Figure 5. Experimental data obtained from batch degradation of phenol (500 mg/L) by *P. aeruginosa*.

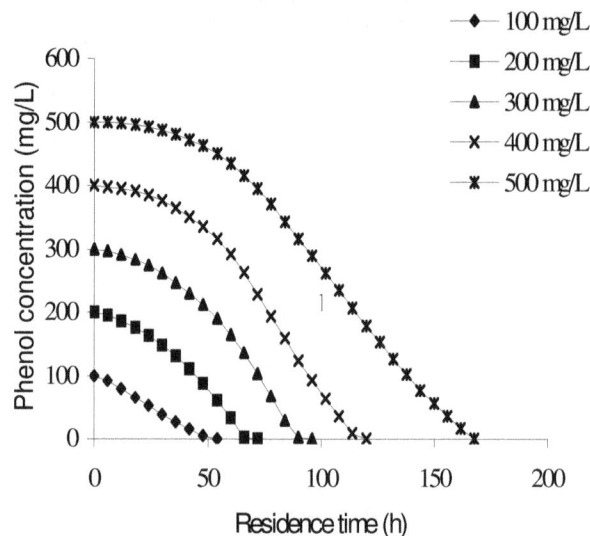

Figure 6. Effect of initial phenol concentration on phenol degradation by *P. aeruginosa*.

Evaluation of biokinetic parameters

Batch phenol degradation was carried out with free suspended cells of indigenous monoculture of *P. aeruginosa* under different initial phenol concentrations as stated above. In this work, phenol well known as an inhibitory substrate under different concentrations (100 – 500 mg/L) was completely degraded by the monoculture of *P. aeruginosa* as shown in Figure 6. According to Prpich and Daugulis (2005), the rate of substrate consumption was suggested to be the most important measure of microbe performance. Zilli et al. (1993) have similar results but relatively less data exists in the literature on this parameter. Most of the data available concerns specific growth rate. It was on this basis that the specific phenol (substrate) consumption rate was calculated and plotted against phenol concentration as shown in Figure 7. As seen from this Figure, the specific phenol consumption rate (r_s) decreases as the phenol concentration (S) decreased. Therefore, it seems that there is also an influence of the initial phenol concentration on the specific phenol consumption rate. Hinteregger et al. (1992) and Abd-El Hameidshalaby (2003) have reported similar observations.

According to Layokun et al. (1987), the growth of microorganisms corresponds to the degradation (consumption) of the substrate. Hence, the growth of microorganisms on phenol can be described by the most commonly used kinetic models. Posten has proposed that these models can be based on specific substrate consumption rates (Solomon et al., 1994), which have been also used by Zilli et al. (1993) and Schroder et al. (1997). The classic method of obtaining kinetic parameters (constants) is to linearize kinetic models.

Figures 3 - 5). It is evident from Figure 6, which compares the time course for phenol substrate consumption of all the five batches that the rate of degradation decreases with increase in the initial phenol concentration. Bandyopadhyay et al. (1998); Ruiz-ordaz et al. (2001); Agarry and Solomon (2008) reported similar observations for *P. putida*, *C. tropicalis* and *Pseudomonas fluorescence* grown on phenol, respectively.

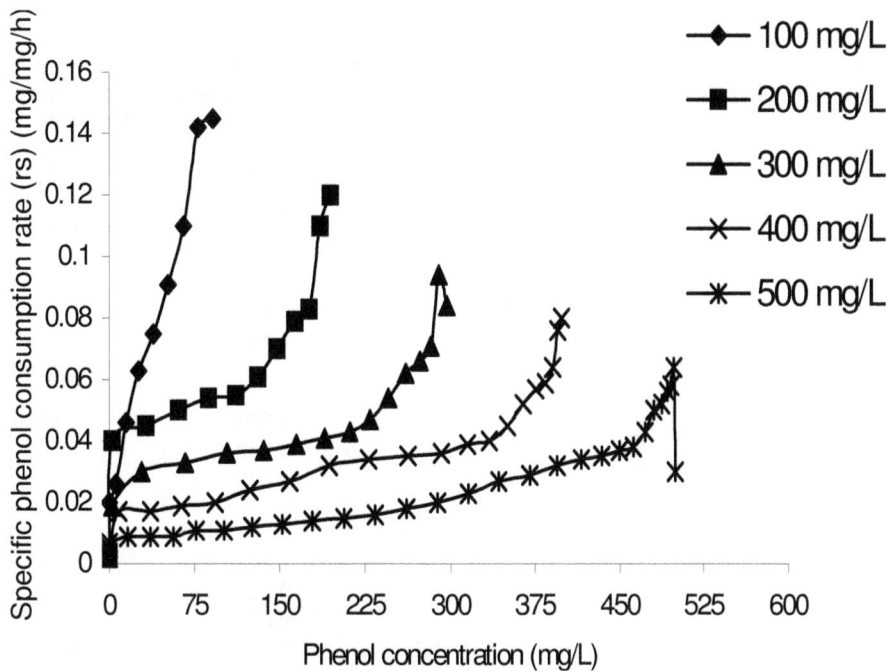

Figure 7. Specific phenol consumption rate vs phenol concentration for monoculture of *P. aeruginosa*.

However, non-linear least squares computer fitting of data to model equations are being used (Reardon et al., 2000; Schroder et al., 1997; Saravanan et al., 2008). The non-linear least square fitting routine of MATLAB 6.5 software package was used to fit the Eckenfelder, Monod, Moser and the adapted Miura models to the different batch experimental data. The parameters of these models (K_s and $r_{s\,max}$) were fitted to the experimental calculated specific phenol consumption rate and the corresponding phenol concentration under the constraint that r_s never exceed the maximum obtainable specific consumption rate ($r_{s\,max}$). The results from Table 1 have revealed that for initial phenol concentration (S_o) of 100 mg/L, the adapted Miura (R^2 = 0.9311, RMSE = 0.0130) and Eckenfelder (R^2 = 0.9036, RMSE = 0.0144) models show a better fit as compared to other models. However, amongst the two models, the adapted Miura model showed the best fit. For initial phenol concentration (S_o) of 200 mg/L, once again, the adapted Miura (R^2 = 0.6290, RMSE = 0.0187) and Eckenfelder (R2 = 0.6290, RMSE = 0.0192) models, show a better fit. This indicates that the mode of 200 mg/L phenol utilization is well represented by the two models. Nonetheless, based on the lower RMSE value, the adapted Miura model showed the best fit. For initial phenol concentration (S_o) of 300 mg/L, the adapted Miura (R^2 = 0.7592, RMSE = 0.0120) and Eckenfelder (R^2 = 0.7504, RMSE = 0.0118) models show a better fit but the adapted Miura model showed the best fit. For initial phenol concentration of 400 mg/L, the

adapted Miura (R^2 = 0.8220, RMSE = 0.0014) and Eckenfelder (R^2 = 0.8007, RMSE = 0.0091) models indicated a better fit. Yet again the adapted Miura model showed the best fit (having a higher R^2 value). The adapted Miura (R^2 = 0.8593, RMSE = 0.0011) and a strong function of initial phenol concentration (S_o). The variation of $r_{s\,max}$ with S_o has been indicated in Figure 8. It is also fitted by the fourth order polynomial trendline from which $r_{s\,max}$ at any value of S_o within the range of 100 - 500 mg/L of phenol concentration can be predicted. However, the observation of substrate inhibition due to phenol can be modeled using substrate inhibition models described in literature (Schroder et al., 1997). The experimental results of specific phenol consumption rate variation with initial phenol concentration were fitted to five inhibition models namely Haldane (1968); Yano and Koga (1969); Aiba et al. (1968); Teissier (Edward, 1970); Webb (Edward, 1970) shown in Figure 9. The model with the best fit was selected on the basis of highest correlation coefficient (R^2) and the least root mean square error (RMSE). The kinetic parameters of the models ($r_{s\,max}$, K_s and K_i) were estimated using the non-linear regression routine of MATLAB 6.5. The results shown in Table 2 revealed that between the five models, Haldane and Yano and Koga models have a correlation coefficient (R^2) greater than 0.90 and a root mean square error (RMSE) less than 1%. This indicates a very good fit to the batch

Table 1. Kinetic constants obtained from the fitting of batch experimental runs data of phenol degradation by *P. aeruginosa* to substrate utilization kinetic models.

Model	S_o (mg/L)	K_s (mg/L)	$r_{s\,max}$ (mg/mg/h)	RMSE	R^2
Monod		23.8	0.145	0.0188	0.8347
Moser		853.4	0.143	0.0178	0.8701
Adapted Miura	100	0.91	0.145	0.0130	0.9311
Eckenfelder		0.0017	-	0.0144	0.9036
Monod		79.8	0.120	0.0203	0.5845
Moser		905.3	0.073	0.0242	0.4623
Adapted Miura	200	1.63	0.110	0.0187	0.6290
Eckenfelder		0.0005	-	0.0192	0.6290
Monod		139.8	0.094	0.0134	0.6808
Moser		1015.9	0.053	0.0191	0.3928
Adapted Miura	300	4.41	0.079	0.0120	0.7592
Eckenfelder		0.0003	-	0.0118	0.7504
Monod		208	0.080	0.0113	0.6973
Moser		11460	0.055	0.0131	0.6086
Adapted Miura	400	13.8	0.065	0.0014	0.8220
Eckenfelder		0.0002	-	0.0091	0.8007
Monod		331.2	0.064	0.0098	0.6682
Moser		13590	0.038	0.0119	0.5277
Adapted Miura	500	40.6	0.051	0.0011	0.8593
Eckenfelder		0.0001	-	0.0073	0.8177

experimental data. The difference in the R^2 and RMSE values between the two models is statistically insignificant. Thus, both the Haldane and Yano and Koga inhibition models may be proposed as the best models to describe the phenol degradation behaviour of monoculture of *P. aeruginosa*. Yang and Humphrey (1975); Agarry and Solomon (2008) have reported similar observations with Haldane's equation and two other models in describing phenol degradation by *P. putida*, *T. cutaneum* and *Pseudomonas fluorescence*, respectively.

Assessment of performance

Phenol has been used widely as a model inhibitory substrate and its biodegradation kinetics have been determined for many microorganisms (Bandyopadhyay et al., 1998; Oboirien et al., 2005; Saravanan et al., 2008; Agarry and Solomon, 2008) The performance of this indigenous monoculture of *P. aeruginosa* is being compared with well known effective degraders of phenol with emphasis on maximum specific substrate consumption rate. Reported values of the maximum specific substrate consumption rate ($r_{s\,max}$) varied from 0.001 to 2.6 h^{-1} (Zilli et al., 1993; Folsom et al., 1990; Schroder et al., 1997). Folsom et al. (1990) and Schroder

et al. (1997) reported a $r_{s\,max}$ value of 2.6 and 0.4 h^{-1} for *Burkholderia cepacia* G4, respectively. Whereas, Zilli et al. (1993) reported a value of 0.0016 h^{-1} for *P. putida* NCIMB 10015. The $r_{s\,max}$ value of 0.294 mg/mg/h (using the value obtained for Yano and Koga model) for the monoculture of *P. aeruginosa* was comparatively lower than the value obtained by Schroder et al. (1997) for *B. cepacia* G4, however, higher than the value for *P. putida* NCIMB 10015. Using the Haldane model, for equivalent initial phenol concentrations, the phenol degradation efficiencies obtained in this work ($r_{s\,max}$ = 0.457) were higher than those reported by Agarry and Solomon (2008) for the monoculture of indigenous *P. fluorescence* ($r_{s\,max}$ = 0.357). More also, the performance of the indigenous monoculture of Pseudomonas aeruginosa in the degradation of pure phenol and phenol present in the refinery waste water effluents are compared as shown in Table 3. The results revealed that local isolates of P. aeruginosa was more effective in the degradation of pure phenol than phenol present in the refinery waste water effluents. This showed that the biodegradation of phenol present in refinery waste water effluents is being inhibited by other compounds in the waste effluents. This corroborates the report of Reardon et al. (2000) that degradation or the removal of one compound can be inhibited by another compound in the mixture.

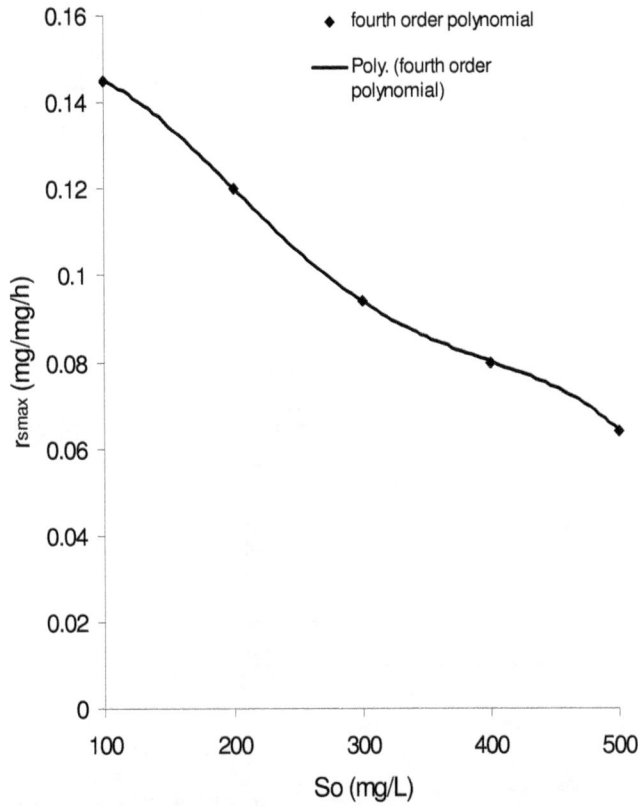

Figure 8. Variation of $r_{s\,max}$ with So for phenol degradation by monoculture of *P. aeruginosa*.

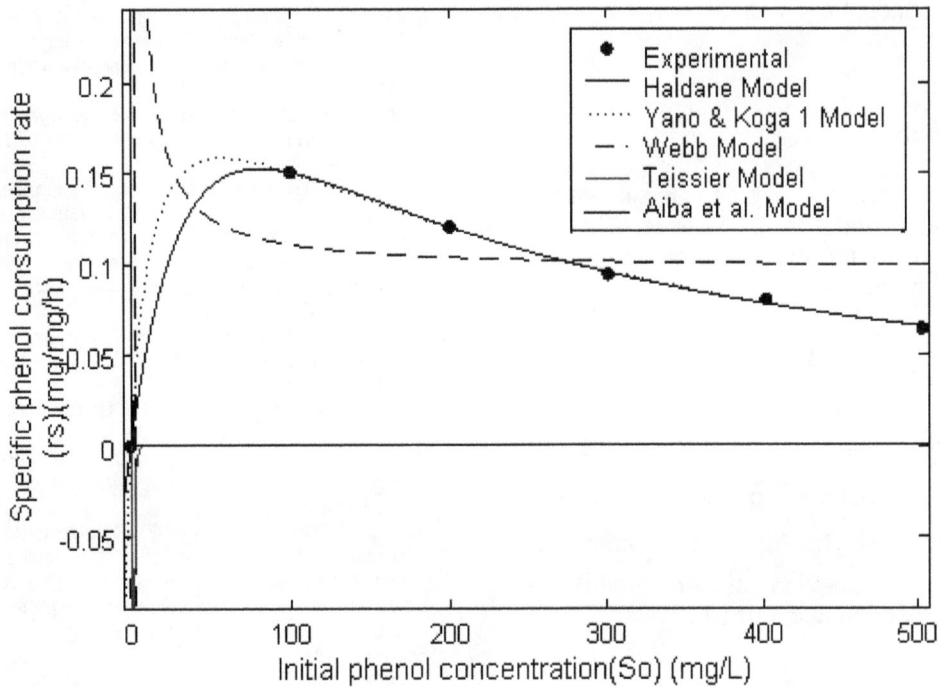

Figure 9. Experimental and predicted specific phenol consumption rate of *P. aeruginosa* due to some kinetic models.

Table 2. Kinetic parameters value obtained from five inhibition models fitted to the biodegradation data of *P. aeruginosa*.

Model	$r_{s\,max}$ (mg/mg/h)	K_s (mg/L)	K_1 (mg/L)	K_2 (mg/L)	K_i (mg/L)	R^2	RMSE
Yano and Koga 1	0.294	42.7	172	678	-	0.9994	0.0019
Teissier	0.565	0.441	-	-	0.605	-3.349	0.1351
Aiba et al	0.565	0.441	-	-	0.605	-3.35	0.1351
Webb	4.821	-1.631	0.543	-	29	0.8073	0.0348
Haldane	0.458	99.9	-	-	86.1	0.9993	0.0017

Table 3. Comparison of the biodegradation of pure phenol and phenol present in refinery waste water by indigenous monoculture of *P. aeruginosa*.

Organism	Type of waste	Residence time (h)	% Phenol degradation	References
P. aeruginosa	Phenol in refinery waste water (28 mg/L)	48	82.6	Aremu (2003)
P. aeruginosa	Phenol in refinery waste water (30 mg/L)	48	90	Ojumu et al. (2005)
		60	100	,,
P. aeruginosa	Pure phenol (100 mg/L)	48	94.4	This study
		54	100	,,

Conclusion

The present study shows the potential of the isolated indigenous monoculture of *P. aeruginosa* for phenol wastewater treatment. The performance of the indigenous strain in biodegradation of phenol in the nutrient medium is excellent. The parameter K_s increased, while $r_{s\,max}$ decreased with the higher values of initial phenol concentration, indicating an inhibition effect of phenol.

ACKNOWLEDGMENT

Prof. B. O. Solomon wishes to express his sincere thanks to the International Foundation for Science (IFS) for the financial support used for the procurement of all the chemicals needed for this work.

NOMENCLATURE

K_s, Half-saturation constant (mg/L); K_i, Inhibition constant (g/l); r_s, Specific phenol (substrate) consumption rate (mg/mg/hr); $r_{s\,max}$, Maximum specific phenol (substrate) consumption rate (mg/mg/hr); S, C_s, Substrate (phenol) concentration (mg/L).

REFERENCES

Abd-El H, El-s M (2003). Biological degradation of substrate mixtures composed of phenol, benzoate and acetate by *Burkholderia cepacia* G4. Ph.D Thesis. Gesellschaft fur Biotechnologische Forschung mbH, MascheroderWegl, D – 38124 Braunschweig, Germany.

Agarry SE, Solomon BO (2008). Kinetics of batch microbial degradation of phenols by indigenous *Pseudomonas fluorescence*. Int. J. Environ. Sci. Tech. 2(5): 244 – 253.

Aiba S, Shoda M, Nagatami M (1968). Kinetics of product inhibition in alcohol fermentation. Biotechnol. Bioeng. 10: 845-864.

Andrews JF (1968). A mathematical model for the continuous culture of microorganisms utilizing inhibitory substance. Biotechnol. Bioeng. 10: 707 - 723.

Annadurai G, Balan SM, Murugesan T (2000). Design of experiments in the biodegradation of phenol using immobilized *Pseudomonas pictorium* (NICM-2077) on activated carbon. Bioprocess Eng. 22: 101 -107.

Aremu MO (2003). A study of the biodegradation of phenol in refinery liquid effluent in batch process. M.Sc.Thesis, Obafemi Awolowo University, Ile-ife, Nigeria.

ATSDR (2003) Agency for Toxic Substances and Disease Registry. Medical Management Guidelines for Phenol. http://www.atsdr.cdc.gov/MHM 1/mmg 115.html.

Bandyopadhyay K, Das D, Maiti BR (1998). Kinetics of phenol degradation using *Pseudomonas putida* MTCC 1194. Bioprocess Eng. 18: 373 - 377.

Bettman H, Rehm HJ (1984). Degradation of phenol by polymer entrapped microorganisms. Appl. Microbiol. Biotechnol. 20: 285 - 290.

Calabrese EJ, Kenyon EM (1991). Air toxics and Risk Assessment. Lewis publishers, Chelsea, MI.

Chang YH, Li CT, Chang MC, Shieh WK (1998). Batch phenol degradation by *Candida tropicalis* and its fusant. Biotechnol. Bioeng. 60: 391 - 395.

Collins LD, Daugulis AJ (1997). Biodegradation of phenol at high initial concentration in two-phase partitioning batch and fed-batch bioreactors. Biotechnol. Bioeng. 55: 155 - 162.

Edwards VH (1970). The influence of high substrate concentrations on microbial kinetics, Biotechnol. Bioeng. 12: 679 - 712.

Environmental Protection Agency (EPA) (1979). Phenol ambient water quality criteria. Office of planning and standards. Washington, D. C. BB296786.

Fava F, Armenante PM, Kafkewitz D, Marchetti L (1995). Influence of organic and inorganic growth supplements on the aerobic biodegradation of chlorobenzoic acid. Appl. Microbiol. Biotechnol. 43: 171 - 177.

Folsom BR, Chapman PJ, Pritchard PH (1990). Phenol and trichloroethylene degradation by *Pseudomonas cepacia* G4: Kinetics and interactions between substrates. Appl. Environ. Microbiol. 57: 1279 - 1285.

Hao O, Kim M, Seagren E, Kim H (2002). Kinetics of phenol and chlorophenol utilization by *Acinetobacter isolates*. Chemosphere 46: 797 - 807.

Hill GA, Robinson CW (1975). Substrate inhibition kinetics: phenol degradation by *Pseudomonas putida*. Biotechnol. Bioeng. 17: 599 - 615.

Hinteregger C, Leitner R, Loidl M, Fershl A, Streichsbier F (1992). Degradation of phenol and phenolic compounds by *Pseudomonas putida* EK 11. Appl. Environ. Microbiol. 37: 252 - 259.

Hughes EJ, Bayly RC, Skurray RA (1984). Evidence for isofunctional enzymes in the degradation of phenol, m – and p – toluate, and p – cresol via catechol metacleavage pathways in *Alcaligenes eutrophus*. J. Bacteriol. 158: 79 - 83.

Kobayashi H, Rittman BE (1982). Microbial removal of hazardous organic compounds. Environ. Sci. Technol. 16: 170 - 183.

Kotturi G, Robinson CW, Inniss WE (1991). Phenol degradation by a psychrotrophic strain of *Pseudomonas putida*. Appl. Microbiol. Biotechnol. 34: 539 - 543.

Layokun SK, Umoh EF, Solomon BO (1987). A kinetic model for the degradation of dodecane by *P. fluorescens* isolated from the oil polluted area, Warri in Nigeria. J.Nsche. 16: 48 - 52.

Leonard D, Lindley ND (1998). Carbon and energy flux constraints in continuous cultures of *Alcaligenes eutrophus* grown on phenol. Microbiol. 144: 241 - 248.

Mahadevaswamy M, Mall ID, Prasad B, Mishra IM (1997). Removal of phenol by adsorption on coal fly ash and activated carbon. Poll. Res. 16(3): 170 – 175.

Miura Y (1978). Mechanism of liquid hydrocarbon uptake by microorganisms and growth kinetics. Adv. Biochem. Eng. 9: 31.

Monod J (1949). The growth of bacterial cultures. Ann. Rev. Microbiol. 3: 371 - 394.

Nikakhtari H, Hill GA (2006). Continuous bioremediation of phenol-polluted air in an external loop airlift bioreactor with a packed bed. J. Chem. Tech. Biotechnol. 81(6):1029 - 1038.

Oboirien BO, Amigun B, Ojumu TV, Ogunkunle OA, Adetunji OA, Betiku E, Solomon BO (2005). Substrate inhibition kinetics of phenol degradation by *Pseudomonas aeruginosa* and *Pseudomonas fluorescence*. Biotechnol. 4(1): 56 - 61.

Ojumu TV, Bello OO, Sonibare JA, Solomon BO (2005). Evaluation of microbial systems for bioremediation of petroleum refinery effluents in Nigeria. Afr. J. Biotechnol. 4(1): 31-35.

Paller G, Hommel RK, Kleber HP (1995). Phenol degradation by *Acinetobacter calcoaceticus* NCIB 8250. J. Basic Microbiol. 35: 325 - 335.

Pirt SJ (1975). Principles of microbe and cell cultivation. Blackwell scientific publication, Oxford, United Kingdom.

Prpich GP, Daugulis AJ (2005). Enhanced biodegradation of phenol by a microbial consortium in a solid-liquid two-phase partitioning bioreactor. Biodegradation 16: 329 - 339.

Reardon KF, Mosteller DC, Rogers JD (2000). Biodegradation kinetics of benzene, toluene and phenol and mixed substrates for *Pseudomonas putida* F1. Biotechnol. Bioeng. 69: 385 - 400.

Ruiz-ordaz N, Ruiz-Lagunez JC, Castanou-Gonzalez JH, Hernandez-Manzano E, Cristiani-Urbina E, Galindez-Mayer J (1998). Growth kinetic model that describes the inhibitory and lytic effects of phenol on *Candida tropicalis* yeast. Biotechnol. Prog. 14: 966 - 969.

Ruiz-ordaz N, Ruiz-Lagunez JC, Castanou-Gonzalez JH, Hernandez-Manzano E, Cristiani-Urbina E, Galindez-Mayer J (2001). Phenol biodegradation using a repeated batch culture of *Candida tropicalis* in a multistage bubble column, Revista Latinoamericana de Microbiogia 43: 19 - 25.

Saravanan P, Pakshirajan K, Saha P (2008). Growth kinetics of an indigenous mixed microbial consortium during phenol degradation in a batch reactor. Bioresource Technology 99: 205 - 209.

Schroder M, Muller C, Posten C, Deckwer WD, Hecht V (1997). Inhibition kinetics of phenol degradation from unstable steady state data. Biotechnol. Bioeng. 54: 567 - 576.

Sokol W (1988). Dynamics of continuous stirred-tank biochemical reactor utilizing inhibitory substrate. Biotechnol. Bioeng. 31: 198 - 202.

Solomon BO, Posten C, Harder MPF, Hecht V, Deckwer WD (1994). Energetics of *Pseudomonas cepacia* growth in a chemostat with phenol limitation. J. Chem. Technol. Biotechnol. 60: 275 - 282.

Yang RD, Humphrey AE (1975). Dynamic and steady state studies of phenol biodegradation in pure and mixed cultures. Biotechnol. Bioeng. 17: 1211 - 1235.

Yano T, Koga S (1969). Dynamic behaviour of the chemostat subject to substrate inhibition. Biotechnol. Bioeng. 11: 139 - 153.

Zilli M, Converti A, Lodi A, DelBorghi M, Ferraiolo G (1993). Phenol removal from waste gases with a biological fitter by *Pseudomonas putida*. Biotechnol. Bioeng. 41: 693 - 699.

Appendix

Equations for kinetic models according to Tables 1 and 2

Monod (1949): $r_s = \dfrac{r_{s,\max}\, S}{K_s + S}$

Adapted Miura (Layokun et al., 1987): $r_s = \dfrac{r_{s,\max}\, S\!/\!X}{K_s + S\!/\!X}$

Moser (Layokun et al., 1987): $r_s = \dfrac{r_{s,\max}\, S^2}{K_s + S^2}$

Eckenfelder (Layokun et al., 1987): $r_s = KS$

Haldane (Andrews, 1968): $r_s = \dfrac{r_{s\max}\, S}{K_s + S + \dfrac{S^2}{K_i}}$

Aiba et al. (1968): $r_s = r_{s_{\max}} \dfrac{C_{s_{\exp}}\left(-C_s\!/\!K_i\right)}{K_s + C_s}$

Teissier (Edwards, 1970): $r_s = r_{s_{\max}} \left[\exp\left(-C_s\!/\!K_i\right) - \exp\left(-C_s\!/\!K_s\right) \right]$

Webb (Edwards, 1970): $r_s = r_{s_{\max}} \dfrac{C_s\left(1 + C_s\!/\!K_i\right)}{K_s + C_s + C_s^2\!/\!K_1}$

Yano and Koga (1969): $r_s = r_{s_{\max}} \dfrac{C_s}{K_s + C_s + C_s^2\!/\!K_1 + C_s^3\!/\!K_2^2}$

9

Application of subspecies-specific marker system identified from *O. sativa* to *O. glaberrima* accessions and *O. sativa* × *O. glaberrima* F₁ interspecific progenies

Isaac Kofi Bimpong[1,2], Joong Hyoun Chin[2*], Joie Ramos[2] and Hee-Jong Koh[3]

[1]Africa Rice Centre, BP 96, St Louis, Senegal, West Africa.
[2]International Rice Research Institute (IRRI), DAPO Box 7777, Metro Manila, Philippines.
[3]Dept of Plant Science, College of Agriculture and Life Sciences, Seoul National University, Seoul, 151-921, Korea.

Interspecific hybrids (F₁'s) between Asian rice (*Oryza sativa* 2n=24 AA) and African rice (*Oryza glaberrima* 2n=24 AA) are almost completely sterile. This hybrid sterility barrier is mainly caused by an arrest of pollen development at the microspore stage. Intersubspecific F₁ hybrid sterility is mainly caused by cryptic chromosomal aberrations and allelic interaction between *indica* and *japonica*. To identify *O. glaberrima* specific loci, 67 subspecies-specific (SS) sequenced-tagged site (STS) marker were used to evaluate 30 *O. glaberrima* accessions, which could be classified into sub eleven groups. SPI (subspecies-prototype index) of *O. glaberrima* accessions ranged from 51.67 to 60.00, suggesting intermediate subspecific type based on whole-genome. Some informative markers for classifying O. *glaberrima* accessions, called reference markers, S01054, S01160, S02085, S02140, S03041, and S08107, showed *indica* alleles, which might have contributed to genomic diversification of *O. glaberrima*. Ten (14.9%) SS markers generated *glaberrima*-specific alleles, implying loci adjacent with these markers could be a key for interspecific hybrid sterility. Only 40 (59.7%) SS markers might be useful in *O. glaberrima* analysis, as other markers did not amplify heterozygous alleles in F₁ of *O.sativa* x *O. glaberrima*.

Key words: Subspecies-specific marker (SS), STS markers, indels, subspecies-prototype (SP), *Oryza sativa*, *Oryza glaberrima*.

INTRODUCTION

The genus *Oryza* is known to consist of two cultivated species, Asian rice (*Oryza sativa* 2n=24=AA) and African rice (*Oryza glaberrima* 2n=24=AA) and 22 wild species (2n=24, 48) representing 10 genomic types namely, AA, BB, CC, BBCC, CCDD, EE, FF, GG, HHJJ and HHKK (Vaughan, 1994; Aggarwal et al., 1997).Unlike *O. sativa*, *O. glaberrima* has no known subspecies.

It might have arose from an African wild species, *O. barthii* independently of the origin of *O. sativa* from the Asian form of *O. perennis* (Semon et al., 2005).The two species are adapted to diverse environments and has its own ecologically adapted and useful traits (Glaszmann,

1987; Sarla et al., 2005).

A number of different markers such as isozyme (Glaszmann, 1987), protein (Bi et al., 1997), RFLP (Qian et al., 1995) RAPD (Chin et al. 2003;), simple sequence repeat SSR (McCouch et al., 2002; Chen et al., 2002; Ni et al., 2002), AFLP Cho et al., 1999), STS (Chin et al., 2007; Edwards et al., 2004), SNPs (McNally et al., 2009; Feltus et al., 2004), and chloroplast DNA (Sun et al., 2002) have been utilized to estimate the extent of genetic diversity in *O. sativa*. In *O. glaberrima*, estimates of genetic diversity based on molecular markers are comparatively few, markers such as isozyme, RFLP SSR and SNPs have been used to estimates genetic diversity in *O. glaberrima* and its close genetic relationship to *O. barthii* (Lorieux et al., 2000; Semon et al., 2005) Even though diversity in *O. glaberrima* are significantly lower than those

*Corresponding author. E- mail: kofibimpong@yahoo.com.

than those in *O. sativa,* it has been shown to harbors genes that have allowed the species to survive and prosper in West Africa with minimal human intervention (Barry et al., 2006; Wang et al., 1992).

Even though *O. glaberrima* and *O. sativa* share the same genome, with minor sub-genomic differences which do not hinder normal chromosome pairing and gamete formation in the hybrids (Nayar, 1973); yet, F_1 hybrids between them shows complete sterility irrespective of the combinations of parental varieties (Pham and Bougero, 1993). Various causes such as meiotic irregularities (Heuer et al., 2003), low proportion of viable pollen, low pollen germination, cytoplasm and its interaction effects from male side and early elimination of female gametes and zygotes from female side (Porteres, 1956; Kitampura, 1962) have been ascribed for sterility. Other causes of sterility are due to segregation distortion (Causse et al., 1994; Lorieux et al., 2000), presence of sterility loci in O. glaberrima, (Koide et al., 2008; Sano 1986; Doi et al., 1999; Li et al., 2008), hybrid breakdown (Li et al., 1997; Kubo and Yoshimura, 2005) and suppressed recombination (Ikehashi, 1982; Neiman and Linksvayer, 2006); hindering easy transfer of useful genes between the two species. Some QTLs and epistatic interaction controlling hybrid-sterility have also been identified (Li et al., 2008).

It is of interest to understand the genetic structure of *O. glaberrima* as information on its diversity and structure is expected to assist plant breeders in the selection of parents for hybridization and also to identify materials that harbor alleles of value for plant improvement. Molecular markers have increasingly become useful tools for evaluating genetic diversity and determining cultivar identity. Compared to morphological markers, molecular markers can reveal differences among accessions at the DNA level and thus provide a more direct, reliable, and efficient tool for germplasm conservation and management.

Subspecies-specific (SS) or species-specific genomic regions could be inherited in a conserved manner to each of subspecies and species from which the SS regions were originated in the progenies of inter-subspecific or inter-specific crosses (Tanksley et al., 1992; Wang et al., 2001). Thus SS regions may provide a clue in understanding the mechanisms for reproductive barriers including inter-subspecific hybrid sterility and for the differentiation of rice subspecies.

OBJECTIVES

The purpose of this study was to evaluate the extent of genetic differentiation between diverse collections of *O. glaberrima* accessions using 67 subspecies-specific (SS) markers. We were interested in developing molecular markers in identifying *O. sativa* and/or *O.glaberrima* loci, and it usefulness in interspecific crosses.

MATERIALS AND METHODS

Plant material

Thirty accessions of *O. glaberrima* were obtained from the germplasm collection at International Rice Research Institute (IRRI) in the Philippines and Africa Rice Centre, Benin in West Africa, 12 accessions of *O. sativa*, representing both *indica* and *japonica* subspecies and 16 F_1 progenies from cross between *O. sativa* × *O. glaberrima* were used. The F_1s were produced by making crosses in the screenhouse of IRRI between 4 elite indica cultivars (IR64, PSBRc 18 -irrigated, IR 69502-6-SRN-3-UBN-1-B – rainfed and IR55423-01-upland cultivar) and several accessions of *O. glaberrima* referred to as RAM which were received from Mali in West Africa and have been field tested as drought tolerance. *O. sativa* was used as female parent in crosses with *O. glaberrima*. The F_1 plants were intermediate in morphological characteristics but were highly sterile. Variety names source/origin are given in Table 1.

Primer designing

A set of 67 STS markers used in this study were design by Chin et al. (2007) using an online-service software primer3 (http://frodo.wi.mit.edu/cgi-bin/primer3/primer3_www.cgi) to detect the insertion/deletion (InDel) polymorphism between the genome sequence of Nipponbare (*japonica*) and 9311 (*indica*). The amplicon size for each primer set was determined so that the amplicon contained at least 5% InDel difference of its whole size, 100 to 400 bp. These markers covers the whole chromosomes at an 2 to 3 cm interval based on the sequence information available at RGP for *japonica* and NCBI for *indica* and are distributed throughout the 12 chromosomes

PCR amplification

The protocols for PCR amplification and detection for STS markers were similar as described in Temnykh et al. (2000) with some modifications. Each 25 µl reaction mixture contained 50 ng DNA, 5 pmol of each primer, 2 µl PCR buffer [100 mM Tris (pH 8.3), 500 mM KCl, 15 mM $MgCl_2$, 2 µg gelatin], 250 µM of each dNTPs and 0.5 unit Taq polymerase. The thermocycler profile was: 5 min at 94°C, 35 cycles of 1 min at 94°C, 1 min at 48°C or 55°C, 2 min at 72°C, and 5 min at 72°C for final extension using the MJ research PCR system. PCR amplicons were resolved by electrophoresis in 3% agarose gels and marker bands were revealed using the silver-staining protocols as described by Panaud et al. (1996).

Scoring of the SS –STS markers

The SS STS markers were scored as 'a' (*japonica* allele) or 'b' (*indica* allele) for each marker locus. The total number of 'a' from *japonica* varieties and 'b' from *indica* were counted. Since some markers showed variation in generating SS alleles among varieties within and inter-subspecies, the concept of subspecies-specificity (SS) was employed as follows:

Subspecies-specificity (SS) score of each marker = (Total number of expected alleles in each subspecies) / (Total number of varieties/accessions tested) × 100 (%)

For example, if a marker has a SS score of 100%, it means that the SS marker generated SS alleles for all the accessions without

Table 1. Plant materials in this study.

Species/ subspecies	Entry No.	Name	Source	Entry No.	Cross combination*	Source
Indica	1	IR55423-01	IRRI	43	IR64 × RAM54	IRRI
	2	IR60080-46-A		44	IR64 × RAM86	
	3	IR64		45	IR64 × RAM90	
	4	IR68703-AC-24-1		46	IR64 × RAM120	
	5	IR69502-6-SRN		47	IR64 × RAM134	
	6	PSBRC18		48	IR64 × RAM131	
	7	PSBRC82		49	PSBRC18 × RAM111	
Japonica	8	Hwacheongbyeo	Korea	50	IR55423-01 × RAM3	
	9	Ilpumbyeo		51	IR55423-01 × RAM24	
	10	Jinmibyeo		52	IR55423-01 × RAM163	
	11	Junambyeo		53	IR69502 × RAM118	
	12	TR22183	China	54	IR69502 × RAM121	
O. glaberrima	13	RAM3	Mali	55	IR69502 × RAM163	
	14	RAM24		56	IR60080-46-A × IG10	
	15	RAM54		57	IR68703-AC-24-1 × CG14	
	16	RAM86		58	IR60080-46-A × CG14	
	17	RAM90				
	18	RAM111				
	19	RAM118				
	20	RAM120				
	21	RAM121				
	22	RAM131				
	23	RAM134				
	24	RAM152				
	25	RAM163				
	26	IG10	Ivory coast			
	27	CG14				
	28	CG17				
	29	CG20				
	30	Acc.103477				
	31	TOG5674				
	32	TOG5681				
	33	TOG5860	Africa			
	34	TOG6472				
	35	TOG6508				
	36	TOG6589				
	37	TOG6597	Ivory coast			
	38	TOG6629				
	39	TOG6631	Africa			
	40	TOG7235				
	41	TOG7291				
	42	TOG7442				

Entry no. 43- 58 are F_1 progenies between *O. sativa* × *O. glaberrima*.

exception. A marker with SS scores equal to or higher than 93.3 (up to 2 exceptions out of the total number of accessions) was regarded as SS marker. In addition, the Subspecies-Prototype (SP) degree for each accession was calculated in order to describe the relative genomic inclination of each accession toward either subspecies as follows:

Subspecies-prototype (SP) degree = Total number of *japonica* SS alleles in each accession - Total number of *Indica* SS alleles in each accession of each accession / Total number of SS markers tested

If a variety has a SP degree close to 1 or -1, the variety is estimated to have the genomic constitution close to the prototype of *japonica* or *indica*, respectively.

RESULTS

Genotyping by subspecies-specific (SS) markers

The information of 67 SS STS markers used in this study is summarized in supplementary Table 1. For a marker to be confirmed as SS, a threshold of 93.3% was set. There was only one SS markers detected on chromosome 6, while 11 SS markers were identified on chromosome 3. The average number of SS markers was 5.6 per chromosome The BAC/PAC clones from which STS markers were originated and the marker location within BAC/PAC clones were denoted in a sequence order of base pairs. The SS markers which showed perfect SS scores were S01022, S02026, S02140, S03020, S03041, S04128, S06001, S07011, S09026B, S10003A, S11004A, S11006A and S12011B.

Classification of *O. glaberrima* accessions by SS markers

Figure 1 show the gel profile of an SS- STS marker applied to amplify 12 *O.sativa* varieties, 30 *O. glaberrima* accessions, and 16 F_1 progenies between *O.sativa* × *O. glaberrima*. As expected, most of the SS markers detected *O. sativa* alleles with only 7% (10 markers) detecting *O. glaberrima*-specific allele (Table 2). Estimated size of alleles present in only *O. glaberrima* ranged from 160 bp in SS marker S10003A to 610 bp in marker S11004A. Two SS markers S02085 and S02140 did not detect any *indica-japonica* alleles among the *O. glaberrima* accessions (Table 2).

The average value of *Indica*-prototype index which is similar to *indica* varieties of *O .sativa* (IPI) was about 50% for each *O. glaberrima* accessions and between 80 to 90% among *indica* varieties from IRRI (Figure 2). No IPI was observed in the *japonica* varieties of Korean origin while the IRRI type had about 15%. The 2 *japonicas* and the 5 *indica* varieties were similar in allelic composition to the IRRI varieties, even though they might have different plant types (Figure 2, Supplementary Tables 2 and 3); The subspecies-prototype index (SPI) of *O. glaberrima* accessions ranged between 51.67- 60.00, while the japonica species had very low SPI (0 to 13.24) (Supplementary table 2).

A total of 10 subgroups were identified based on 6 informative markers, called reference markers, S01054, S01160, S02085, S02140, S03041, and S08107 (Table 3). Each of the 10 subgroups revealed different markers showing the kind of mutation occurring at that specific locus (either as an *indica/japonica* allele mutating to *japonica, indica* or *O. glaberrima* alleles). For example in group IV, the *O. glaberrima* allele mutated from *japonica* allele as revealed by marker S01160. Also *O. glaberrima*

accession TOG5674 could be distinguished from CG14 by the presence of additional *indica* allele revealed by marker S02085 and specific allele by S02140. Twenty-nine of the 30 *O. glaberrima* accessions (except TOG 6629) were observed to be segregating for different alleles (Table 3).

Forty-two percent SS markers detected heterozygous alleles between *japonica/glaberrima* in the F_1 progenies; whilst 34% markers also detected heterozygous alleles between *indica/glaberrima* in the F_1 progenies (Table 4 and Supplementary Tables 3). Some makers (13%) did not detect heterozygous alleles in the F_1 between *O.sativa* and *O. glaberrima* species; whilst others such as S09093A could not distinguish the heterozygous alleles between *indica and glaberrima.*

Comparative view of genome of *O. glaberrima* based on *O. sativa* spp *japonica* genome

A total of 38 loci among the *O. glaberrima* accessions had only *indica* alleles and 26 loci had only *Japonica* alleles, whilst only 1 loci showed both *indica* and *japonica* alleles (Figure 3). Some non-*sativa* alleles were detected on chromosome 1, 2, 9, 10, 11, and 12. Heterozygous alleles of *indica* and *glaberrima* (G+I) were identified on 3 loci on chromosomes 1, 2 and 3. Markers on inter-sub specific hybrid sterility QTLs, S05014B and RM413 on chromosome 5 and S08066 on chromosome 8, showed *indica* alleles in 29 *O. glaberrima* accessions.

DISCUSSION

Allele frequency of 30 *O. glaberrima* accessions

A small proportion of the SS-STS markers tested (10 in all=14.9% 10 in 67) did not amplify *O. sativa* allele but rather *O. glaberrima* specific alleles, and consist of 6 to 7 glaberrima specific alleles. Polymorphism between *O. glaberrima* at the DNA level has been reported to be low; few polymorphisms (37 to 41%) could be detected by Enriquez et al. (2001) using SSR markers. Further, Bimpong et al. (2004) observed 38% polymorphism between *O. sativa* × *O. glaberrima* parents using SSR markers. Those SS markers that detected *O. glaberrima* alleles might be related to the evolution of *O. glaberrima*. Very few STS markers have been used to detect polymorphism among *O. glaberrima* species. SSR have been used widely in genetic diversity studies (Semon et al., 2005; Garris et al., 2004; Senior, 1998); however, much work has not been done on the use of STS to detect genetic diversity in *O. glaberrima*. Bimpong et al. (2009) detected 9.9% (16 out of 162 STS markers) polymorphism between 10 accessions of *O. glaberrima* using STS markers. The other primers (54.5%) amplified *indica, japonica* or unspecific alleles in some genotypes. The lack of amplification of products in some SS markers

Supplementary Table 1. List of subspecies-specific primers.

Chromosome	Marker	Physical location in Nipponbare pseudomolecule(bp)		Expected size of amplicon (bp)		Primer sequence		BAC clone 1)	SS score2 (%)
		start	stop	Japonica	Indica	Forward	Reverse		
1	S01022	4384676	4384975	300	312	catggatgatgcttccctct	ttgacagtggctccacaaag	AP002484	100
	S01054	10309451	10309687	237	266	gcgaagcctgctttttgat	cggagatttttccctaaaacaa	AP002070	96.7
	S01140	35147646	35147820	175	187	gctaggcagactctagctcatca	tggaacaagtagaagcagaagtca	AP003411	93.3
	S01157B	39802962	39803196	235	223	ccctcaatcatcgcaactgt	cagatgcagaaaagcgcata	AP006531	93.3
	S01160	40802478	40802660	183	179	ttgcgatttatttgccagtg	ccaggcatccaatgcttatt	AP004672	96.7
2	S02026	5345560	5345726	167	180	tggtccatcatattgccaac	tcctctcagatccgatttca	AP004184	100
	S02052	12020182	12020373	192	201	gcagtcggttcaattggt	gattttccagcccattctca	AP005743	93.3
	S02054	14117145	14117316	172	157	tttgaagcacgagggatctt	ataaagaaccgatgcaaacg	AP004856	93.3
	S02057B	17440500	17440729	230	241	agcctcttcccctcctcac	tgcaaacaccataacaaccaa	AP004999	93.3
	S02081B	20964659	20964883	225	201	agcggcatatttgcatagc	tgttttgcaggacgcagtag	AP004876	96.7
	S02085	21636396	21636559	164	153	gcgagagtgtacccctttga	tgtgtaccttgcaccctgaa	AP006068	96.7
	S02140	32850429	32850633	205	220	tgggaggagagatattgttgga	tgacaggttgatgtgatggaa	AP005538	100
3	S03010B	2098371	2098585	215	203	gtgcggatttggttctgtt	gagggagggccagattctt	AC118132	93.3
	S03020	4302802	4302984	183	168	tttctagttacatttaagcaagca	catgaatttgaagctgcgagta	AC126223	100
	S03027	5713283	5713531	249	232	tgaacattttggtcgtctg	ttgacgaagtcaccatagacg	AC105928	96.7
	S03041	8900833	8901024	192	201	gctgacattgtccgaggtt	ccgacgtccaacctaagc	AC139168	100
	S03046	10137125	10137381	257	248	tcacagtttacaggcggaatc	gcaccatgtatagaccattcca	AC137634	93.3
	S03048	10754658	10754836	179	159	gggatgggagaagggaataa	gccagctaggatgttgaagg	AC137267	96.7
	S03096	24299548	24299716	169	183	cacttgcaagctaagcacca	ccttcctgcttgacgagaaa	AC120505	96.7
	S03099	24995662	24995883	222	233	ctcccaggatgctcactcag	ataatccaaggcacagcac	AL731878	96.7
	S03120	27366848	27367089	242	254	tgtgcgctcgtgattatttt	aaggggagcagataatgcag	AC092779	96.7
	S03136	30109023	30109222	200	219	gcattaaggcacacaaagca	tgtttgtaatcgcatggaa	AC118133	96.7
	S03145	32174684	32174922	239	251	tcacctacaggaagcagcag	gccgcgttgaagaagtagc	AC091494	93.3
4	S04058	20162588	20162832	245	226	gatccatgcagttgattgtga	tcgtcttatctaaaagaaaatttga	AL662947	96.7
	S04060	20474915	20475135	221	203	tatggttttatccgccaacc	gctacaactaaaaacaagaaaacgtga	AL606598	96.7
	S04077B	24949310	24949483	174	201	atgtggatggtggtcctat	agggtcatcgctaatgctg	AL606604	93.3
	S04077A	24958459	24958724	266	247	tcccaggtgaactacggact	cagcattttcagtggaagca	AL606604	93.3
	S04087A	27761378	27761633	256	248	atgtttggcaatccgctaag	aaagatgggttgagcggaaga	AL606682	96.7
	S04097B	29346635	29346813	179	189	tccacagtctgtcgtgaaa	ctccttgtcgtgtcgcagaattg	AL662957	93.3
	S04128	34569925	34570087	163	181	tcacggaaagctttgtat	aacttatgcagccaccatcc	AL606456	100
	S04129B	35102075	35102256	182	203	aatcgattcattcgcacaaa	ctttcatgctctgccattga	AL606637	93.3

Supplementary Table 1. Contd.

5	S05064	16966554	16966786	245	257	aaagcaagtcacaaacacaaataaa	tgcctcgatttcataagca	AC104272	93.3
	S05080A	20663155	20663383	229	254	tggccaacttgggaattta	aagagtcgtgcaaatgaaaaga	AC109595	96.7
6	S06001	546207	546437	231	244	agctcaatatcaggcaagcag	aaatgacacagttgacctttgaa	AP000616	100
7	S07011	2543283	2543511	229	205	ctggatccaaggcatcattc	cttcgctctcaccatcaaca	AP004263	100
	S07048	8487589	8487745	157	172	catggcacctgagagttga	acacatggagctggcttctc	AP005824	96.7
	S07050C	13437934	13438142	209	225	ctccacttatggcagcgaat	caagtgaagtgggagcaggt	AP003745	93.3
	S07050A	14531440	14531638	199	211	tacacgaacgaacgacaagg	cgctgatttgggtaggtctc	AP005200	96.7
	S07101	26848149	26848350	202	216	gcatgccaggatatggtctc	tcggtacacacctcctgtga	AP003832	93.3
	S07103	27558599	27558809	211	223	agcatggatccttcatccaa	actccgatttttgcacttcg	AP005182	93.3
8	S08066	18904657	18904874	218	238	ttgttccgttgtgtgtcaact	gatgcagcgacgtgaaatc	AP003947	96.7
	S08090	23079842	23080054	213	231	gcgtgtggaagaggagaaag	cagtgagaatctgcagtcg	AP004693	96.7
	S08106	25773305	25773524	220	194	ttacggattgtcacggtttt	ggaattgtcactggtttcca	AP005509	96.7
	S08107	25956924	25957152	229	240	ttggtaatgcccatgctaga	cacgattcggtcatttcaga	AP003888	93.3
9	S09000A	244321	244528	208	221	ccaattcacggtttaacaagg	gccatgaagcttcgttagga	AP006058	96.7
	S09026B	9142928	9143141	214	189	gggaggcagaggaactact	ttatcaggccaggtcctttg	AP005780	100
	S09040B	12641376	12641601	226	214	taatatcgcatggcaagacg	actttgcagaggcgacaaac	AP005637	96.7
	S09058	15942709	15942930	222	233	cgtgagaagtccagtccaca	attgatcgattggggattt	AP005551	93.3
	S09062B	16864607	16864856	250	236	acgcataccgaatgtgacag	gttgcactccgattaaaa	AP005559	93.3
	S09065	17914403	17914639	237	246	tgtgttcgacgtttgaccat	gggccaggtacattgaata	AP005574	96.7
	S09073	19077948	19078180	233	250	accacctgaaccacaacat	tcactggttctgtgtccaa	AC099403	96.7
	S09075B	19519638	19519866	229	211	gactaacgaacgggcctat	ggcagcccacactattagg	AC108753	96.7
	S09075A	19575874	19576047	174	154	cctcactcacctggagagg	cgtccacactaacggacaca	AC108753	93.3
	S09093A	22803693	22803950	258	232	caccgctccactgtcattc	tccctcagccataaaaccag	AP006162	96.7
10	S10001	992379	992586	208	229	atcgtgtcgggattatgag	gcatcatggctttgttg	AC078891	96.7
	S10003A	1715981	1716214	234	246	ataagacgacggtcaaacg	atctcttgtgggctttgtg	AC025098	100
	S10013A	5180767	5180949	183	170	agtcgggtcatttcttagcc	ctacgtctccgtttcacaa	AC083944	93.3
	S10019	10299169	10299319	151	163	atgcatctacatggcatttg	gatgctgagatgcgattgaa	AC123594	93.3
	S10026C	13594825	13595071	247	227	tacgtgtccttgtgcctgaa	tttcaccccactgtaaagg	AC021893	93.3
	S10071	20926684	20926850	167	158	tatggctcaaccctggaaac	cgtcagtttgttcactgga	AC051633	96.7
	S10072	21129266	21129444	179	203	tgagtgttcgttgtcttcc	tggtaaggccttgaagatgg	AC020666	96.7
11	S11004A	1081615	1081787	173	157	tctctggccttctactcatgg	ttgtgtttctaacttggactctttt	AC136970	100
	S11006A	1270331	1270591	261	248	atgcgcgctccaacttatac	tggtgcaaaggaatgaacaa	AC123525	100
	S11028	5463772	5463946	175	186	attccctgggggtagctaga	atgggtgaattgcagagaat	AC123523	96.7

Supplementary Table 1. Contd.

12	S12011B	1884649	1884804	156	177	tgggggagttctgaaatctg	ttaagttcggtgcccataa	AL935154	100
	S12030	3843516	3843732	217	235	tcccacatgtaaaccgctgaa	tgagtgatataacaacacacaacca	AL732376	96.7
	S12109B	27415607	27415770	164	173	ggactcggataaccgcatta	ggaacgcagcgaaagaat	AL732378	93.3

1BAC clone information is available at International Rice Genome Sequencing Project (IRGSP). g Threshold of SS score for identification of SS marker was 93.3 (%) (See Materials and Methods).

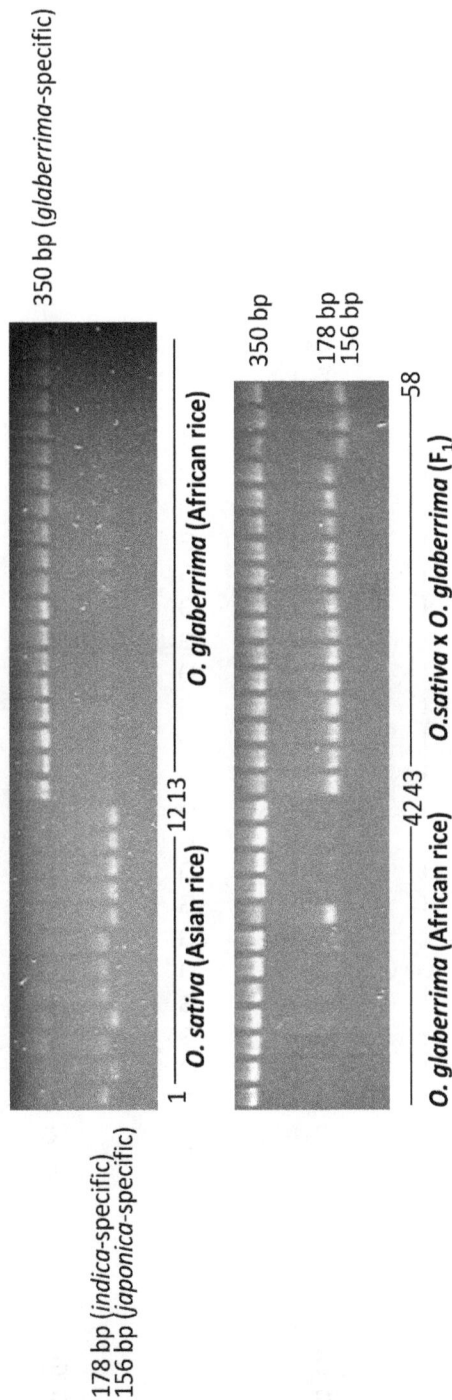

Figure 1. Genotyping of *O. glaberrima* accessions by subspecies-specific (SS) STS markers. (a) 1 to 12 : *O. sativa* (*indica* allele : 178bp and *japonica* allele : 156 bp). 13 to 42: *O. glaberrima* (350 bp non-*O.sativa* allele). (b) 43 to 58 : showed both the alleles of *sativa* and *glaberrima*, but the band size of F1's were different, implying the amplified regions of *O. sativa* and *O. glaberrima* were neighbored.

markers has been a common obser-vation in the STS markers (Wang et al., 2009; Perry et al., 1999) and it may reflect divergences in the sequences flanking the SS STS loci, leading to the production of possible null alleles, or totally restricting amplification.

The informative markers (called reference markers) used to classify O. glaberrima accessions into 10 subgroups (S01054, S01160, S02085, S02140, S03041, and S08107), might have contributed to genomic diversification of *O. glaberrima*, as they were able to show the kind of mutation occurring at that specific locus (either as an

indica/japonica allele mutated to japonica, indica or O. glaberrima alleles); suggesting a continuous mutation of some SS markers were associated in terms of inheritance; and might have contributed to genomic diversification of *O. glaberrima.*. For example, 'TOG5674' can be distinguished from 'CG14' by additional *indica* allele of S02085 and specific allele of S02140.

Whole genome analysis has revealed the structural similarities between *O sativa* and *O. glaberrima* species, (Park et al., 2003,) but due to the high frequency of polymorphism in subspecies-specific (SS) loci, it is assumed that

there is a relationship between *sativa* × *glaberrima* F1 hybrid sterility and SS loci. *O. glaberrima* had *indica* alleles at two loci associated with inter-subspecific F₁ hybrid sterility on chromosome 5 and chromosome 8 (Figure 3).

Application of SS-STS markers to study the relations within *O. glaberrima* species

The SS STSs markers used in the study were able to revealed different alleles both from *japonica* and *indica* sources among the *O. glaberrima* accessions. The efficiency of STS

Table 2. Subspecies-specific STS markers generating *glaberrima* (G)-specific alleles.

Name of varieties/lines	S01160	S02085	S02140	S03145	S09093A	S10003A	S10013A	S11004A	S1201
IR55423-01	J[1]	I	I	I	I	I	I	J	I
IR60080-46-A	I	J	J	J	J	J	I	J	J
IR64	I	I	I	I	I	I	I	I	I
IR68703-AC-24-1	I	J	J	J	J	J	I	J	J
IR69502-6-SRN	I	I	I	I	I	I	I	I	I
PSBRC18	J	I	I	I	I	I	I	I	I
PSBRC82	I	I	I	I	I	I	I	I	I
Hwacheongbyeo	J	J	J	J	J	J	J	J	J
Ilpumbyeo	J	J	J	J	J	J	J	J	J
Jinmibyeo	J	J	J	J	J	J	J	J	J
Junambyeo	J	J	J	J	J	J	J	J	J
TR22183	J	J	J	G+J	J	J	J	J	J
RAM3	G	G	I	G+I	G	G	G	G	G
RAM24	G	G	I	G+I	G	G	G	G	G
RAM54	G	G	I	G+I	G	G	G	G	G
RAM86	G	G	I	G+I	G	G	G	G	G
RAM90	G	G	I	G+I	G	G	G	G	G
RAM111	G	G	I	G+I	G	G	G	G	G
RAM118	G	G	I	G+I	G	G	G	G	G
RAM120	G	G	I	G+I	G	G	G	G	G
RAM121	G	G	I	G+I	G	G	G	G	G
RAM131	G	G	I	G+I	G	G	G	G	G
RAM134	G	G	I	G+I	G	G	G	G	G
RAM152	G	G	I	G+I	G	G	G	G	G
RAM163	G	G	I	G+I	G	G	G	G	G
IG10	G	G	I	G+I	G	G	G	G	G
CG14	G	G	I	G+I	G	G	G	G	G
CG17	G	G	I	G+I	G	G	G	G	G
CG20	J	G	I	G+I	G	G	G	G	G
Acc.103477	G	G	I	G+I	G	G	G	G	G
TOG5674	I	G+I	G	G+I	G	G	G	G	G
TOG5681	I	G+I	I	G+I	G	G	G	G	G
TOG5860	I	G	I	G+I	G	G	G	G	G
TOG6472	I	G	I	G+I	G	G	G	G	G
TOG6508	G+I	G	I	G+I	G	G	G	G	G
TOG6589	G+I	G	I	G+I	G	G	G	G	G
TOG6597	G+I	G	I	-	G	G	G	G	G
TOG6629	G+I	G+I	I	-	I	G+I	G+I	J	G+I
TOG6631	I	G	I	G+I	G	G	G	G	G
TOG7235	I	G	I	G+I	G	G	G	G	G
TOG7291	I	G	G	G+I	G	G	G	G	G
TOG7442	I	G	I	G+I	G	G	G	G	G
IR64 × RAM54	G+I	G+I	I	G+I	I	G+I	G+I	G+I	G+I
IR64 × RAM86	G+I	G+I	I	G+I	I	G+I	G+I	G+I	G+I
IR64 × RAM90	G+I	G+I	I	G+I	I	G+I	G+I	G+I	G+I
IR64 × RAM120	G+I	G+I	I	G+I	I	G+I	G+I	G+I	G+I
IR64 × RAM134	G+I	G+I	I	G+I	I	G+I	G+I	G+I	G+I
IR64 × RAM131	G+I	G+I	I	-	I	G+I	G+I	G+I	G+I
PSBRC18 × RAM111	G+J	G+I	I	G+I	I	G+I	G+I	G+I	G+I
IR55423-01 × RAM3	G+J	G+I	I	G+I	I	G+I	G+I	G+J	G+I
IR55423-01 × RAM24	G+J	G+I	I	G+I	I	G+I	G+I	G+J	G+I

Table 2. Contd.

IR55423-01 × RAM163	G+J	G+I	I	G+I	I	G+I	G+I	G+J	G+I
IR69502 × RAM118	G+I	G+I	I	G+I	I	G+I	G+I	G+I	G+I
IR69502 × RAM121	G+I	G+I	I	G+I	I	G+I	G+I	G+I	G+I
IR69502 × RAM163	G+I	G+I	I	G+I	I	G+I	G+I	G+I	G+I
IR60080-46-A × IG10	G+I	G+J	H	G+J	G+J	G+J	G+I	G+J	G+J
IR68703-AC-24-1 × CG14	I	G+J	H	G+J	G+J	G+I	G+I	G+J	G+J
IR60080-46-A × CG14	I	G+J	H	G+J	G+J	G+J	G+J	G+J	G+J
Alleles in *glaberrima*[2] (bp)	176	NULL	NULL	270 and 290	240	300	160	610	350

[1]J: *japonica*-specific allele, I: *indica*-specific allele, G: alleles-present in *O. glaberrima* accessions, G+I: alleles in glaberrima and indica allele, G+J: alleles in glaberrima and japonica allele. [2]Estimated size of alleles only found in *O. glaberrima* not in *O. sativa* in basepair (bp). 'NULL' represents no amplification of *indica-japonica* alleles in *O. glaberrima* accessions.

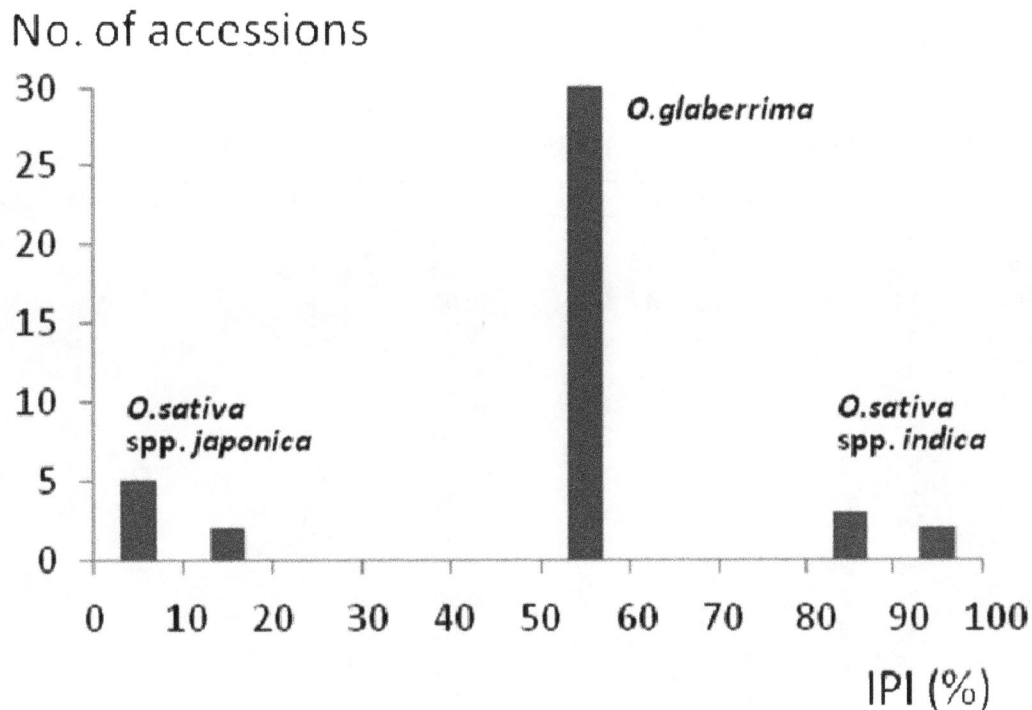

Figure 2. IPI (*Indica*-prototype index: similarity to *indica* varieties of *O.sativa*) of 30 *O. glaberrima* accessions.

Table 3. Successful polymorphic markers between *O. glaberrima* and *O. sativa*.

Subspecies of *O.sativa*[1]	Chromosome													Marker frequency[2]
	1	2	3	4	5	6	7	8	9	10	11	12	Total	
indica	3	2	4	1	0	0	3	1	4	3	1	1	23	34.33%
japonica	1	3	5	6	2	1	3	1	5	0	0	1	28	41.79%
indica/japonica	1	1	1	0	0	0	0	0	0	2	1	1	7	10.45%
-	0	1	1	1	0	0	0	2	1	2	1	0	9	13.43%

[1]Two bands from parents represent hetero alleles were successfully amplified when *O.glaberrima* accessions were crossed with corresponding subspecies of *O.sativa*. [2]Total number of markers out of total of 67 subspecies-specific STS markers.

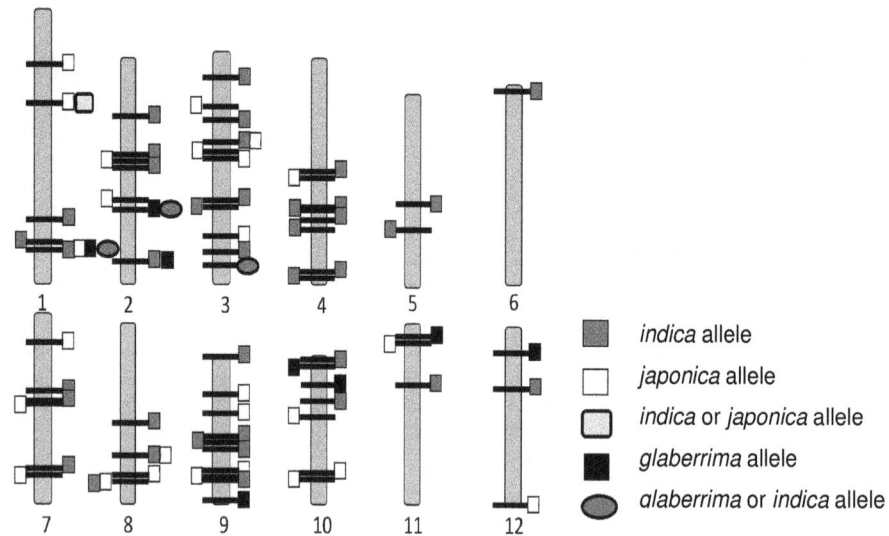

Figure 3. Comparative view of alleles of *O.glaberrima* based on Nipponbare genome.

Table 4. Reference markers classifying 30 *O.glaberrima* accessions.

Group	Name	I	J	-	G	H	G+I	G+J	SPI=I/(I+J+H)	Reference markers		Allele change from G1[1]
G1	RAM86	36	24	0	7	0	1	0	60.00			
	RAM90	36	24	0	7	0	1	0	60.00			
	RAM111	36	24	0	7	0	1	0	60.00			
	RAM118	36	24	0	7	0	1	0	60.00			
	RAM120	36	24	0	7	0	1	0	60.00			
	RAM121	36	24	0	7	0	1	0	60.00			
	RAM131	36	24	0	7	0	1	0	60.00			
	RAM134	36	24	0	7	0	1	0	60.00			
	RAM152	36	24	0	7	0	1	0	60.00			
	RAM163	36	24	0	7	0	1	0	60.00			
	IG10	34	24	2	7	0	1	0	58.62			
	CG14	36	24	0	7	0	1	0	60.00			
	CG17	36	24	0	7	0	1	0	60.00			
	TOG6472	35	25	1	6	0	1	0	58.33			
	TOG7235	36	24	1	6	0	1	0	60.00			
G2	RAM3	35	25	0	7	0	1	0	58.33	S08107		I->J
	RAM24	35	25	0	7	0	1	0	58.33			
	RAM54	35	25	0	7	0	1	0	58.33			
G3	Acc.103477	35	25	0	7	0	1	0	58.33	S03041		I->J
G4	CG20	36	25	0	6	0	1	0	59.02	S01160		G->J
G5	TOG5681	35	25	1	5	0	2	0	58.33	S02085		G->G+I
G6	TOG5674	34	25	1	6	0	2	0	57.63	S02085	S02140	G->G+I, I->G
G7	TOG6508	34	25	1	6	0	2	0	57.63	S01160		I->G+I
	TOG6589	34	24	2	6	0	2	0	58.62			
G8	TOG5860	35	23	2	6	1	1	0	59.32	S01054		J->H
	TOG6631	36	24	0	6	1	1	0	59.02			
	TOG7442	36	24	0	6	1	1	0	59.02			
G9	TOG6597	33	22	5	6	1	1	0	58.93	S01054	S01160	J->H, G->G+I
G10	TOG7291	35	24	0	7	1	1	0	58.33	S01054	S02140	J->H, I->G

[1]*O. glaberrima* accessions in different groups can be distinguished using corresponding reference markers by observation of allele change. For example, 'TOG5674' can be distinguished from 'CG14' by additional *indica* allele of S02085 and specific allele of S02140.

Supplementary Table 2. Genotyping results with 67 SS-STS markers in this study.

Accession name	Entry No.	S01022	S01054	S01140	S01157B	S01160	S02026	S02052	S02054	S02057B	S02081B	S02085	S02140	S03010B	S03020	S03027	S03041	S03046	S03048	S03096	S03099	S03115	S03120	S03136
IR55423-01	1	—	—	—	—	J	—	—	J	—	—	—	—	—	—	—	J	J	J	—	—	J	J	—
IR60080-46-A	2	—	—	—	—	J	J	J	J	J	J	J	J	J	J	J	—	J	J	—	—	J	J	J
IR64	3	J	J	J	—	J	—	—	J	J	—	—	—	—	—	J	—	J	J	—	—	J	J	J
IR68703-AC-24-1	4	—	—	—	—	—	—	—	—	J	—	—	—	—	—	J	J	J	J	—	—	—	J	J
IR69502-6-SRN	5	J	J	J	—	—	—	—	—	J	—	—	—	—	—	—	J	J	J	—	—	J	J	J
PSBRC18	6	—	—	—	—	J	—	—	—	J	—	—	—	—	—	—	J	J	J	—	—	J	J	—
PSBRC82	7	—	—	J	—	J	J	J	J	P	—	—	—	J	J	J	J	J	J	J	J	J	J	J
Hwacheongbyeo	8	—	—	—	—	J	J	J	J	—	—	—	—	J	J	J	J	J	J	J	J	J	J	J
Ilpumbyeo	9	J	J	-	J	J	J	J	J	J	J	J	J	J	J	J	J	J	J	J	J	J	J	J
Jinmibyeo	10	J	J	J	J	J	J	J	J	J	J	J	J	J	J	J	J	J	J	J	J	J	J	J
Junambyeo	11	J	J	J	J	J	J	J	J	J	J	J	J	J	J	J	J	J	J	J	J	J	J	J
TR22183	12	J	J	J	J	J	—	—	J	—	J	J	J	J	J	J	J	J	J	—	—	J	J	—
RAM3	13	J	J	J	J	G	J	J	J	J	J	G	J	J	J	J	J	J	J	—	—	J	J	—
RAM24	14	J	J	J	J	G	J	J	J	J	J	G	J	J	J	J	J	J	J	—	—	J	J	—
RAM54	15	J	J	J	J	G	J	J	J	J	J	G	J	J	J	J	J	J	J	—	—	J	J	—
RAM86	16	J	J	J	J	G	J	J	J	J	J	G	J	J	J	J	J	J	J	—	—	J	J	—
RAM90	17	J	J	J	J	G	J	J	J	J	J	G	J	J	J	J	J	J	J	—	—	J	J	—
RAM111	18	J	J	J	J	G	J	J	J	J	J	G	J	J	J	J	J	J	J	—	—	J	J	—
RAM118	19	J	J	J	J	G	J	J	J	J	J	G	J	J	J	J	J	J	J	—	—	J	J	—
RAM120	20	J	J	J	J	G	J	J	J	J	J	G	J	J	J	J	J	J	J	—	—	J	J	—
RAM121	21	J	J	J	J	G	J	J	J	J	J	G	J	J	J	J	J	J	J	—	—	J	J	—
RAM131	22	J	J	J	J	G	J	J	J	J	J	G	J	J	J	J	J	J	J	—	—	J	J	—
RAM134	23	J	J	J	J	G	J	J	J	J	J	G	J	J	J	J	J	J	J	—	—	J	J	—
RAM152	24	J	J	J	J	G	J	J	J	J	J	G	J	J	J	J	J	J	J	—	—	J	J	—
RAM163	25	J	J	J	J	G	J	J	J	J	J	G	J	J	J	J	J	J	J	—	—	J	J	—
IG10	26	J	J	J	J	G	J	J	J	J	J	G	J	J	J	J	J	J	J	—	—	J	J	—
CG14	27	J	J	J	J	G	J	J	J	J	J	G	J	J	J	J	J	J	J	—	—	J	J	—
CG17	28	J	J	J	J	G	J	J	J	J	J	G	G	J	J	J	J	J	J	—	—	J	J	—
CG20	29	J	J	J	J	J	J	J	J	J	J	J	J	J	J	J	J	J	J	—	—	J	J	—
Acc.103477	30	J	J	J	J	—	J	J	J	J	J	G+I	G	J	J	J	J	J	J	—	—	J	J	—
TOG5674	31	J	J	J	J	—	J	J	J	J	J	G+I	—	J	J	J	J	J	J	—	—	J	J	—
TOG5681	32	J	J	J	J	G	J	J	J	J	J	J	—	J	J	J	J	J	J	—	—	J	J	—
TOG5860	33	J	H	J	J	J	J	J	J	J	-	G	—	J	J	J	J	J	J	—	—	J	J	G
TOG6472	34	J	J	—	J	—	J	J	J	—	J	G	—	J	J	J	J	J	J	—	—	J	J	—

Supplementary Table 2. Genotyping results with 67 SS-STS markers in this study (contd).

Entry No.		S03145	S04058	S04060	S04077A	S04077B	S04087A	S04097B	S04128	S04129B	S05064	S05080A	S06001	S07011	S07048	S07050C	S07050A	S07101	S07103	S08066	S08090	S08106	S08107
TOG6508	35	J	J	J	—	G+I	—	—	J	—	—	J	G	G	H	—	—	J	J	—	—	J	—
TOG6589	36	J	J	J	—	G+I	—	—	J	—	—	J	G	H	H	—	—	J	J	—	—	J	—
TOG6597	37	J	J	H	—	G+I	—	—	J	—	—	J	G	H	H	—	—	J	H	—	—	J	—
TOG6629	38	J	H	H	—	G+I	—	—	H	—	—	H	G+I	H	H	—	—	H	H	—	—	J	—
TOG6631	39	H	J	J	—	—	—	—	J	—	—	J	G	—	H	—	—	J	J	—	—	J	—
TOG7235	40	J	J	H	—	—	—	—	J	—	—	J	G	H	H	—	—	J	H	—	—	J	—
TOG7291	41	J	J	—	—	—	—	—	J	—	—	J	G	G	H	—	—	H	H	—	—	J	—
TOG7442	42	J	J	J	—	—	—	—	J	—	—	J	G	H	H	—	—	J	H	—	—	J	—
IR64×RAM54	43	H	H	H	G+I	—	—	H	H	—	—	H	G+I	H	H	—	—	H	H	—	H	J	—
IR64×RAM86	44	H	H	H	G+I	—	—	H	H	—	—	H	G+I	H	H	—	—	H	H	—	H	J	—
IR64×RAM90	45	H	H	—	G+I	—	—	H	H	—	—	H	G+I	H	H	—	—	H	H	—	H	J	—
IR64×RAM120	46	H	H	—	G+I	—	—	H	H	—	—	H	G+I	H	H	—	—	H	H	—	H	J	—
IR64×RAM134	47	H	J	—	G+I	—	—	H	J	—	—	J	G+I	H	H	—	—	H	H	—	H	J	—
IR64×RAM131	48	H	H	H	G+I	—	—	H	H	—	—	H	G+I	H	H	—	—	H	H	—	H	J	—
PSBRC18×RAM111	49	H	H	H	G+I	—	—	H	H	—	—	H	G+I	H	H	—	—	H	H	—	H	J	—
IR55423-01×RAM3	50	H	H	H	G+I	—	—	H	H	—	—	H	G+I	H	H	—	—	H	H	—	H	J	—
IR55423-01×RAM24	51	H	H	H	G+J	—	—	H	H	—	—	H	G+I	H	H	—	—	H	H	—	H	J	—
IR55423-01×RAM163	52	H	H	H	G+J	—	—	H	H	—	—	H	G+I	H	H	—	—	H	H	—	H	J	—
IR69502×RAM118	53	H	H	—	G+I	—	—	H	H	—	—	H	G+I	H	H	—	—	H	H	—	H	J	—
IR69502×RAM121	54	H	H	—	G+I	—	—	H	H	—	—	H	G+I	H	H	—	—	H	H	—	H	J	—
IR69502×RAM163	55	H	H	H	G+I	—	—	H	H	—	—	H	G+I	H	H	—	—	H	H	—	H	J	—
IR60080-46-A×IG10	56	J	J	H	G+I	—	H	H	J	—	—	J	G+I	H	H	—	—	H	G+J	H	—	J	—
IR68703-AC-24-1×CG14	57	J	J	H	—	I	—	H	J	—	—	J	G+J	H	H	—	—	H	G+J	H	H	J	—
IR60080-46-A×CG14	58	J	J	H	—	—	—	H	H	—	—	H	G+J	H	H	—	—	H	G+J	—	H	J	J
Specific alleles (Neither I or J)					G=176		I=H	P=260	N	N	I=H							I=H		Hetero G			

* Alleles: I:*indica*; J:*japonica*; H: hetero (I and J); G: *glaberrima*-specific; N: non-amplified allele of *O.glaberrima*; P: TR22183 specific; S: smear bands

Supplementary Table 2. Genotyping results with 67 SS-STS markers in this study (continued).

Accession Name	Entry No.	S03145	S04058	S04060	S04077A	S04077B	S04087A	S04097B	S04128	S04129B	S05064	S05080A	S06001	S07011	S07048	S07050C	S07050A	S07101	S07103	S08066	S08090	S08106	S08107
IR55423-01	1	J	J	J	J	J	-	J	J	J	J	J	J	J	J	J	-	J	J	J	J	J	J
IR60080-46-A	2	J	J	J	J	J	J	J	J	J	J	J	J	J	J	J	J	J	J	J	J	J	J

Supplementary Table 2. Genotyping results with 67 SS-STS markers in this study (continued).

IR64	3	–	–	J	J	–	–	–	–	–	–	–	–	–	–	–	–	–
IR68703-AC-24-1	4	–	J	J	J	J	J	J	J	J	J	J	J	J	J	J	J	J
IR69502-6-SRN	5	–	–	–	–	–	–	–	–	–	–	–	–	–	–	–	–	–
PSBRC18	6	–	–	–	J	–	–	–	–	–	–	–	–	–	J	–	–	–
PSBRC82	7	–	J	J	J	J	–	J	J	–	J	–	–	J	J	–	–	J
Hwacheongbyeo	8	J	J	J	J	J	J	J	J	J	J	J	J	J	J	J	J	J
Ilpumbyeo	9	J	J	J	J	J	J	J	J	J	J	J	J	J	J	J	J	J
Jinmibyeo	10	J	–	J	J	J	–	J	J	J	J	J	J	J	J	J	J	J
Junambyeo	11	J	J	J	J	J	J	J	J	J	J	J	J	J	J	J	J	J
TR22183	12	G+J	J	J	J	J	J	J	J	J	J	J	J	J	J	J	J	–
RAM3	13	G+I	J	J	J	J	J	J	J	J	J	J	J	J	J	J	J	J
RAM24	14	G+I	J	J	J	J	J	J	J	J	J	J	J	J	J	J	J	J
RAM54	15	G+I	J	J	J	J	J	J	J	J	J	J	J	J	J	J	J	J
RAM86	16	G+I	J	J	J	J	J	J	J	J	J	J	J	J	J	J	J	J
RAM90	17	G+I	J	J	J	J	J	J	J	J	J	J	J	J	J	J	J	J
RAM111	18	G+I	J	J	J	J	J	J	J	J	J	J	J	J	J	J	J	J
RAM118	19	G+I	J	J	J	J	J	J	J	J	J	J	J	J	J	J	J	J
RAM120	20	G+I	J	J	J	J	J	J	J	J	J	J	J	J	J	J	J	J
RAM121	21	G+I	J	J	J	J	J	J	J	J	J	J	J	J	J	J	J	J
RAM131	22	G+I	J	J	J	J	J	J	J	J	J	J	J	J	J	J	J	J
RAM134	23	G+I	J	J	J	J	J	J	J	J	J	J	J	J	J	J	J	J
RAM152	24	G+I	J	J	J	J	J	J	J	J	J	J	J	J	J	J	J	J
RAM163	25	G+I	J	J	J	J	J	J	J	J	J	J	J	J	J	J	J	J
IG10	26	G+I	J	J	–	J	–	–	J	J	J	J	J	J	J	J	J	J
CG14	27	G+I	J	J	J	J	J	–	J	J	J	J	J	J	J	J	J	J
CG17	28	G+I	J	J	J	J	J	J	J	J	J	J	J	J	J	J	J	J
CG20	29	G+I	J	J	J	J	J	J	J	J	J	J	J	J	J	J	J	J
Acc.103477	30	G+I	J	J	J	J	J	J	J	J	J	J	J	J	J	J	J	–
TOG5674	31	G+I	J	J	J	J	J	J	J	J	J	J	J	J	J	J	J	–
TOG5681	32	G+I	J	J	J	J	J	J	J	J	J	J	J	J	J	J	J	–
TOG5860	33	G+I	J	J	J	J	J	J	J	J	J	J	J	J	J	J	J	–
TOG6472	34	G+I	J	J	J	J	J	J	J	J	J	J	J	J	J	J	J	–
TOG6508	35	G+I	J	J	J	J	J	J	J	J	J	J	J	J	J	J	J	–
TOG6589	36	G+I	J	J	–	J	–	J	–	J	J	J	J	J	J	J	–	–
TOG6597	37	–	J	J	J	–	–	–	–	–	–	–	–	–	–	–	–	–
TOG6629	38	–	H	H	J	H	H	H	H	H	–	–	–	H	H	–	H	–
TOG6631	39	G+I	J	J	–	J	J	J	J	J	J	J	J	J	J	J	J	–

Supplementary Table 2. Contd.

		S09000A	S09026B	S09040B	S09058	S09062B	S09065	S09073	S09075A	S09075B	S09093A	S10001	S10003A	S10013A	S10019	S10026C	S10071	S10072	S11004A	S11006A	S11028	S12011B	S12030	S12109B
TOG7235	40	G+I	—	—	J	—	—	—	—	—	—	—	—	—	J	—	J	—	—	—	—	—	—	J
TOG7291	41	G+I	—	—	J	—	—	—	—	—	—	—	—	—	J	—	J	—	—	—	—	—	—	J
TOG7442	42	G+I	—	—	J	—	—	—	—	—	—	—	—	—	J	—	J	—	—	—	—	—	—	J
IR64×RAM54	43	G+I	—	—	H	—	—	—	—	—	—	—	—	H	H	—	H	H	—	—	—	—	—	—
IR64×RAM86	44	G+I	—	—	H	—	—	—	—	—	—	—	—	—	H	—	H	H	—	—	—	—	—	—
IR64×RAM90	45	G+I	—	—	H	—	—	—	—	—	—	—	—	H	H	—	H	H	—	—	—	—	—	—
IR64×RAM120	46	G+I	—	—	H	—	—	—	—	—	—	—	—	—	H	-	H	H	—	—	—	—	—	—
IR64×RAM134	47	G+I	—	—	H	—	—	—	—	—	—	—	—	H	H	—	H	H	—	—	—	—	—	—
IR64×RAM131	48	-	—	—	H	—	—	—	—	—	—	—	—	—	H	—	H	H	—	—	—	—	—	—
PSBRC18×RAM111	49	G+I	—	—	H	—	—	—	—	—	—	—	—	H	H	—	H	H	—	—	—	—	—	—
IR55423-01×RAM3	50	G+I	—	—	H	—	—	—	—	—	—	—	—	H	H	—	H	H	—	—	—	—	—	—
IR55423-01×RAM24	51	G+I	—	—	H	—	—	—	—	—	—	—	—	—	H	—	H	H	—	—	—	—	—	—
IR55423-01×RAM163	52	G+I	—	—	H	—	—	—	—	—	—	—	—	H	H	-	H	H	—	—	—	—	—	—
IR69502×RAM118	53	G+I	G	—	H	—	—	—	—	—	—	—	—	H	H	—	H	H	—	—	—	—	—	—
IR69502×RAM121	54	G+I	G	—	H	—	—	—	—	—	—	—	—	H	H	—	H	H	—	—	—	—	—	—
IR69502×RAM163	55	G+I	G	—	H	—	—	—	—	—	—	—	—	—	H	—	H	H	—	—	—	—	—	—
IR60080-46-A×IG10	56	S	G	G	H	H	H	H	H	H	H	H	H	—	J	H	J	H	H	J	J	G+H	H	J
IR68703-AC-24-1×CG14	57	S	S	S	H	H	H	H	H	H	-	H	H	H	J	-	J	J	J	J	J	G+H	J	J
IR60080-46-A×CG14	58	S	S	S	H	H	H	H	H	H	H	H	H	H	J	H	J	H	H	H	—	G+H	H	J
Specific alleles (Neither I nor J)		G=270,290	Hetero G																					

Supplementary Table 2. Genotyping results with 67 SS-STS markers in this study (continued).

Accession Name	Entry No.	S09000A	S09026B	S09040B	S09058	S09062B	S09065	S09073	S09075A	S09075B	S09093A	S10001	S10003A	S10013A	S10019	S10026C	S10071	S10072	S11004A	S11006A	S11028	S12011B	S12030	S12109B
IR55423-01	1	J	—	J	—	J	—	—	J	—	—	J	—	J	—	J	—	—	—	—	—	J	—	J
IR60080-46-A	2	J	J	J	J	J	J	J	J	J	J	J	J	J	J	J	J	J	J	J	J	J	J	J
IR64	3	—	—	—	—	—	—	—	—	—	—	—	—	—	—	—	—	—	—	—	—	—	—	—
IR68703-AC-24-1	4	J	J	J	J	J	J	J	J	J	J	J	J	J	J	J	J	J	J	J	J	J	J	J
IR69502-6-SRN	5	—	—	—	—	—	—	—	—	—	—	—	—	—	—	—	—	—	—	—	—	—	—	—
PSBRC18	6	—	—	—	—	—	—	—	—	—	—	—	—	—	—	—	—	—	—	—	—	—	—	—

Supplementary Table 2. Genotyping results with 67 SS-STS markers in this study (continued).

No.	Sample
7	BRC82
8	Hwacheongbyeo
9	Ilpumbyeo
10	Jinmibyeo
11	Junambyeo
12	TR22183
13	RAM3
14	RAM24
15	RAM54
16	RAM86
17	RAM90
18	RAM111
19	RAM118
20	RAM120
21	RAM121
22	RAM131
23	RAM134
24	RAM152
25	RAM163
26	IG10
27	CG14
28	CG17
29	CG20
30	Acc.103477
31	TOG5674
32	TOG5681
33	TOG5860
34	TOG6472
35	TOG6508
36	TOG6589
37	TOG6597
38	TOG6629
39	TOG6631
40	TOG7235
41	TOG7291
42	TOG7442
43	IR64×RAM54

Supplementary Table 2. Genotyping results with 67 SS-STS markers in this study (continued).

Crosses	Entry No.																			
IR64×RAM86	44	I	I	H	H	H	H	—	H	—	G+I	H	G+I	H	—	J	H	H	J	G+I	H
IR64×RAM90	45	I	I	H	H	H	H	—	H	—	G+I	H	G+I	H	H	J	H	H	J	G+I	H
IR64×RAM120	46	I	I	H	H	H	H	—	H	—	G+I	H	G+I	H	H	J	H	H	J	G+I	H
IR64×RAM134	47	I	I	H	H	H	H	—	H	—	G+I	H	G+I	H	H	J	H	H	J	G+I	H
IR64×RAM131	48	I	I	H	H	H	H	—	H	—	G+I	H	G+I	H	H	J	H	H	J	G+I	H
PSBRC18×RAM111	49	I	I	H	H	H	H	—	H	—	G+I	H	G+I	H	H	J	H	H	J	G+I	H
IR55423-01×RAM3	50	I	I	H	H	H	H	H	H	—	G+I	H	G+I	H	H	J	H	H	J	G+I	H
IR55423-01×RAM24	51	I	I	H	H	H	H	H	H	—	G+I	H	G+I	H	H	J	H	H	J	G+I	H
IR55423-01×RAM163	52	I	I	H	H	H	H	H	H	—	G+I	H	G+I	H	H	J	H	H	J	G+I	H
IR69502×RAM118	53	I	I	H	H	H	H	H	H	—	G+I	H	G+I	H	H	J	H	H	J	G+I	H
IR69502×RAM121	54	I	I	H	H	H	H	H	H	—	G+I	H	G+I	H	H	J	H	H	J	G+I	H
IR69502×RAM163	55	I	I	H	H	H	H	H	H	—	G+I	H	G+I	H	H	J	H	H	J	G+I	H
IR60080-46-A×IG10	56	I	J	J	J	H	J	H	—	G+J	G+J	H	G+J	G+J	J	J	J	J	J	G+J	J
IR68703-AC-24-1×CG14	57	J	J	J	J	H	J	H	H	G+J	G+J	H	G+J	G+J	J	J	J	J	J	G+J	J
IR60080-46-A×CG14	58	J	H	J	J	H	J	H	—	G+J	G+J	H	G+J	G+J	J	J	J	J	G+J	H	J

Specific alleles
(Neither I nor J) G=240 G=300 G=160 G=610 G=350

*Alleles: I: *indica*; J: *japonica*; H: hetero (I and J); G: *glaberrima*-specific; N: non-amplified allele of *O. glaberrima*; P: TR22183 specific; S: smear bands.

Supplementary Table 3. Allele constitution of parents and F₁ progenies to elucidate useful polymorphic markers in *O. sativa* × *O. glaberrima* breeding programs.

Crosses	Entry No.	Description	S01022	S01054	S01140	S01157B	S01160	S02026	S02052	S02054	S02057B	S02081B	S02085	S02140	S03010B	S03020	S03027	S03041	S03046	S03048	S03096	S03099	S03120	S03136	S03145
Indica × *Glaberrima*																									
	3	IR64	—	—	—	—	G	—	—	—	—	—	G	—	—	—	—	—	—	J	—	—	J	—	G+I
	15	RAM54	—	—	—	—	G+I	—	—	—	—	—	G+I	—	—	—	—	—	—	J	—	—	J	—	G+I
	43	IR64×RAM54	H	H	—	H	G+I	—	—	H	—	H	G+I	—	—	H	—	H	H	H	—	—	H	—	G+I
	3	IR64	—	J	—	J	—	—	—	J	—	J	—	—	—	J	—	J	J	J	—	—	J	—	—
	16	RAM86	—	—	—	—	G	—	—	—	—	—	G	—	—	—	—	—	—	H	—	—	H	—	G+I
	44	IR64×RAM86	H	H	—	H	G	—	—	H	—	H	G	—	—	H	—	H	H	H	—	—	H	—	G+I
	3	IR64	—	J	—	J	—	—	—	J	—	J	—	—	—	J	—	J	J	J	—	—	J	—	—
	17	RAM90	H	H	—	H	G+I	—	—	H	—	H	G+I	—	—	H	—	H	H	H	—	—	H	—	G+I
	45	IR64×RAM90	J	—	H	—	G	—	—	H	—	H	G	—	—	J	—	J	H	—	—	—	—	—	G+I
	3	IR64	—	J	—	J	—	—	—	J	—	J	—	—	—	J	—	J	J	J	—	—	J	—	—
	20	RAM120	J	J	—	J	G	—	—	J	—	J	G	—	—	J	—	J	J	J	—	—	J	—	G+I

Indica × Glaberrima

No.	Name																				
46	IR64×RAM120	I	-	I	H	-	I	J	-	H	J	-	H	J	-	H	-	H	-	-	G+I
3	IR64	-	-	G	J	-	J	J	-	G	J	-	J	J	-	J	-	J	-	-	G+I
23	RAM134	I	-	H	J	-	H	H	-	I	H	-	H	H	-	H	-	H	-	-	G+I
47	IR64×RAM134	J	-	J	-	J	J	-	J	J	-	J	J	-	J	-	J	J	-	J	-
3	IR64	I	-	H	J	-	G	J	-	I	J	-	H	J	-	H	-	H	-	J	G+I
22	RAM131	-	-	G	J	-	G	J	-	G	J	-	G	J	-	G	-	G	-	-	-
48	IR64×RAM131	I	-	H	J	-	G+I	J	-	I	J	-	H	J	-	H	-	H	-	J	G+I
6	PSBRC18	I	-	H	J	-	G	J	-	I	J	-	H	J	-	H	-	H	-	J	G+I
18	RAM111	-	-	G	J	-	G	J	-	G	J	-	G	J	-	G	-	G	-	-	G+I
49	PSBRC18×RAM111	I	-	H	J	-	G+J	J	-	I	J	-	H	J	-	H	-	H	-	J	G+I
1	IR55423-01	I	-	H	-	I	G	J	-	I	J	-	H	-	I	H	-	H	-	J	G+I
13	RAM3	-	-	G	J	-	J	J	-	G	J	-	G	J	-	G	-	G	-	J	G+I
50	IR55423-01×RAM3	I	-	H	J	-	G+J	J	-	I	J	-	H	J	-	H	-	H	-	J	G+I
1	IR55423-01	-	-	G	J	-	J	J	-	G	J	-	G	J	-	G	-	G	-	J	G+I
14	RAM24	I	-	H	J	-	G+J	J	-	I	J	-	H	J	-	H	-	H	-	J	G+I
51	IR55423-01×RAM24	I	-	H	J	-	G+J	J	-	I	J	-	H	J	-	H	-	H	-	J	G+I
52	IR55423-01×RAM163	H	-	H	J	-	G+J	J	-	I	J	-	H	J	-	H	-	H	-	J	G+I
25	RAM163	J	-	G	J	-	G	J	-	J	J	-	J	J	-	J	-	J	-	J	G+I
5	IR69502-6-SRN	H	-	I	J	-	G+I	J	-	H	J	-	H	J	-	H	-	H	-	J	G+I
19	RAM118	J	-	H	J	-	G	J	-	J	J	-	J	J	-	J	-	J	-	J	G+I
53	IR69502×RAM118	H	-	H	J	-	G+I	J	-	H	J	-	H	J	-	H	-	H	-	J	G+I
5	IR69502-6-SRN	J	-	H	J	-	G	J	-	J	J	-	J	J	-	J	-	J	-	J	G+I
21	RAM121	H	-	H	J	-	G	J	-	H	J	-	H	J	-	H	-	H	-	J	G+I
54	IR69502×RAM121	H	-	H	J	-	G+I	J	-	H	J	-	H	J	-	H	-	H	-	J	G+I
5	IR69502-6-SRN	J	-	H	J	-	-	J	-	J	J	-	J	J	-	J	-	J	-	J	G+I
25	RAM163	H	-	H	J	-	G	J	-	H	J	-	H	J	-	H	-	H	-	J	G+I
55	IR69502×RAM163	H	H	H	H	H	G+I	H	I	H	H	H	H	H	H	H	H	H	H	H	G+I

Japonica × Glaberrima

No.	Name																				
2	IR60080-46-A	J	J	J	J	J	G	J	J	J	J	J	J	J	J	J	J	J	J	J	G+I
26	IG10	J	J	J	-	G	J	-	J	J	J	J	J	J	-	H	J	J	J	J	G+I
56	IR60080-46-A×IG10	J	J	J	H	G+I	J	-	J	J	H	J	J	J	H	H	J	H	J	H	S
4	IR68703-AC-24-1	J	J	J	-	J	-	I	J	J	-	J	J	J	-	J	J	-	J	J	J
27	CG14	J	J	J	J	J	G	J	-	J	J	J	J	J	-	J	J	-	J	J	G+I
57	IR68703-AC-24-1×CG14	J	J	J	H	G+J	J	-	J	J	H	J	J	J	H	G+J	J	H	J	J	G+I
2	IR60080-46-A	J	J	J	-	J	J	J	J	J	-	J	J	J	-	J	J	-	J	J	S
27	CG14	J	J	J	J	G	J	J	J	J	J	J	J	J	J	J	J	J	J	J	G+I
58	IR60080-46-A×CG14	J	J	H	-	G	-	J	J	H	-	H	J	G+J	H	H	J	H	J	H	S

Supplementary Table 3. Allele constitution of parents and F_1 progenies to elucidate useful polymorphic markers in *O. sativa* × *O. glaberrima* breeding programs (continued).

Crosses	Entry No.	Description	S04058	S04060	S04077A	S04077B	S04087A	S04097B	S04128	S04129B	S05064	S05080A	S06001	S07011	S07048	S07050C	S07050A	S07101	S07103	S08066	S08090	S08106	S08107	S09000A	S09026B
Indica × Glaberrima	3	IR64	—	—	—	—	—	—	—	—	—	—	H	C	—	—	C	—	C	—	—	C	—	—	C
	15	RAM54	—	H	—	—	—	—	—	—	—	—	—	—	—	—	—	—	—	—	—	—	—	—	—
	43	IR64×RAM54	—	C	—	—	—	—	—	—	—	—	C	H	—	—	H	—	H	—	—	H	—	—	H
	3	IR64	—	—	—	—	—	—	—	—	—	—	—	C	—	—	—	—	C	—	—	C	—	—	C
	16	RAM86	—	H	—	—	—	—	—	—	—	—	—	—	—	—	—	—	—	—	—	—	—	—	—
	44	IR64×RAM86	—	C	—	—	—	—	—	—	—	—	—	H	—	—	—	—	H	—	—	H	—	—	H
	3	IR64	—	—	—	—	—	—	—	—	—	—	—	C	—	—	—	—	C	—	—	C	—	—	C
	17	RAM90	—	H	—	—	—	—	—	—	—	—	—	—	—	—	—	—	—	—	—	—	—	—	—
	45	IR64×RAM90	—	C	—	—	—	—	—	—	—	—	—	H	—	—	—	—	H	—	—	H	—	—	H
	3	IR64	—	—	—	—	—	—	—	—	—	—	—	C	—	—	—	—	C	—	—	C	—	—	C
	20	RAM120	—	H	—	—	—	—	—	—	—	—	—	—	—	—	—	—	—	—	—	—	—	—	—
	46	IR64×RAM120	—	C	—	—	—	—	—	—	—	—	—	H	—	—	—	—	H	—	—	H	—	—	H
	3	IR64	—	—	—	—	—	—	—	—	—	—	—	C	—	—	—	—	C	—	—	C	—	—	C
	23	RAM134	—	H	—	—	—	—	—	—	—	—	—	—	—	—	—	—	—	—	—	—	—	—	—
	47	IR64×RAM134	—	C	—	—	—	—	—	—	—	—	—	H	—	—	—	—	H	—	—	H	—	—	H
	3	IR64	—	—	—	—	—	—	—	—	—	—	H	C	—	—	C	—	C	—	—	C	—	—	C
	22	RAM131	—	H	—	—	—	—	—	—	—	—	—	—	—	—	—	—	—	—	—	—	—	—	—
	48	IR64×RAM131	—	C	—	—	—	—	—	—	—	—	C	H	—	—	H	—	H	—	—	H	—	—	H
	6	PSBRC18	—	—	—	—	—	—	—	—	—	—	H	C	—	—	C	—	C	—	—	C	—	—	C
	18	RAM111	—	H	—	—	—	—	—	—	—	—	—	—	—	—	—	—	—	—	—	—	—	—	—
	49	PSBRC18×RAM111	—	C	—	—	—	—	—	—	—	—	C	H	—	—	H	—	H	—	—	H	—	—	H
	1	IR55423-01	—	—	—	—	—	—	—	—	—	—	H	C	—	—	C	—	C	—	—	C	—	—	C
	13	RAM3	—	H	—	—	—	—	—	—	—	—	—	—	—	—	—	—	—	—	—	—	—	—	—
	50	IR55423-01×RAM3	—	C	—	—	—	—	—	—	—	—	C	H	—	—	H	—	H	—	—	H	—	—	H
	1	IR55423-01	—	—	—	—	—	—	—	—	—	—	H	C	—	—	C	—	C	—	—	C	C	—	C
	14	RAM24	—	H	—	—	—	—	—	—	—	—	—	—	—	—	—	—	—	—	—	—	—	—	—
	51	IR55423-01×RAM24	—	C	—	—	—	—	—	—	—	—	C	H	—	—	H	—	H	—	—	H	H	—	H
	1	IR55423-01	—	—	—	—	—	—	—	—	—	—	H	C	—	—	C	—	C	—	—	C	C	—	C
	25	RAM163	—	H	—	—	—	—	—	—	—	—	—	—	—	—	—	—	—	—	—	—	—	—	—
	52	IR55423-01×RAM163	—	C	—	—	—	—	—	—	—	—	C	H	—	—	H	—	H	—	—	H	H	—	H
	5	IR69502-6-SRN	—	—	—	—	—	—	—	—	—	—	H	C	—	—	C	—	C	—	—	C	C	—	C
	19	RAM118	—	C	—	—	—	—	—	—	—	—	C	—	—	—	—	—	—	—	—	—	—	—	—

Japonica × *Glaberrima*

Entry No.	Description	S09040B	S09058	S09062B	S09065	S09073	S09075A	S09075B	S09093A	S10001	S10003A	S10013A	S10019	S10026C	S10071	S10072	S11004A	S11006A	S11028	S12011B	S12030	S12109B
53	IR69502×RAM118	H	—	H	H	H	H	H	H	H	—	—	J	—	—	H	—	H	J	H	J	H
5	IR69502-6-SRN	—	—	—	—	—	—	—	—	—	—	—	J	—	—	—	—	J	J	I	J	J
21	RAM121	—	J	J	—	J	J	J	J	J	J	J	J	J	—	J	J	J	J	J	J	J
54	IR69502×RAM121	H	—	H	H	H	H	H	—	H	—	H	J	H	H	H	—	H	J	J	J	H
5	IR69502-6-SRN	—	J	—	—	—	—	—	—	—	—	—	J	—	—	J	—	J	J	—	J	—
25	RAM163	—	—	—	—	—	—	—	—	—	—	—	H	—	—	—	—	H	J	H	J	J
55	IR69502×RAM163	H	—	H	H	H	H	H	H	H	—	H	H	H	H	H	—	H	J	—	J	H
2	IR60080-46-A	J	J	J	H	J	J	—	H	J	J	H	H	J	J	J	J	—	J	J	J	H
26	IG10	—	J	J	—	J	J	—	J	—	—	—	J	J	J	J	J	—	J	J	J	J
56	IR60080-46-A×IG10	S	S	H	J	H	H	H	H	H	—	H	J	H	H	—	J	—	J	G+H	J	—
4	IR68703-AC-24-1	J	J	J	J	J	J	J	—	J	J	J	J	J	J	J	J	J	J	J	J	J
27	CG14	—	H	H	H	H	H	—	H	H	—	H	H	H	H	H	H	—	J	G+H	J	J
57	IR68703-AC-24-1×CG14	S	S	J	J	J	J	J	—	J	—	J	J	J	J	J	J	—	J	G+H	J	J
2	IR60080-46-A	—	J	J	J	J	J	J	J	J	J	J	J	J	J	J	J	—	J	J	J	J
58	IR60080-46-A×CG14	S	H	H	H	H	H	H	H	H	—	—	J	H	H	J	J	H	J	G+H	J	H
27	CG14	—	J	J	H	J	J	—	H	J	J	H	H	J	J	J	J	—	J	—	J	H

Crosses

Entry No.	Description	S09040B	S09058	S09062B	S09065	S09073	S09075A	S09075B	S09093A	S10001	S10003A	S10013A	S10019	S10026C	S10071	S10072	S11004A	S11006A	S11028	S12011B	S12030	S12109B
3	IR64	—	—	H	—	H	H	H	—	—	—	G+I	—	H	—	H	G	H	—	G	—	J
15	RAM54	—	—	—	—	—	—	—	—	—	G+I	G+I	—	J	—	J	G+I	H	—	G+I	—	—
43	IR64×RAM54	H	—	H	—	H	H	H	G	—	G	G	—	H	H	H	G	H	—	G	—	H
3	IR64	—	—	—	—	—	—	—	—	—	G	G	—	J	J	J	G	J	—	G	—	J
16	RAM86	J	—	J	—	J	J	J	G	—	G	G	—	H	J	J	G	H	—	G	—	—
44	IR64×RAM86	J	—	H	—	H	H	H	—	—	G+I	G+I	—	H	H	H	G+I	H	—	G+I	—	H
3	IR64	H	—	—	—	J	J	J	G	—	G	G	—	J	J	J	G	J	—	G	—	J
17	RAM90	J	—	H	—	H	H	H	—	—	G+I	G+I	—	J	J	H	G	H	—	G	—	H
45	IR64×RAM90	J	—	—	—	J	J	J	—	—	G+I	G+I	—	H	J	J	G+I	H	—	G+I	—	J
3	IR64	H	—	H	—	H	H	H	—	—	G	G	—	J	J	J	G	J	—	G	—	—
20	RAM120	J	—	—	—	J	J	J	G	—	G	—	—	J	J	J	G	J	—	G	—	J

indica×glaberrima

indica×glaberrima

No.	Cross															
46	IR64×RAM120	—	H	H	J	J	H	—	J	—	G+I	—	G+I	G	—	H	J
3	IR64	H	—	H	J	J	—	—	—	—	—	—	—	J	H	J	H
23	RAM134	—	J	H	J	J	H	G	—	G	—	G	—	H	J	G	J
47	IR64×RAM134	J	—	H	J	J	—	—	J	—	G+I	—	G+I	J	J	J	—
3	IR64	H	—	H	J	J	H	G	—	G	—	G	—	H	H	G	J
22	RAM131	—	J	H	J	J	J	—	J	—	G+I	—	G+I	J	J	J	J
48	IR64×RAM131	J	—	H	J	J	—	G	—	G	—	G	—	H	J	G	—
6	PSBRC18	H	—	H	J	J	H	—	J	—	G+I	—	G+I	H	J	—	H
18	PSBRC18	—	H	H	J	J	J	G	—	G	—	G	—	J	J	G	J
49	RAM111	J	—	H	H	H	—	—	J	—	G+I	—	G+I	H	H	J	—
1	PSBRC18×RAM111	H	—	H	J	J	H	G	—	G	—	G	—	H	J	G	H
13	RAM3	—	H	H	J	J	J	—	J	—	G+I	—	G+I	J	J	J	J
50	IR55423-01×RAM3	J	—	H	J	J	—	G	—	G	—	G	—	H	J	G	—
1	IR55423-01	H	—	H	J	J	H	—	J	—	G+I	—	G+I	H	J	J	H
14	RAM24	—	H	H	J	J	J	G	—	G	—	G	—	J	J	G	J
51	IR55423-01×RAM24	J	—	H	J	J	—	—	J	—	G+I	—	G+I	H	H	J	—
1	IR55423-01	H	—	H	J	J	H	G	—	G	—	G	—	H	J	G	H
52	IR55423-01×RAM163	—	H	H	J	J	J	—	J	—	G+I	—	G+I	J	J	J	J
25	RAM163	J	—	H	J	J	—	G	—	G	—	G	—	H	—	G	—
5	IR69502-6-SRN	H	—	H	J	J	H	—	J	—	G+I	—	G+I	H	H	J	H
54	IR69502×RAM121	—	H	H	J	J	J	G	—	G	—	G+I	—	J	J	G	J
21	RAM121	J	—	H	J	J	—	—	J	—	G+I	—	G+I	H	J	J	—
5	IR69502-6-SRN	H	—	H	J	J	H	G	—	G	—	G	—	H	J	G	H
53	IR69502×RAM118	—	H	H	J	J	J	G+J	—	G+I	—	G+I	—	J	J	G+J	J
19	RAM118	J	—	H	J	J	—	—	J	—	G+I	—	G+I	H	H	J	—
5	IR69502-6-SRN	H	—	H	J	J	H	G	—	G	—	G	—	H	J	G	H
55	IR69502×RAM163	H	—	H	J	J	H	—	J	—	G+I	—	G+I	H	J	G+I	J
25	RAM163	J	—	H	J	J	—	G	—	G	—	G	—	J	J	G	J

Japonica × Glaberrima

No.	Cross															
2	IR60080-46-A	J	J	J	J	J	J	G	J	G	J	G	J	J	J	G	J
26	IG10	J	—	—	J	J	J	—	—	—	—	—	—	J	J	—	J
56	IR60080-46-A×IG10	J	—	J	J	J	J	G+J	G+I	G	G+J	—	G+J	J	—	G+J	J
4	IR68703-AC-24-1	J	—	J	J	J	J	J	J	J	J	J	J	J	—	J	J
27	CG14	J	J	J	J	J	J	G	G	G	G	G	G	J	J	G	J
57	IR68703-AC-24-1×CG14	J	H	H	J	J	J	G+J	H	G+I	G+I	G+J	G+J	H	H	G+J	J
2	IR60080-46-A	J	—	—	J	J	J	—	—	J	—	J	J	—	J	—	J
27	CG14	J	J	J	J	J	J	G	J	G	J	G	J	J	J	G	J
58	IR60080-46-A×CG14	H	H	H	J	J	H	G+J	—	G+J	G+J	G+J	G+J	H	J	G+J	H

markers to determine relations within the AA genome species is well documented. Robeniol et al. (1996) using only 14 STS markers accurately determined the genome composition of O. *meridionalis as* an AA genome species and most distantly related specie to O. *sativa*, and O. *longistaminata* the second most distantly related.

The SS markers which detected *glaberrima*-specific alleles suggest that loci adjacent to these markers could be a key for interspecific hybrid sterility. It may be interesting to compare these SS markers with other alleles of other wild rice species. The detection of heterozygous alleles between *japonica/glaberrima* and between *indica/glaberrima* in the F1s, suggest caution when applying some SS markers to other rice species and implying their distinguished association to O. *glaberrima* genome. Only 40 (59.7%) of the SS markers might be useful in the O. *glaberrima* analysis, as other markers did not detect any amplification of heterozygous alleles in F₁ progenies between O.*sativa* × O. *glaberrima*. This might be due to minute genomic differences between O.*sativa* and O. *glaberrima (*Ohmido and Fukui, 1995; Park et al., 2003*).* Also, some markers did not generate heterozygous allele in the F₁'s, suggesting that those loci are unique in O.*sativa* or O. *glaberrima* (S01160, S02052, S03099, S07048, S07050C, S08090, S08107, S09000A and S09058). Minor difference in the sequence of some markers might have affected the recombination in PCR amplicon region of some markers such as S02054, S02081, S04060, and S08106), and are allelic-specific (S03020 and S03046). Some small cryptic changes and mutations in PCR amplification region of some markers might have caused some markers not align well during PCR amplification, that is, S03048.

O. *glaberrima* had *indica* alleles at two loci associated with intersubspecific F₁ hybrid sterility on chromosome 5 and chromosome 8. Interspecific hybrids (F₁'s) between O.*sativa* and O. *glaberrima* are almost completely sterile. This hybrid sterility barrier is mainly caused by an arrest of pollen development at the microspore stage (Heuer et al., 2003; Peltier, 1953). Intersubspecific F₁ hybrid sterility is mainly caused by cryptic chromosomal aberrations and allelic interaction between *indica* and *japonica* (Chin et al., 2007). The SS (subspecies-specific) STS marker were able to classify the O. *glaberrima accessions* into 10 sub-groups. Subspecies-prototype index (SPI) of O. *glaberrima* accessions ranged from 51.67 to 60.00, suggesting intermediate subspecific type based on whole-genome.

Comparative view of genome of O. *glaberrima* based on O. *sativa* spp. *japonica* genome

A total of 23 and 22 loci showed only *indica* and *japonicas* alleles respectively whilst 4 loci showed both *indica* and *japonica* alleles. Some non-sativa alleles which were detected on chromosomes 1, 2, 3, 9, 10, 11, and 12 might be O. *glaberrima* specific alleles (Figure 3),

The heterozygous alleles of indica and O. *glaberrima* (G+I) identified on 3 loci on chromosomes 1, 2 and 3, suggests that non-sativa regions might be located on aligned BAC clones of O. *glaberrima*. This information can be useful in further studies involving the F₁ hybrid sterility between O.*sativa* and O. *glaberrima*.

Conclusion

The informative markers identified in this study might be very useful in studying the diversification of O. *glaberrima*; Loci adjacent to the SS markers which detected *glaberrima*-specific alleles could be a key for interspecific hybrid sterility between O. *sativa* × O. *glaberrima*. The detection of heterozygous alleles between *japonica* and *glaberrima* and between *indica* and *glaberrima* by some SS markers suggest that caution must be taken when applying some SS markers to other rice species and implying their distinguished association to O. *glaberrima* genome.

ACKNOWLEDGEMENT

Isaac Kofi Bimpong and Joong Hyoun Chin contributed equally to the research.

REFERENCES

Barry MB, Pham JL, Noyer JL, Billot C, Courtois B, Ahmadi N (2007). Genetic diversity of the two cultivated rice species (O. sativa & O. glaberrima) in Maritime Guinea. Evidence for interspecific recombination. Euphytica, 154: 127-137.

Bi XZ, Xiao YH, Liu WF (1997). Studies on subspecies differentiating protein markers in Oryza sativa by two-dimensional polyacrylamide gel electrophoresis. Rice Genetics Newsletter, 14: 31-33.

Bimpong IK, Mendoza EMT, Hernandez JE, Mendioro MS, Brar DS (2009). Identification and Mapping of QTLs for Drought Tolerance Introgressed from Oryza glaberrima Steud. into Indica Rice (Oryza. sativa L). PhD thesis submitted to the University of the Philippines. Los Banos Philippines.

Bimpong IK, Carpena AL, Borromeo TH, Mendioro MS, Brar DS (2004). Nematode resistance of backcross derivatives of Oryza sativa L crosses with Oryza glaberrima Steud. and molecular characterization of introgression. Thesis submitted to the University of the Philippines. Los Banos Philippines

Cause MA, Fulto TM, Cho YG, Ahn SN, Chuncongse J (1994). Saturated molecular map of the rice genome based on an interspecific backcross population. Genet. 138: 1251–1274.

Chin JH, Kim JH, Jiang W, Chu SH, Woo MO, Han L, Brar D, Koh HJ (2007). Identification of Subspecies-specific STS Markers and Their Association with Segregation Distortion in Rice (Oryza sativa L.) J. Crop Sci. Biotech. 10(3): 175-184

Chin JH, Kim JH, Kwon SW, Cho YI, Piao ZZ, Han LZ, Koh HJ (2003). Identification of subspecies-specific RAPD markers in rice. Korean J. Breed., 35(2): 102-108

Cho YC, Shin YS, Ahn SN, Gregorio GB, Kang KH, Brar D, Moon HP (1999). DNA fingerprinting of rice cultivars using AFLP and RAPD markers. Korean J. Crop Sci., 44(1): 26-31.

Enriquez EC, Rosario TL, Brar DS, Mendioro MS, Hernandez JE, Barrion AA (2001). Production of doubled haploids from Oryza sativa L. × O. glaberrima Steud. and their characterization using microsatellite markers. PhD thesis submitted to the University of the Philippines. Los Banos Philippines.

Feltus FA, Wan J, Schulze SR, Estill JC, Jiang N, Paterson AH (2004).

An SNP resource for rice genetics and breeding based on subspecies *indica* and *japonica* genome alignments. Genome Res., 14: 1812-1819.

Glaszmann JC (1987). Isozymes and classification of Asian rice varieties. Theor. Appl. Genet., 74: 21–30.

Heuer SM, Meizan KM (2003). Assessing hybrid sterility in *O. glaberrima x O. sativa* hybrid progenies by PCR marker analysis and crossing with wide compatibility varieties. Theory Appl. Genet., 107: 902–909.

Kitampura E (1962). Studies on cytoplasmic sterility of hybrids in distantly related varieties of rice *O. sativa* L. In Fertility of F1 hybrids between strains derived from certain Philippine and Japanese variety crosses and Japanese varieties. Jpn. J. Breed., 12: 81–84.

Koide Y, Onishi K, Kanazawa A, Sano Y (2008). Genetics of speciation in rice. In Rice Biology in the Genomics Era. Edited by Hirano H, Sano Y, Hirai A, Sasaki T. Biotechnol. Agric. For. Springer-Verlag. pp: 247-259.

Kubo T, Yoshimura A (2005). Epistasis underlying female sterility detected in hybrid breakdown in a *japonica-indica* cross of rice (*Oryza sativa* L.). Theor. Appl. Genet., 110: 346-355.

Li J, Xu P, Deng X, Zhou J, Hu F, Wan J, Tao D (2008). Identifcation of four genes for stable hybrid sterility and an epistatic QTL from a cross between *Oryza sativa* and *Oryza glaberrima*. Euphytica., 164: 699–708.

Lorieux M, Ndjionjop N, Ghesquire A (2000). A first interspecific *Oryza sativa* × *Oryza glaberrima* microsatellite-based genetic linkage map. Theor. Appl. Genet., 100: 593-601.

McCouch SR, Teytelman L, Xu Y, Lobos KB, Clare K, Walton M, Fu B, Maghirang R, Li, Z, Xing Y, Zhang Q, Kono I, Yano M, Fjellstrom R, DeClerck G, Schneider D, Cartinhour S, Ware D, Stein L (2002). Dvelopment and mapping of 2240 new SSR markers for rice (*Oryza sativa* L.). DNA Res., 9: 199-207.

McNally K, Childs KL, Bohnert R, Davidson RM, Zhao K, Ulat VJ, Zeller G, Clark RM, Hoen DR, Bureau TE, Stokowski R, Ballinger DG, Frazer KA, Cox DR, Padhukasahasram B, Bustamante CD, Weigel D, Mackill DJ, Bruskiewich RM, Ra tsch G, Buell CR, Leung H, Leach JE (2009). Genomewide SNP reveals relationships among landraces and modern varieties of rice. PNAS. 106(30): 12273-12278.

Ohmido N, Fukui K (1995). Cytological studies of African cultivated rice. *Oryza glaberrima*. Theor. Appl. Genet., 91: 212–217.

Park KC, Kim NH, Cho YS, Kang KH, Lee JK, Kim NS (2003). Genetic variations of AA genome *Oryza* species measured by MITE–AFLP. Theor. Appl. Genet., 107: 203–209.

Perry DJ, Isabela N, Bousquet J, (1999). Sequence-tagged-site (STS) markers of arbitrary genes: the amount and nature of variation revealed in Norway spruce. Heredity, 83: 239-248.

Ni J, Colowit PM, Mackill DJ (2002). Evaluation of genetic diversity in rice subspecies using microsatellite markers. Crop Sci. 42: 601-607.

Neiman M, Linksvayer TA (2006). The conversion of variance and the evolutionary potential of restricted recombination. Heredity, 96: 111-121.

Porteres R (1956). Taxonomie agrobotanique des riz cultives *O. sativa* L. et *O. glaberrima*. S. J. Agric. Trop. Bot. Appl., 3: 341–384, 541–580, 627–700, 821–856

Panaud O, Chen X, MCcouch SR (1996). Development of microsatellite markers and characterization of simple sequence length polymorphism (SSLP) in rice (*Oryza sativa* L.). Mol. Gen. Genet., 252: 597–607.

Pham J, Bougerol B (1993). Abnormal segregation in crosses between two cultivated rice species. Heredity, 70: 447–466.

Qian HR, Zhuang JY, Lin HX, Lu J, Zheng KL (1995). Identification of a set of RFLP probes for subspecies differentiation in *Oryza sativa* L. Theor. Appl. Genet., 90: 878-884.

Ren F, Lu BR, Li S, Huang J, Ying G (2003). Theor. Appl. Genet. 108(1): 113-120.

Robeniol JA, Constantino SV, Resurreccion AP, Villareal CP, Ghareyazie B, Lu BR, Katiyar SK, Menguito CA, Angeles ER, Fu H, Reddy YS, Park W, McCouch SR, Khush GS, Bennett J (1996). Sequence-tagged sites and low-cost DNA markers for rice. : [IRRI] International Rice Research Institute. 1996. Rice genetics III. Proc. 3rd International Rice Genetics Symposium, 16-20 Oct 1995. Manila (Philippines).

Sarla AN, Mallikarjuna SPB (2005). *Oryza glaberrima*: A source for the improvement of *Oryza sativa*. Cur. Sci., 89: 955-963.

Semon M, Nielsen R, Jones MP, MCcouch SR (2005). The population structure of African cultivated rice *Oryza glaberrima* (Steud.): Evidence for elevated levels of linkage disequilibrium caused by admixture with *O. sativa* and ecological adaptation. Genet. 169: 1639–1647.

Sun CQ, Wang XK, Yoshimura A, Doi K (2002). Genetic differentiation for nuclear, mitochondrial and chloroplast genomes in common wild rice (*Oryza rufipogon* Griff.) and cultivated rice (*Oryza sativa* L.). Theor. Appl. Genet. 104: 1335-1345.

Tanksley SD, Genal MW, Prince JP, de Vicente MC, Bonierbale MW, Broun P, Fulton TM, Giovannoni JJ, Grandillo S, Martin GB, Messeguer R, Miller JC, Miller L, Paterson AH, Pineda O, Roder MS, Wing RA, Wu W, Young ND (1992). High density molecular linkage maps of the tomato and potato genomes. Genet. 132: 1141-1160.

Temnykh S, Park WD, Ayres N, Cartinhour S, Hauck N, Lipovtiesich L, Cho YG, Ishii T, McCouch SR (2000). Mapping and genome organization of microsatellite sequences in rice (*Oryza sativae*).Theor. Appl. Genet. 100: 697–712.

Vaughan DA.(2003). Genepools in the genus Oryza. In: Nanda JS, Sharma SD, editors. Monograph on the genus *Oryza*. Enfield, N.H. (USA): Science Publishers, Inc. pp: 113-138.

Wang CM, Li LH, Zhang XT, Gao Q, Wang RF, An DG (2009). Development and Application of EST-STS Markers Specific to Chromosome 1RS of *Secale cereal*. Cereal Res. Comm., 37(1): 13–21.

Wang RRC, Li X, Chatterton J (2001). A proposed mechanism for loss of heterozygosity in rice hybrids. Euphytica, 118: 119-126.

10

Chemical fractionation and heavy metal accumulation in maize (*Zea mays*) grown on chromated copper arsenate (CCA) contaminated soil amended with cow dung manure

S. O. P. Urunmatsoma*, E. U. Ikhuoria and F. E. Okieimen

Department of Chemistry, Geochemical Research Laboratory, University of Benin, Benin City, Nigeria.

Cow dung used as soil amendments and a sequential chemical speciation (six steps) procedure were used to predict the uptake of Cr, Cu and As by maize (*Zea mays*) plant in chromated copper arsenate (CCA) contaminated soil. A pot experiment containing the contaminated soil samples with different percentage levels of amendments and control (no amendment) was set up. The relative concentrations of the metals in the CCA contaminated soil were established as Cr 265.84 mg/kg, Cu 155.82 mg/kg and As 33.09 mg/kg. However, with the use of speciation and calculations based on mobility factor (M_f), the relative toxicity of the metals in the soil was established as As (60%) > Cr (19%) > Cu (8%). The amendment, rich in organic matter raised the pH level of the soil, demobilized the metals rendering them unavailable through bounding resulting into relatively lower uptake by plants in soils with amendment when compared with plants in the control pots.

Key words: Chromated copper arsenate CCA contaminated soil, amendment, copper, maize (*Zea mays*).

INTRODUCTION

The air we breathe, the water we drink, and the soil we rely on to grow plants for food are all being contaminated as a direct result of human activities. Metal-rich mine tailings, metal smelting, electroplating, gas exhausts, energy and fuel production, downwash from power lines, intensive agriculture, and sludge dumping are the most important human activities that contaminate soils with large quantities of toxic metals (Seward et al., 1990). Soil may also be contaminated by heavy metals such as arsenic, chromium, copper, lead and zinc due to improper waste disposal practices, and spillage of chemicals such as wood preserving agents and petroleum products (USEAP, 1997; Sun et al., 2001., Peters, 1991).

Maize (*Zea mays*) native to tropical America is widely grown in Nigeria. It is a shallow rooted plant and possesses prop roots above the ground and fibrous roots underground. Maize may be classified into the followings:

1. Sweet maize (*Z. mays sacharata*). The grains are soft and sweet; contains more of sugar with little starch.
2. Flint maize (*Z. mays indurate*). The grains consist of hard starch; used for making flour.
3. Dent maize (*Z. mays indentata*). Used for making flour.

Maize is harvested green 12 - 14 weeks after planting or dry after 15 - 17 weeks. It can be eaten boiled, roasted or used as pap. Flour can be obtained from maize grains and it can be used for alcoholic drinks. The yield of maize seed in Nigeria is 4.5 tons/ha for hybrid maize (Ekohwo, 2007).

Phytoremediation is a method that utilizes plants to clean up pollutants in soil, water and air. An estimated 350 species of plants naturally take up toxic materials. Sunflower plants have been found to effectively remove radioactive cesium and strontium from ponds at the Chernobyl nuclear power plant in Ukraine and water hyacinth has been used to remove arsenic from water supplies in Bangladesh, India (William and Michael, 2009). Because high concentrations of pollutants often kill most plants, phytoremediation tends to work best at

*Corresponding author. E-mail: sunnyrunmatsoma@yahoo.com.

low pollutant concentrations. The basis of phytorem-ediation is pollutant uptake or bounding by plants. A phytoremediation of metal contaminated soil encom-passes two different stratifies; phytostabilization and phytoextraction (Cunningham et al., 1995; Salt et al., 1998).

In earlier times, the energy used in the farm is derived from man through the use of human muscles. Later, animal power was employed. Animals, mostly pair of work bulls are used for tilling of grounds (Ekohwo, 2007). Another major benefit derived by farmers from this method is the fertilization of the farm from the animal's wastes. These wastes go a long way to improve the physical condition of the soil and supplies N-P-K and other nutrients to plants. The water holding capacity of the soil is also greatly increased. This old method of using animal waste is still employed today through the use of amendment.

Amendment or fertilization also called nutrient enrich-ment is a phytoremediation approach. This approach in which fertilizers are added to a contaminated soil to stimulate the growth of microorganisms that can degrade pollutants helps to sustain the life of the plant through nutrient enrichment of the soil, protection or curing of the plants against the toxic nature of pollutants. Also by adding amendment to the soil, microorganism replicates, increase in number, and grow rapidly and thus increase the rate of biodegradation of the pollutants (William and Michael, 2009). Some of the products of biodegradation are useful plant nutrient and organic matter. Thus the level of pollutant toxicity is reduced. Organic fertilizers do not destroy beneficial microorganisms and earthworms.

Composting, a natural biological process is the controlled decay of organic matter in a warm moist environment by the action of bacteria, fungi and other organisms (Salvator and Sabee, 1995). The process can either be anaerobic or aerobic. Organic waste materials mainly of animal and plant origin are potential sources of organic matter and plant nutrient (Adeniran et al., 2003). Processing of organic waste by compost provide an opportunity to reduce bulk and oduor while increasing the nutritive values of the materials. Using compost as an organic soil amendment stimulates microorganisms to take nitrogen from the air and fix it in the soil where plants can use it. Also a plant rich in decomposing organic matter provides a much higher level of CO_2 in the air just above the soil for the plant use.

The aim of this work is to study the efficiency and effectiveness of cow dung manure as a soil amendment in the phytoremediation of CCA contaminated soil.

MATERIALS AND METHODS

Study site

Our study site is the premises of Bendel Wood Factory, Benin City, Edo State, Nigeria. The factory is located along Ekenwan road in Benin City and was established in 1963. Their main function is the treatment of wood used as poles for distributing electricity. The main chemical used by the factory is chromated copper arsenate (CCA).

Sampling

Soil

Five soil samples were collected from areas of known contamination (Uwumarongie et al., 2008) in the premises of Bendel Wood Factory, Benin City, Edo state, Nigeria. Plastic spade was used to collect soil from a depth not deeper than topsoil (0 – 15 cm) into polythene bags. A composite of all the samples was made, thoroughly mixed in a large polythene spread. It was then taken to the laboratory in two polythene bags. A laboratory sample of 20 g was taken from the composite sample, air dried, and crushed to pass through a 2 mm sieve and stored in a polythene bag. This was used for the various analyses.

Cow dung

The cow dung manure was collected with a plastic spade into a plastic bucket from a pen at Kwale, Delta State, Nigeria. All non compostable materials in the waste were sorted out and thrown away and not included in the compost preparation. Slurry of the cow dung was made by adding enough water into it, and properly stirred with hand using hand gloves. It was then spread out in a large polythene sheet in an aerated shade, occasionally turned and allowed to dry. A powder of the dry cake was made and stored in a polythene bag and used for the experiment. Strictly ambient condition was used for the compost.

Maize grain

The maize grain used for the study was obtained from Edo State Ministry of Agriculture, Sapele Road, Benin City.

Pot experiment/germination studies

2 kg of CCA polluted soil containing 2, 5, 10 and 20% of cow dung amendment were placed in plastic pots. Mixed thoroughly, watered and left for 2 weeks to stabilize before maize was planted. Control was set up without amendment. Maize seedlings (Zea mays) were soaked in water for 5 h and the viable ones are sown in the plastic pots. Maintenance was carried out by watering using tap water when necessary.

Total concentration of As, Cr and Cu in CCA contaminated soil

5 ml of aqua regia and 1 ml of perchloric acid were added to 1 g of soil sample in a 150 ml digestion tube and digested on a heating digester until white fumes of perchloric acid appeared. The tube was cooled and the sides rinsed with distilled water and then filtered through a Whatman 1 filter paper into a 100 ml volumetric flask. The volume was made up with distilled water (Tessier et al., 1979). The concentrations of the heavy metals in the various extracts were determined in a pre-calibrated AAS.

Sequential chemical speciation (Salbu and Oughton, 1998)

The extraction scheme used here is based on six operationally defined fractions (Salbu and Oughton, 1998). It is a modification of sequential extraction procedure (Tessier et al., 1979). 2 g of the prepared soil sample was weighed and placed in a 100 ml polypropylene bottle. The sequential extractions were made into six various fractions as shown below.

Soluble fractions

20 ml of distilled water was added to the soil sample in the polypropylene bottle and the mixture was shaken for 1 h. The mixture was then centrifuged at 1500 rpm for 15 min. The supernatant was filtered into a polypropylene bottle for metal analysis, while the residue was used for the next extraction below.

Exchangeable fractions

20 M of 1 ml NH_4OA_C was added to the residue obtained from the soluble fractions obtained above and the pH adjusted to 7 with ammonium hydroxide solution and agitated for 2 h. The mixture was then centrifuged at 1500 rpm for 15 min. The supernatant was filtered into a polypropylene bottle for metal analysis, while the residue was used for the next extraction.

Carbonate-bound fractions

20 ml of 1 M NH_4OA_C was added to the residue obtained from the exchangeable fractions obtained above and adjusted to pH 5 with concentrated acetic acid and agitated for 2 h. The mixture was then centrifuged at 1500 rpm for 15 min. The supernatant was filtered into a polypropylene bottle for metal analysis, while the residue was used for the next extraction.

Fe-Mn oxides bound fractions

20 ml of 0.04 M $NH_2OH.HCl$ in 25% HOA_C was added to the residue obtained from the carbonate bound fraction obtained above and placed in a water bath for 6 h at 60 °C. The mixture was brought out and centrifuged at 1500 rpm for 15 min. The supernatant was filtered into a polypropylene bottle for metal analysis, while the residue was used for the next extraction.

Organically bound fractions

15 ml of 30% H_2O_2 adjusted with HNO_3 to pH 2 was added to the residue obtained from the step above and heated for 5.5 h in a water bath at 80 °C. After cooling, 5 ml of 3.2 MNH_4OAC in 20% HNO_3 was added; sample was shaken for 30 min and finally diluted to 20 ml with distilled water. The mixture was centrifuged at 1500 rpm for 15 min. The supernatant was filtered into a polypropylene bottle for metal analysis, while the residue was used for the last stage.

Residual fraction

5 ml of nitric acid and 1 ml of perchloric acid were added to 1 g of residue obtained from the step above in a conical flask and heated on a hot plate at 60 °C for 6 h. After evaporation, 1 ml of 2 M HNO_3 was added and the residue after dissolution was filtered through Whatman No 1 filter paper and into a 100 ml volumetric flask and diluted with distilled water to the mark.

Note: All the solid phases were washed with 10 ml distilled water before the next extraction step. The washings were filtered with Whatman No 1 filter paper and added to the previous supernatant fraction and analyzed.

Uptake of As, Cr and Cu by maize

Plants were uprooted 20 days after germination, rinsed with deionized water, cut into pieces, dried for two days at 80 °C. It was then ashed in a Muffle furnace at 500 °C for 6 h. The ash was dissolved in 20% nitric acid. The concentrations (mg/Kg) of the metals in the dry weight of plant samples were determined by AAS Bulk Scientific VGP 210.

RESULT AND DISCUSSION

Table 1 shows the physicochemical properties of the soils (control and soil with different percentage level of amendment). The pH and organic carbon increased with the level of amendment. The   use of amendment especially at 20% level raised the pH level of the soil sample from 6.20 to 6.60. It was established that near neutral pH generally results in micronutrient cations to be soluble enough to satisfy plant needs without becoming soluble enough as to be toxic (Nyle and Ray, 2005). The increase in pH brought about by the amendment helps to bound the metals. The nutrient content of the soil increased if values at control are compared with 20% amendment (Ca: 5.68 to6.09, K: 0.57 to 068P: 44.74 to 908.74, N: 0.34to 0.45)

Table 2 shows the total concentration of the metals in the soil as compared with their intervention values. Though total metal concentration do not necessarily correspond with metal availability and mobility, nations and corporate bodies around the world have placed standards for target and intervention levels based on total concentrations. Intervention values indicate that remediation action should be triggered, if soil metal concentration exceeds limit specified. From the values, it is clear that the soil is polluted with regard to the three metals under study as the concentration for chromium, copper, and arsenic are all higher than their intervention values. The equation shown below was used to calculate the intervention value for the soil (Department of Petroleum Resources guideline, Lagos, 1991).

$$Ic = \frac{Ist \times A + B \times \% CLAY + C \times \% OM}{A + B \times 25 + C \times 10} \qquad (1)$$

Where:
Ic = Intervention value applying for the soil being evaluated in mg/kg, Ist = Intervention value for standard soil [55mg/kg for As, 380 mg/kg for Cr and 190 mg/kg for Cu], %Clay = measured % clay in the soil being evaluated = 24.80% (Table 1), % Organic matter (OM) = Measured % organic matter in the soil being evaluated = 2.18% (Table 1), A, B and C = Constants which depends on the substances, As, A = 15, B = 0.4 and C 0.4, Cr, A = 50, B = 2 and C = 0.0, Cu, A = 15, B = 0.6 and C = 0.6.

Table 1. Physicochemical properties of the soils.

Parameter	Control (no amendment)	2% amendment	5% amendment	10% amendment	20% amendment
pH	6.20 ± 0.40	6.43 ± 0.80	6.48 ± 0.1.20	6.57 ± 1.10	6.60 ± 1.10
OC%	1.26 ± 0.50	1.60 ± 0.70	2.12 ± 0.00	3.90 ± 0.90	5.70 ± 1.00
OM%	2.18 ± 0.50	2.77 ± 0.70	3.67 ± 0.00	6.75 ± 0.90	9.86 ± 1.00
Calcium(Meq/100g)	5.68 ± 0.40	5.72 ± 1.60	5.77 ± 1.30	5.86 ± 1.00	6.09 ± 1.70
Magnesium (Meq/100g)	1.96 ± 0.30	1.96 ± 0.60	1.99 ± 0.40	2.05 ± 1.00	2.17 ± 1.00
Sodium (Meq/100g)	0.19 ± 0.10	0.20 ± 0.00	0.22 ± 0.10	0.25 ± 0.00	0.31 ± 0.12
Potassium (Meq/100g)	0.57 ± 0.10	0.58 ± 0.20	0.60 ± 0.10	0.63 ± 0.20	0.68 ± 0.20
CEC (Meq/100g)	8.40 ± 0.20	8.46 ± 1.20	8.58 ± 0.60	8.79 ± 0.50	9.25 ± 0.90
Phosphorus (mg/Kg)	44.74 ± 3.73	131.14 ± 27.00	260.74 ± 41.00	476.74 ± 30.00	908.74 ± 42.00
Nitrogen %	0.34 ± 0.08	0.35 ± 0.14	0.37 ± 0.10	0.40 ± 0.16	0.45 ± 0.20
Clay %	24.80				
Silt %	2.10				
Sand %	73.10				

OC = Organic carbon; OM = Organic matter; CEC = Cations exchange capacity.

Table 2. Total concentration of the metals in soil sample/intervention values set by DPR

Metals	Total concentration (mg/Kg)	Intervention values (mg/Kg)
Chromium	265.84 ± 33.0	190.52
Copper	155.82 ± 12.98	79.61
Arsenic	32.09 ± 2.48	28.82

Table 3. Extractants used in a six step sequential speciation (Salbu and Oughton, 1998). A modified method Tessier et al. (91979).

Step	Soil phase	Extractant	Agitation time
1	Soluble fractions	20 ml distilled water	1 h 20 °C
2	Exchangeable	20 ml NH$_4$OAc (pH 7)	2 h
3	Carbonate-bound	20 ml NH$_4$OAc (pH5)	2 h
4	Fe-Mn oxide bound	20 ml NH$_2$OH. HCl	6 h at 60°C
		15 ml of 30% H$_2$O$_2$ (pH 2 HNO$_3$)	
		After cooling,	5.5 h at 80° C
5	Organic bound	5 ml^3.2MNH4OAci	
		In 20% HNO$_3$	30 min
		Then dilute 20 ml with water	
6	Residual	5 ml HNO$_3$+1 ml HClO	6 h
		After cooling + 2 M HNO$_3$	

To calculate the intervention value for arsenic metal the figures should be computed as follows:

$$Ic = \frac{55 \times 15 + 0.4 \times 24.80 + 0.4 \times 2.18}{15 + 0.4 \times 25 + 0.4 \times 10}$$

From equation (1)

When the above calculation is resolved, it gives a value of 28.82 mg/kg

Total concentration helps to estimate the effects and potential risks associated with elevated elemental concentrations. The concentrations of the metals in the soil under study need clean-up if intended for agricultural purposes.

Table 3 summarizes the various chemical extractants used in the fractionation. From the perspective of risk assessment, the chemical forms or species, in which a

Table 4. Geochemical forms of the metals in the CCA contaminated soil.

Fraction	As (mg/Kg)		Cr (mg/Kg)		Cu (mg/Kg)	
	Mean	Percent	Mean	Percent	Mean	Percent
Water soluble (F₁)	4.0 ± 0.3	12.9	13.1 ± 0.7	5.21	1.0 ± 0.1	0.66
Exchangeable (F₂)	9.75 ± 0.15	31.4	19.83 ± 0.28	7.9	3.48 ± 0.08	2.3
Carbonate (F₃)	5.0 ± 0.1	16.1	15.1 ± 0.5	6	8.8 ± 0.2	5.8
Fe-Mn oxide (F₄)	3.3 ± 0.2	10.63	8.5 ± 0.7	3.38	12.5 ± 0.3	8.24
Organic (F₅)	2.15 ± 0.25	6.92	38.8 ± 0.4	15.43	26.6 ± 0.3	17.54
Residual (F₆)	6.85 ± 0.35	22.1	156.18 ± 4.03	62.1	99.3 ± 0.4	65.47
Total	31.05		251.57		151.68	

Table 5. Geochemical forms of arsenic metal in soil after 20 days phyto-remediation.

Fractions	Without amendment	With 2% amendment	With 5% amendment	With 10% amendment	With 20% amendment
Water soluble	1.10 ± 0.30	1.20 ± 0.10	1.24 ± 0.00	1.30 ± 0.30	1.40 ± 0.30
Exchangeable	1.85 ± 0.20	1.90 ± 0100	1.98 ± 0.00	2.10 ± 0.60	2.10 ± 0.60
Carbonate	1.80 ± 0.40	1.90 ± 0.90	2.02 ± 0.00	2.10 ± 0.10	2.50 ± 1.00
Fe-Mn oxide	4.40 ± 0.10	4.50 ± 0.40	4.65 ± 0.20	4.76 ± 0.00	4.90 ± 0.00
Organic	3.40 ± 0.00	3.48 ± 0.40	3.54 ± 0.10	3.60 ± 0.30	3.70 ± 0.20
Residual	9.60 ± 0.20	9.65 ± 0.20	9.70 ± 0.00	9.70 ± 0.60	9.80 ± 0.00
Sum of fractions	22.15	22.63	23.13	23.51	24.40
Total	26.03 ± 1.00	26.42 ± 1.20	26.65 ± 1.10	26.96 ± 1.60	25.20 ± 0.00

metal is found in the environment, provides predictive insights on the bioavailability, mobility, and fate of the metal contaminant. In order to estimate effects and potential risk associated with elemental species and association, we must identify the fractions that are bioavailable for incorporation into biota (bioaccumulation).

Table 4 above shows the geochemical forms of the metals in the CCA contaminated soil without amendment. Geochemical forms of heavy metals in soil affect their solubility which directly influences their bioavailability (Xian, 1987). Therefore, metals in water soluble and exchangeable fractions would be readily bioavailable to the environment, whereas the metals in the residual fraction are tightly bound and would not be expected to be released under natural conditions (Xian, 1989; Clevenger and Mullins, 1982). Metal species associated with organic, Fe-Mn oxide fractions are also not readily bioavailable. They are tightly held and bound. Their release into the soil solution depends on strong depletion of minerals content of the soil solution, decomposition and oxidation of organic matter. The identification and quantification of the forms in which a metal is present in soil helps to establish its potential and actual mobility and toxicity in the soil.

Arsenic has its highest concentration in the exchangeable phase (9.75 mg/kg). The exchangeable fraction is most likely to cause a release into the soil solution due to ion exchange. When exchanged with other cations, it

goes into solution. It is then available for plant uptake through movement of element from soil solution to plant root. Thus arsenic can be bioavailable and mobile in the soil.

The specie of As associated with organic matter is low (2 mg/kg or 7%). Metals associated with organic matter are either complex or adsorbed. Thus they are tightly held and their release into the soil solution is slow. Only 7% of total arsenic is in this fraction and this means that most of the arsenic is in the form that can easily go into solution. Arsenic concentration in the residual fraction is 6.85 mg/kg or 22%. At low pH this could be released. The pH of the CCA contaminated soil is 6.20 (Table 1). The specie of chromium that is associated with the soluble, exchangeable and Fe- Mn oxide fraction is low as shown in the Table 4. Thus they may not be readily available and mobile. The bulk of it is in residual 156 mg/kg or 62% and organic 38.8 mg/kg or 15%.

Most species of copper like chromium are tied to the residual fractions (65%), and organic 18%. However copper is one of the essential micronutrients and are specifically needed by the plants.

Tables 5, 6 and 7 shows the geochemical forms of arsenic, chromium and copper metals, respectively in the amended soil after 20 days of phytoremediation. A comparison of Table 4 with Tables 5, 6 and 7 indicate that after twenty days of germination, the species of the metals associated with soluble and exchangeable fractions in the amended soils reduced. These reductions

Table 6. Geochemical forms of chromium metal in soil after 20 days phytoremediation.

Fractions	Without amendment	With 2% amendment	With 5% amendment	With 10% amendment	With 20% amendment
Water soluble	9.50 ± 0.60	10.10 ± 0.70	10.55 ± 0.30	10.70 ± 0.40	10.90 ±0.00
Exchangeable	14.70 ± 0.70	15.10 ± 0.50	15.60 ± 0.30	15.70 ± 0.90	15.80 ±0.70
Carbonate	14.00 ± 0.60	14.20 ± 0.70	14.60 ± 0.50	14.80 ± 0.80	14.60 ±0.60
Fe-Mn oxide	8.30 ± 0.20	8.30 ± 0.30	8.20 ± 0.70	8.60 ± 0.30	8.60 ± 0.4
Organic	37.00 ± 1.00	35.20 ± 1.30	35.30 ± 1.50	35.80 ± 1.10	35.90 ±1.20
Residual	154.70 ± 1.80	155.90 ± 2.10	155.80 ± 2.00	155.90 ± 2.10 156.10 ± 1.70	156.90 ± 2.00
Sum	239.30	240.05	240.05	240.20	241.70
Total	252.60 ± 2.40	254.30 ± 3.90	254.78 ± 3.00	255.30 ± 1.30	255.91 ± 1.40

Table 7. Geochemical forms of copper metal in soil after 20 days of phytoremediation.

Copper (mg/kg)	Without amendment	With 2% amendment	With 5% amendment	With 10% amendment	With 20% amendment
Water soluble	0.70 ± 0.30	0.80 ± 0.40	0.90 ± 0.00	1.00 ± 0.10	1.10 ± 0.50
Exchangeable	2.50 ± 0.50	2.90 ± 0.40	3.00 ± 0.00	3.10 ± 0.50	3.20 ± 0.40
Carbonate	3.90 ± 0.60	4.08 ± 0.60	4.10 ± 0.00	4.90 ± 0.60	5.40 ± 0.40
Fe-Mn oxide	9.60 ± 1.20	9.90 ± 0.10	10.60 ± 0.00	10.70 ± 0.60	11.50 ± 1.60
Organic	10.10 ±1.00	10.40 ± 1.00	12.20 ± 0.00	12.55 ± 0.80	12.50 ± 1.10
Residual	82.80 ±1.60	84.30 ± 4.00	84.70 ± 1.40	84.60 ± 2.00	86.20 ± 2.00
Sum	112.00	113.70	115.60	115.63	117.30
Total	115.30 ± 1.10	120.70 ± 1.00	122.56 ± 1.90	123.80 ± 0.80	126.40 ± 1.00

Table 8. Metal uptake by plants in cow dung amended soil after 20 days.

Metal (mg/Kg)	Control	2% amendment	5% amendment	10% amendment	20% amendment
Arsenic	6.40 ± 1.30	3.34 ± 0.00	3.26 ± 1.00	3.03 ± 0.50	2.95 ± 0.60
Chromium	8.80 ± 1.00	3.83 ± 0.40	3.18 ± 0.50	2.96 ± 0.80	2.10 ± 1.40
Copper	40.50 ± 2.20	30.86 ± 0.50	27.90 ± 1.00	26.20 ± 0.00	23.90 ± 3.00

are remarkable because these are the fractions that have positive influence on metal bioavailability. A significant point of note is that their rate of reduction increased as the percentage of amendment in the soil increased. Plant uptake is dependent on movement of element from the soil to the plant root through the soil solution; the limiting step for elemental concentration in soil is usually from the soil to the root. The relative mobility and bioavailability of trace metals associated with different fractions has a lot of influence on plant uptake of metals. These reductions are more noticeable with arsenic metal (Table 5). This reduction trend cannot be said of the Fe-Mn, Organic and Residual fractions. As a matter of fact, there is an increase in the fractions (Tables 6 and 7), for arsenic, it is different (Table 5). This is easily expected because incorporation of carbon-rich composts into soils has been shown to increase arsenic metal solubility through formation of soluble metal organic complexes

(Zhou and Wong, 2001). It was established that near neutral pH generally results in the largest diverse bacteria population (Nyle and Ray, 2005). It was also established that pH and microbial activity are most important factors which affect arsenic mobility and bioavailability in soils (Turpeinen et al., 1999; Xu et al., 1991). The amendment apart from enriching the soil a key to effective phytoreme diation, especially phytoextraction, is to enhance pollutant phytoavailability and to sustain adequate pollutant concentrations in soil solution for plant uptake (Lombi et al., 2001).

Table 8 shows the uptake of metals by plants. Generally more metals were consumed by plants in the control pots than in the pots with amendments. This is true for all the metals under investigation. Cationic trace elements normally react with certain organic molecules to form organometallic complexes called chelates. If these complexes are not soluble, the metals are tightly held and

Table 9. Total residual metals in soils after 20 days of phytoremediation.

Metals (mg/Kg)	Control	With 2% amendment	With 5% amendment	With 10% amendment	With 20% amendment
Arsenic	25.20 ± 0.00	26.96 ± 1.60	26.65 ± 1.10	26.42 ± 1.20	28.03 ± 1.00
Chromium	252.60 ± 2.40	255.91 ± 3.90	254.78 ± 3.00	254.30 ± 1.30	255.18 ±1.40
Copper	115.30 ± 1.10	120.70 ± 1.00	122.56 ± 1.90	123.80 ± 0.80	126.40 ±1.00

bound. They are thus not bioavailable to plants. They could only be slowly released through decomposition. Apart from arsenic (Table 5) which recorded reductions in the organic fractions, the other metals recorded an increase in the value of organic fractions (Tables 5 and 6). This indicates that the metals must have gone into reactions with organic materials in the amendment to form complexes which are not soluble rendering them unavailable for plant consumption. Bounding of metals is also a method of soil remediation. The slow release through decomposition of these toxic metals to plants also gives the plants a longer lease of life when compared with the control plants. The plants in the control pot experiment were dying before the expiration of the 20 days experimental period (pictures not shown). As a matter of fact, the 20 days experimental duration was adopted based on the life span of the plants in the control pots.

Table 9 shows the residual metals in the soils after 20 days of phytoremediation. More metals were remaining in pots with different levels of amendment than in control pots indicating that more metals were taken up by plants in control pots (no amendment). Plant growth in the control pots were generally retarded with stunted growth, yellowing of leaves, reduced leaf expansion and dying before the expiration of the 20 days duration when compared to the plants in pots with amendment (picture not shown). This is due to heavy consumption of the toxic metals, while those in the pots with amendment were still alive. The increase in the values of pH, CEC and OM especially at 20% amendment level (Table 1) occasioned by the addition of cow dung amendment did more to bound the metals than make them available for plant uptake. The metals bioavailability of soil depends to a large extent on their distribution between solid and solution phase, which in turn is dependent on soil processes like CEC, OM, and pH. The effect of organic matter amendments on heavy metal solubility depend greatly upon the degree of humification of their OM and their effect upon soil pH (Walker et al., 2003). In general, the concentration of an element in the soil solution is believed to depend on the equilibrium between the soil solution and solid phase, with pH playing the decisive role (Lindsay, WL 1979). The soil's ability to immobilize heavy metals increases with rising pH and peaks under mildly alkaline conditions. Heavy metal mobility is related to their immobilization in the solid phase. (Fuller, WH 1979), in discussing the relatively high mobility of heavy metals with regard to pH, considered that in acid soils (pH 4.2 - 6.6), the elements Cd, Ni, and Zn are highly mobile, Cr is moderately mobile, and Cu and Pb practically immobile. Copper is especially tightly held by organic matter occasioned by the addition of amendment. Its availability is low.

Mobility of arsenic, chromium and copper in the CCA contaminated soil

The bioavailability/mobility of metals in soils is assessed on the basis of absolute and relative content of fractions weakly bound to soil components. The relative index of metal mobility was calculated as a "mobility factor" (Cezary and Bal, 2001) using the equation below:

$$M_f = \frac{F_1 + F_2 + F_3}{F_1 + F_2 + F_3 + F_4 + F_5 + F_6} \times \frac{100}{1} \qquad (2)$$

Where: M_f = Mobility factor, F_1 = Soluble form, F_2 = Exchangeable, F_3 = Carbonate, F_4 = Fe-Mn, F_5 = Organic, F_6 = Residual.

F_1, F_2, F_3, F_4, F_5, and F_6 represents the percentage geochemical forms of the metals in the CCA contaminated soil but here corrected to the nearest whole numbers (Table 4). Values from Table 4 when applied to Equation 2 above, assigned mobility factor (M_f) values of 60 for arsenic, 19 for chromium and 8 for copper.

Metal forms bound to carbonate fractions F_3 are relatively less mobile and soluble than exchangeable fractions.

The result shows that arsenic is potentially mobile and biologically available because of its high M_f value of 60. High M_f values are symptoms of relatively high liability and biological availability of heavy metals in soils (Ahumada et al., 1999; Karczewska, 1996). Chromium is relatively mobile with M_f value of 19 while the mobility of copper is low with an M_f value of 8. The high M_f of As may be attributed to the low organic matter of the soil (Rahman et al., 2004). The organic matter of the soil is 2.5%. The use of a modified Tessier et al. sequential extraction procedure by Salbu and Oughton (1998). (six steps) which partitioned the metals As, Cr and Cu among six operationally defined fractions: F_1 (water soluble), F_2 (exchangeable), F_3 (carbonate), F_4 (Fe-Mn), F_5 (organic)

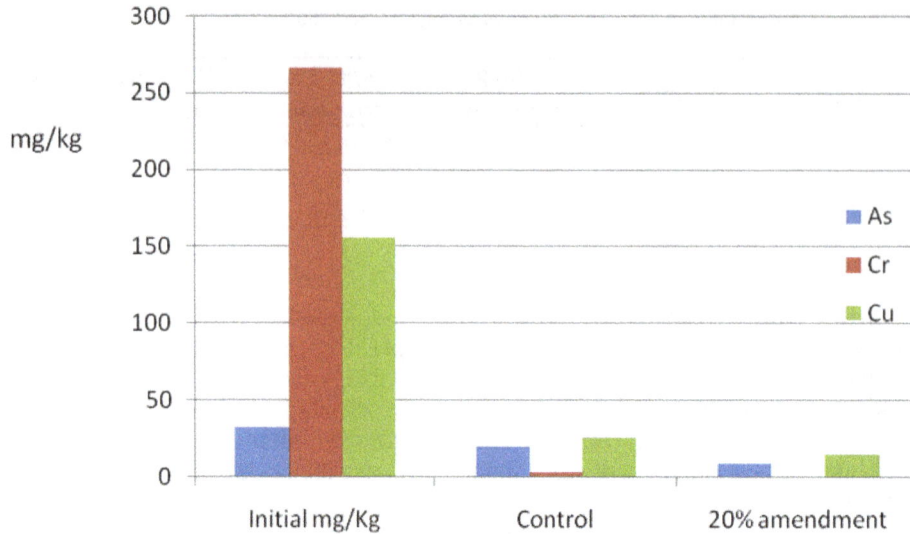

Figure 1. Shows percentage uptake after 20 days of phytoremediation.

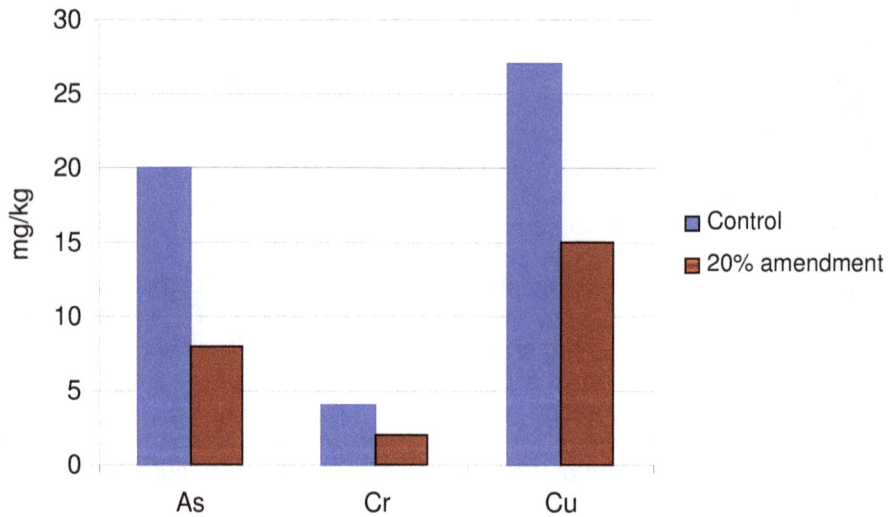

Figure 2. Shows the uptake of the metals by maize plant in both control and soil with 20% amendment.

Equation 2 if calculated). This made it to be highly labile and bioavailable and consequently more dangerous than the other two metals.

Figure 1 compares the percentage uptake of the metals in mg/kg after 20 days of cleanup between the control and soil with 20% amendment. More metals were taken up by plants in the control pots than in the pots with 20% amendment. This results in the plants in the control pots dying before the plants in the pots with amendment.

Figure 2 compares the uptake of the different metals (As, Cr and Cu) after 20 days of phytoremediation in mg/kg between the control and soil with 20% amendment. In both the control pots and in pots with 20%

amendment, copper had the highest uptake. This was followed by arsenic while chromium has the least uptake.

Conclusion

Our studies show that there is a relative advantage in the use of cow dung as soil amendment prior to phyto-remediation of CCA contaminated soil as the plants in soils with amendment out lived those in soil without amendment. Consequently more clean up is expected from living plants than dead plants. Cu and Cr were present in appreciable quantities as organic and residual based forms indicating that the availability of these metals to plants would be less than As.

Cow dung amendment could be used to prolong the life of maize plants growing in soil polluted with As, Cr and Cu. The use of cow dung as amendment also provides a path way towards greener and cleaner planet.

REFERENCES

Adeniran JA, Taiwo LB, Sobulo RA (2003). Effects of organic wastes and method of composting on compost maturity, Nutrient Composition of compost and yields of two vegetable crops, of sustainable Agriculture, 22: 95–101.

Ahumada I, Mendoza J, Asxar L (1999). Sequential extraction of heavy metals in soils irrigated with wastewater. Commun. Soil Sci. Plant Anal., 30: 1507-1519.

Cezary K, Bal RS (2001). Fractionation and mobility of copper, lead and zinc in the vicinity of a copper smelter. J. Environ. Qual., 30: 485-492.

Cunningham SD, Berti SR, Haung JW (1995). In Bioremediation of Inorgaanics. Hinchee R. E. Means J. L., Burries D. R. Eds.; Battelle press: Columbus, O.H., pp.33-54.

Clevenger TE, Mullins W, (1982). The toxic extraction procemental health XVI. Univ. of Missouri, Columbia, MO.

Department of Petroleum Resources, Lagos. (1991). Environmental Guidelines and Standards for the Petroleum Industry in Nigeria (EGASPIN). pp: 278-281.

Fuller WH (1979). Movement of selected metals, asbestos and cyanide in soil: Application to waste disposal problem. EPA-600/2-77-020. Solid and hazardous waste research division, U.S. Environmental protection agency, Cincinnati, OH.

Karczewska A (1996). Metal specie distribution of top and subsoil in an area affected by copper smelter emission API. Geochem., 11: 35-42.

Lindsay WL (1979). Chemical equilibria in soils. John Wiley & Sons, New York, NY,.

Lombi E, Zhao FJ, Dunham SJ, McGrath SP (2001). Phytoremediation of heavy metal conataminated soils: Natural hyperaccumulation versus chemically enhanced phytoremediation. J. Environ. Qual., 30: 1919-1926

Nyle CB, Ray RW (2005). Nature and Properties of Soils. Third Edition pp. 33-34, 663.

Peters RW (1999). Chealant extraction of heavy metals from contaminated soils. J. Hazard. Mater. 66: 151-210.

Rahman FR, Allan DL, Sadowskey MJ (2004). Arsenic Availability from Chromated Copper Arsenate (CCA). treated wood. J. Environ. Qual., 33: 173-180.

Salbu BTK, Oughton DH (1998). Characteristic of radioactive particles in the environment. Analyst 123: 843-849

Salvator K, Sabee WE (1995). Evaluation of Fertilizer Value and Nutrient Release From Corn and Soybean Residues Under Laboratory and Greenhouse. Conditions. Commu. Soil/ Sci., Plant Anal., 26: 469-484

Salt DE, Smith RD, Raskin I (1998). Phutoremediation. Ann. Rev. Plant phys., 49: 643-668.

Seward MRD, Richardson DHS (1990). In Heavy Metal Tolerance in Plants: Evolutionary Aspects; Shaw, A. J., Ed., CRC Press: Boca Raton, FL. pp: 7-19.

Sun B, Zhao FJ, Lombi E, McGrath SP (2001). Leaching of heavy metals from contaminated soils using EDTA. Environ. Pollut. 113: 111-120.10.

Tessier A, Campbell PGC, Bisson M (1979). Sequential extraction procedures for the speciation of particulate trace metals. Anal. Chem., 51(7): 844-851

Turpeinen R, Pantsar-Kallio M, Haggblom M, Kairesaalo T (1999). Influence of microbes on the mobilization, toxicity and biomethylation of arsenic in soil. Sci. Total Environ. 236, 173-180.

US Environmental Protedtion Agency (1997). Cleaning up the nations Waste sites. Markets and Technology Trends, EPA 542-R-96-005. Office of Solid Waste and Emergency Response, Washington, DC.

Uwumarongie EG, Okieimen FE, Uwumarongie OH (2008). Phytoremoval of heavy metals from Chromated Copper Arsenate Contaminated Soil. J. Chem. Soc. Nigeria, 33(1): 126-131.

Uwumarongie EG, Okieimen FE, Uwumarongie OH (2008). Spatial Distribution and Speciation of Arsenic, Chromium and Copper in Contaminated Soil. J. Chem. Soc. Nigeria, 33(1): 112-121.

Walker DJ, Clemente R, Roig A, Bernal MP (2003). The effect of soil amendments on heavy metals bioavailability in two contaminated Mediterranean soils. Environ. Pollut. 122: 303-312.

William JT, Michael A P (2009). Introduction to Biotechonlogy, Second Edition. (p216)

Xu H, Allard B, Grimvall A (1991). Effects of acidification and natural organic materials on the mobility of arsenic in the environment. Water, Air and Soil pollution. 57-58: 269-278.

Xian X (1987). Chemical partitioning of cadmium, zinc, lead, and copper in soils near smelters. J. Environ. Sci. Health A. 6: 527-541.

Xian X (1989). Effect of chemical forms of cadmium, zinc, and lead in polluted soils on their uptake vy cabbage plants. Plant Soil. 113: 257-264.

Zhou LX, Wong JWC (2001). Effect of dissolved organic matter from sludge compost of soil copper sorption. J. Environ. Qual. 30: 878-883.

11

Studies in the graft copolymerization of acrylonitrile onto cassava starch by ceric ion induced initiation

E. U. Ikhuoria*, A. S. Folayan and F. E. Okieimen

Department of Chemistry, University of Benin, Benin City, Nigeria.

Graft copolymers of starch and acrylonitrile were synthesized in aqueous solution. Ceric ammonium ion was used to initiate the graft copolymerization. Ten grades of graft copolymers were synthesized-five by varying the initial concentration of the monomer and the other five by varying the initial concentration of the initiator. Evidence of graft copolymerization of the hydrolyzed products was obtained from the IR analyses. Some grafting parameters such as % grafting ratio and % conversion were favoured by initial increase in the monomer concentration. However, these parameters were observed to decrease at much higher concentrations (>3 M). Evidence of hydrolysis shows that the grafted copolymers could be used as flocculants.

Key words: Acrylonitrile, homopolymer, grafting initiator, starch.

INTRODUCTION

Carbohydrates comprise more than 90% of the dry weight of all biomass and more than 90% of the carbohydrate mass is in the form of carbohydrate polymer (Polysaccharides) (Zohuriaan-Mehr and Pour, 2003). Since polysaccharides are abundant from renewable sources and are relatively inexpensive, safe (non-toxic) and amenable to both chemical and biochemical modifications, it is not surprising that they find widespread and extensive use.

Graft copolymerization is a unique method among the techniques for modifying natural polymers mostly polysaccharides. Polysaccharide graft co-polymers have been prepared in order to add new properties to the natural polymer with a minimum loss of native properties (Fanta and Doane, 1986). Graft co-polymers are prepared by first generating free radicals on polysaccharides and then allowing these free radicals to serve as macro-initiators for the vinyl or acrylic monomer polymerization. Of the vinyl monomers grafted, acrylonitrile has been the most frequently used, mainly due to its highest grafting efficiency (Fanta and Doane, 1986; Athawale and Rathi, 1999; Athawale and Lele, 2000) and the subsequent alkaline hydrolysis of the grafting product to produce

starch - based water absorbent (Athawale and Lele, 2000).

In view of the growing interest and research activity in the use of renewable agriculturally derived products as extenders and replacement for synthetic petroleum - based polymers, incorporation of other monomers/polymers into polysaccharides will not only reduce our dependence on petrochemical derivatives, but also provides improved materials which will biodegrade rapidly in the environment.

Since the last three decades, grafting of various monomers onto starch has been the most frequently attempted method to impart desirable properties on the polysaccharide without sacrificing its biodegradable nature. In the present study, acrylonitrile is grafted onto starch and the effect of varying the concentrations of the monomer and the initiator is examined.

MATERIALS AND METHODS

Materials

Acrylonitrile was extracted with aqueous sodium hydroxide - sodium chloride solution to remove inhibitor. Sodium hydroxide quinol, sodium chloride and methanol were obtained from BDH Ltd (Poole, England). Ammonium nitrate was purchased from Merck (Germany) and was used without purification. The cassava starch was

1. Grafting parameters at constant initiator concentration.

...omer concentration (Mol/l)	Weight of Starch-g-polyacrylonitrile (g)	Weight of homopolymer + grafted polymer (g)	% Monomer conversion	% Grafting ratio (Gr)
1.00	11.01	1.01	12.67	10.01
2.00	12.06	2.06	12.93	20.60
3.00	13.87	3.87	16.19	38.70
4.00	12.64	2.64	8.29	26.40
5.00	12.56	2.46	6.43	25.60

purchased from an open market in Benin City, Nigeria and used without further purification.

Synthesis

Graft copolymerization of acrylonitrile onto starch was carried out using various amounts of the monomer and ceric ions and a constant amount of starch (10 g) dispersed in 100 ml of distilled water at 29°C. The polymerization procedure was based on the method described by Pourjavadi et al. (2006). In a typical experiment, 10 g of starch was dispersed in 100 ml of distilled water in a 250 ml flask. A given amount of monomer was added to the flask and the mixture was stirred for 10 min. Then the initiator solution was added to the mixture and continuously stirred for 3 h. The reaction was stopped by the addition of 2 ml of 5% (w/v) quinol solution to the reaction mixture. The mixture was poured into large excess of methanol with stirring to precipitate the polymer and then filtered. The residue was air dried and weighed.

Hydrolysis of the grafted copolymer

The grafted copolymer produced was hydrolyzed by adding 2MNaOH to the product in a 100 ml flask immersed in thermostated water bath fitted with magnetic stirrer and a reflux condenser. The hydrolysis was on for about 1½ h at 60°C. The pasty mixture was allowed to cool to room temperature and neutralized to pH8 by the addition of 10 wt% aqueous acetic acid solution. The mixture was poured into excess methanol to precipitate out. The precipitate was filtered and air dried.

GRAFTING PARAMETERS (Jideonwo and Okieimen, 2000)

The percent grafting ratio (Gr) is reported as the ratio of the weight of the grafted polymer to the weight of the substrate (starch) multiplied by 100.

$$Gr\% = \frac{weight\ of\ grafted\ polymer}{weight\ of\ starch} \times \frac{100}{1} \qquad (1)$$

The percentage conversion is taken as the ratio of the weight of the grafted polymer to the weight of the monomer.

$$\% \ Conversion = \frac{weight\ of\ grafted\ polymer}{weight\ of\ monomer} \times \frac{100}{1} \qquad (2)$$

SPECTRAL CHARACTERIZATION

The graft copolymer before and after hydrolysis were characterized by IR spectroscopy using KBr pellets on Shimadzu FTIR 4200 spectrophotometer.

RESULTS AND DISCUSSION

The backbone polymer (starch) was grafted with acrylonitrile monomer. The effects of monomer concentration on the level of conversion and quantities of grafted acrylonitrile on starch were investigated. Experiments were performed in the monomer concentration ranges of 1.00 - 5.00 mol/l. The initiator (ceric ammonium ion) concentration of 2M at a reaction temperature of 29°C for 3 h was used. The grafting parameters obtained are given in Table 1.

The results show that the grafting parameters increased initially with increase in monomer concentration and then decreased thereafter 3 M concentration. It has been established that the extent of graft copolymer formation depend on the amount of monomer complexed (Jideonwo and Okieimen, 2000). The increase in grafting ratio and percentage monomer conversion may be probably due to increasing supply of monomers to starch macroradicals and the nonexistence of homopolymer on acrylonitrile (Nayak and Singh, 2001). Maximum values of 38.70 and 16.9% were obtained for percentage grafting ratio and percentage monomer conversion respectively at 3 M monomer concentration. At higher monomer concentration (>3 M), the decrease in grafting parameters may be due to increasing trend of side reaction such as chain transfer to excess molecules in the vicinity of growing ends of grafted chains (Labet et al., 2007). Moreover, large amounts of homopolymer deposits may block the way of monomer molecules to the starch macroradicals resulting in further decrease in percentage monomer conversion and yield. Therefore 3 M was taken as the maximum concentration at which monomer (acrylonitrile) can be complexed. The effect of monomer concentration on the percentage monomer conversion is shown in Figure 1. Table 2 indicates the effect of varying the initiator concentration on some grafting parameter.

The result in Table 2 showed that, the percent grafting ratio and monomer conversion increased initially with an increase in the ceric ion concentration up to 3 M and decreased beyond this initiator concentration. The initial

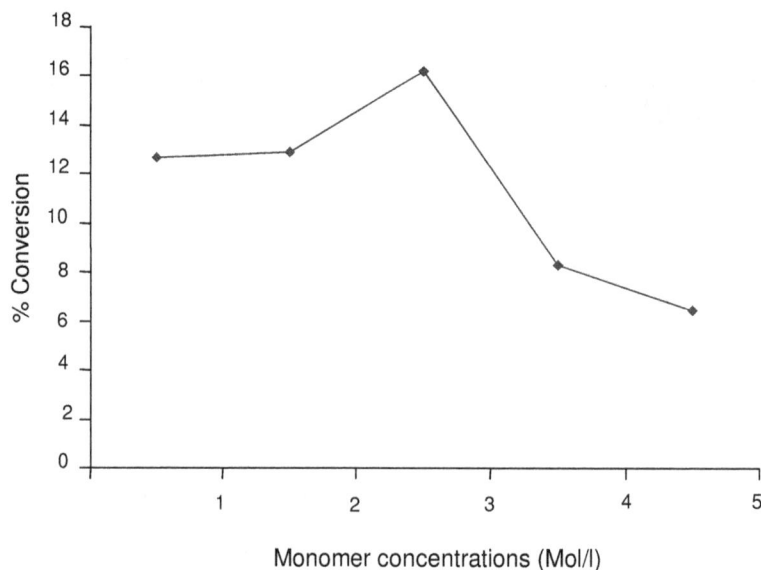

Figure 1. Effect of Monomer concentration on % monomer conversion.

Table 2. Grafting parameters at constant monomer concentration.

Ceric ion concentration (Mol/l)	Weight of starch-g-polyacrylonitrile (g)	Weight of homopolymer + grafted polymer (g)	% Monomer conversion	% grafting ratio (Gr
1.00	11.65	1.16	2.91	11.60
2.00	12.56	2.56	6.43	25.60
3.00	14.23	4.23	10.62	42.30
4.00	14.20	4.20	10.55	42.00
5.00	11.83	1.83	4.59	18.30

increase may be explained in terms of the mechanism of ceric ion initiation which involves the formation of chelate complex that decomposes to generate free radical site on the polymer backbone (Athawale and Rathi, 1999). As the ceric ion concentration increased, the active free radicals on the starch backbone at which the monomer can be grafted also increased and these active free radicals in the presence of monomer generate graft copolymers (Nakason et al., 2004). The average number of grafting sites per backbone molecule depends on the concentration of the ceric ion, and the substrate (Pourjavadi and Zohuriaan-Mehr, 2002; Zohuriaan-Mehr and PourJavadi, 2003). The results also showed that the grafting ratio reached the maximum value of 4.32% at 3 M ceric ion concentration which indicates the reduction equivalent of the polymer backbone (Nakason et al., 2004). The decrease in grafting ratio at 4 M ceric ion concentration may be attributed to the solubility limitation of the starch at higher ceric ion concentration. It may also be due to the termination of the growing grafted chains by excess of ceric ions. The reaction of free radicals on starch backbone to produce oxidized starch is incapable

of initiating polymerization. Figure 2 showed the trend in the percentage monomer conversion with change in ceric ion concentration.

Hydrolysis of the grafted polymer

Starch, on hydrolysis transforms to glucose which is soluble in water and does not precipitate with methanol. However when a solution of the grafted starch was poured in excess of methanol, the precipitate of the hydrolyzed grafted starch was obtained. This shows that the grafted starch could be used as flocculants.

SPECTRAL CHARACTERIZATION

The grafted copolymer and the non grafted starch were characterized by IR spectrophotometer. The spectra of the grafted copolymer showed the existence of a moderate peek at 2240 cm^{-1} as observed in Figure 3 which is an evidence of grafting. This absorption band

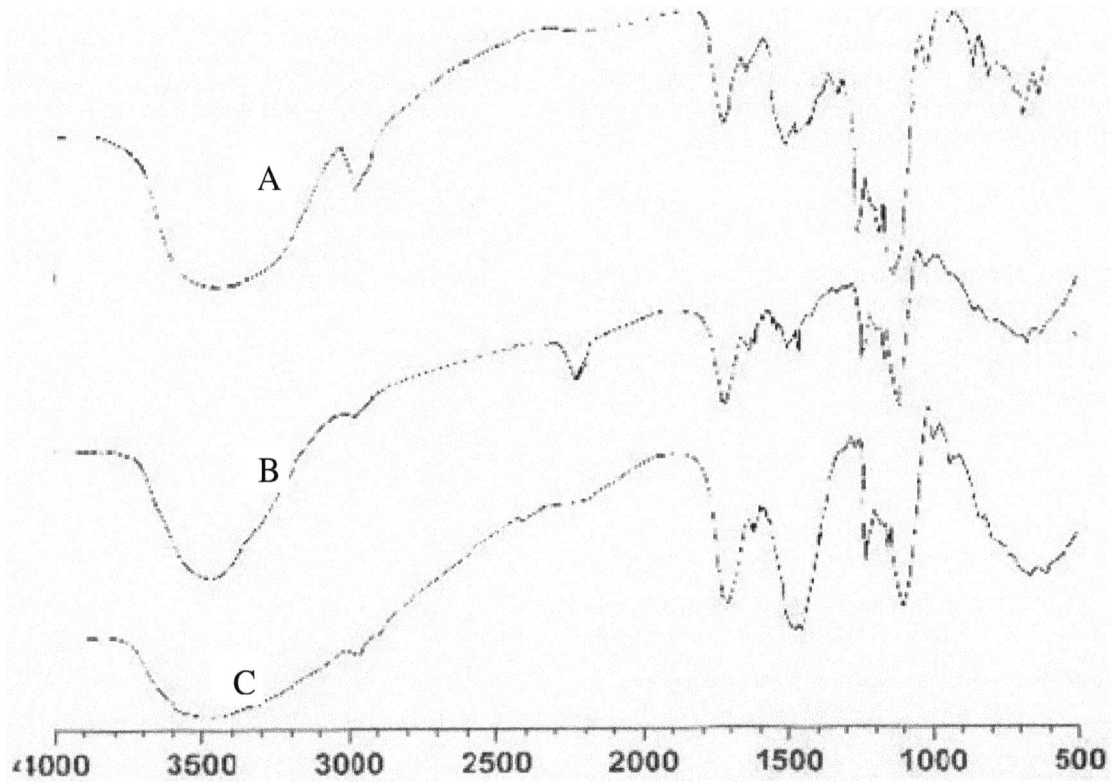

Figure 3. IR spectra of Starch (A), Starch-g- polyacrylonitrile (B) and Hydrolyzed Starch-g- acrylonitrile (C).

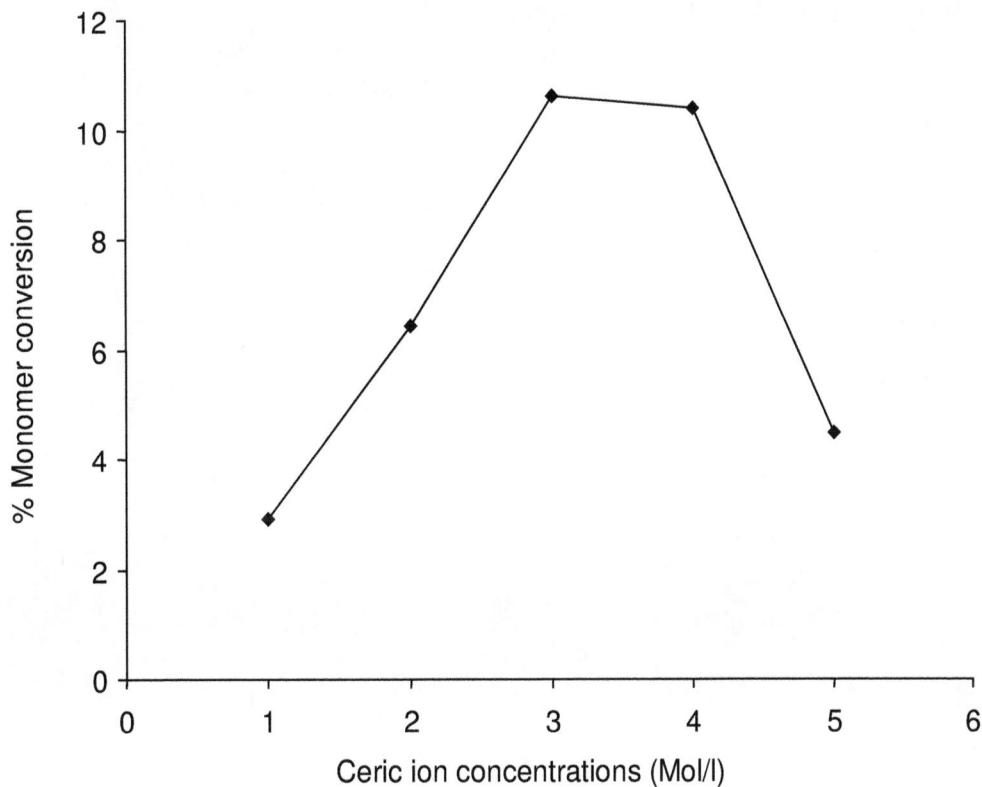

Figure 2. Effect of ceric ion concentration on the % monomer conversion.

arises from the stretching vibration mode of the nitrile groups (B). There is also a small characteristic peak at 2340 cm^{-1} (C) which is a -C≡N- peak, an immediate from the hydrolysis to carboxylic group. Most of the other peeks are related to the polymer backbone (starch).

Conclusion

The results from this study show that the level of grafting is affected by the concentrations of the initiator and the monomer. Study of the IR spectra provides a strong evidence of grafting. The grafted copolymer could be used as flocculants.

REFERENCES

Athawale VD, Lele V (2000). Synthesis and Characterisation of Graft Polymers of maize Starch and Methacrylonitrile. Carbohyr. Polym. 41(4): 407-416.

Athawale VD, Rathi SC (1999). Graft Polymerization: Starch as a model substrate. J. Macromol. Sci. Rev. Macromol. Chem. Phys. C39(3): 445-480.

Fanta GF, Doane WM (1986). In Modified Starches: Properties and Uses, Wurburg-OB (ed). CRC Press: Boca Raton, FL; 149-178.

Jideonwo A, Okieimen FE (2000). Graft copolymerization of methylacrylate onto gum Arabic, Niger. J. Appl. Sci. 18: 109 -114.

Labet M, Thielemans W, Dufresne A (2007). Polymer grafting onto starch nanocrystals, Biomacromolecules 8(9): 2916 - 2927.

Nakason C, Kaesaman A, Supasanthitikul P (2004). The Grafting of meleic Anhydride onto natural rubber, Polymer testing 23: 35-41.

Nayak BR, Singh RO (2001). Development of graft copolymer flocculating agents based on hydroxypropyl guar gum and acrylamide, J. Appl. Polym. Sci. 81(77): 1776 - 1785.

Pourjavadi A, Zohuriaan-Mehr MJ (2002). Modification of carbohydrate polymers via grafting in air, Starch/Starke 54: 140.

Pourjavadi A, Zohuriaan-Mehr MJ, Ghaempoori SN, Hossenzadh H (2007). Modified CMC. V. Synthesis and superswelling behaviour of hydrolysed CMC-g-PAN Hydrogel. J. Appl. Polym. Sci. 103: 877 - 883.

Zohuriaan-Mehr MJ, PourJavadi (2003). New Polysaccharides -g-copolymers: Synthesis and Thermal Characteristics. Polym. Adv. Technol. 14: 508-516.

Zohuriaan-Mehr MJ, PourJavadi (2003). New polysaccharides -g-copolymers: Synthesis and thermal characteristics. Polym. Adv. Technol. 14: 508-516.

12

Effects of harvesting stage and storage duration on postharvest quality and shelf life of sweet bell pepper (*Capsicum annuum* L.) varieties under passive refrigeration system

Dargie Tsegay, Bizuayehu Tesfaye, Ali Mohammed, Haddis Yirga and Andnet Bayleyegn

*Montpellier SupAgro_Centre International d'études Supérieures en Sciences Agronomiques, 2 Place Pierre Viala, 34060 Cedex 2, Montpellier, FRANCE.

A laboratory experiment was carried out to determine the effects of harvesting stages (0, 25, 50, 75 and 100% fruit colourations) and storage durations (0, 1, 2, 3 and 4 weeks) on physicochemical quality and shelf life of sweet pepper varieties (Telmo-Red and Velez-Yellow) under passive refrigeration system (PRS). The aim of the study was to identify the optimum stage of maturity at harvest and storage period under PRS that can ensure better quality and longer shelf life of two greenhouse sweet pepper varieties. The experiment was arranged in 2 x 5 x 5 factorial combinations in complete randomized design (CRD) with three replications. Thirty (30) fruits of sweet pepper were packed in card-board boxes for each treatment and stored under PRS optimum storage conditions. Fruits were assessed for weight loss percentage, fruit firmness, total soluble solids, titratable acidity, postharvest decay percentage and shelf life. Total soluble solids were increased; whereas fruit firmness decreased with increasing harvesting stages. Weight loss percentage, postharvest decay percentage and shelf life increased; while fruit firmness decreased with increasing storage periods. Telmo variety showed significantly better postharvest quality and storability potential than Velez variety.

Key words: Harvesting stage, postharvest, passive refrigeration system, sweet bell pepper.

INTRODUCTION

Sweet bell pepper (*Capsicum annuum* L.) is one of the most commercially important horticultural crops grown in tropical and sub-tropical regions of the world. From the nutritional point of view, peppers are generally considered as a balanced source of most of essential nutrients, high content of vitamins, important antioxidants, rich in flavonoids and phytochemicals (Maria et al., 2010). Sweet peppers are currently the object of much attention due to possible links to prevention of certain types of cardiovascular diseases, atherosclerosis, cancer, haemorrhage, delaying of ageing process, avoiding cholesterol, improving physical resistance and increasing appetite (Marin et al., 2004).

Growing and marketing of fresh produce is complicated by high postharvest losses which are estimated to reach as high as 25-35% of the produced volume for vegetables (Agonafir, 1991). Sweet peppers like other vegetables are quite perishable, about 28.6 and 38.7% postharvest losses were reported during the dry and wet seasons, respectively (Tunde-Akintunde et al., 2005). Optimum temperature and relative humidity can be achieved using passive refrigeration system (PRS) cooling machine, which is a very efficient technique to store and transport products. The system works without ventilation thus assuring shelf life which is better than the active refrigeration system equipment. The thermal autonomy allows the storage and transport without use of power during operations (Nomos, 2008).

However, there is no available scientific literature regarding the effect of harvesting stages and storage durations on retaining the postharvest physicochemical quality properties of sweet bell pepper varieties under passive refrigeration system storage condition. The main objective of the present study was to evaluate the effect of harvesting at different maturity stages and storing in PRS, on shelf life and quality of sweet bell pepper varieties.

MATERIALS AND METHODS

Experimental design and treatments

The treatments were comprised of two varieties of sweet pepper (Telmo and Velez) picked at five harvesting stages (0, 25, 50, 75, 100% colourations) and stored for five storage durations (0, 1, 2, 3, and four weeks) under PRS. The treatments were combined in CRD factorial experiment, resulting in a total of 50 treatment combinations (2x5x5) with three replications and 150 total observations (2x5x5x3). Each treatment consisted of 30 fruits packed in standard card board boxes for storage under PRS.

Experimental procedures

Fruits of two sweet pepper varieties with similar size (160 g) and shape (bell shaped) were harvested from Hawassa Jittu Horticulture PLC greenhouse. Maturity stages of fruits were determined by fruit colouration guide and days from anthesis. Fruits were harvested manually with care to minimize mechanical injuries. After harvest, fruits were immediately transported using standard plastic crates to packing house within 10 min and held at 10°C pre-cooling room overnight. Fruits with bruises, sign of infection or those different from the group were discarded from the samples. Fruits were washed with tap water, surface dried with soft cloth and subdivided, sorted, and weighed in the packinghouse; thereafter stored under PRS (model *DS-TP-001-03*) on three shelves as replication. Samples were taken to food technology laboratory for quality analysis. The treatments were tested at test room environmental conditions (20°C temperature and 70% relative humidity) combined with 24 h lighting to assess the shelf life of fruits after removing from the PRS.

Data collection

Weight loss percentage (WLP)

Five sweet pepper fruits were weighed at day zero and in each storage duration using sensitive balance. The difference between initial and final weight of fruits was considered as total weight loss

during storage interval and expressed as percentage (AOAC, 2007):

$$WLP = \frac{Initial - Final\ Weight}{Initial\ Weght} \times 100\%$$

Fruit firmness

Firmness of three fruits was measured using a computer-controlled automatic fruit texture analyzer (model: *TA-LEVEL-05*) according to Manolopoulou et al. (2010). The firmness measurement was carried out using a cylindrical stainless steel probe of 2 mm in diameter. Puncture tests were taken from the two opposite equatorial sides of the same fruit.

Total soluble solids (TSS)

Juice of sweet pepper fruits was extracted from three fruits in a blender as described by Antoniali et al. (2007). The homogenized sample was filtered using funnel with filter paper in a beaker. The filtrate was taken for TSS determination using digital refractometer (model: RFM-860, Japan) in °Brix by placing a few drops of clear juice on the prism surface.

Titratable acidity (TA)

10 ml of juice was extracted from three fruits and then homogenized and filtered using funnel with filter paper in a beaker. The TA was measured using NaOH (0.1 N) as a standardized titration solution. When the end point of titration was reached at pH 8.2, the amount of NaOH used on the burette was read off and recorded to calculate TA:

$$TA = \frac{Titre \times 0.1N\ NaOH \times 0.67}{1000} \times 100\%$$

Postharvest decay percentage (PDP)

Fruits were visually evaluated for symptoms of decay at the end of each storage interval based on the method prescribed by El-Mougy et al. (2012). Samples having symptoms of chilling injury and of diseases were counted. Pathogens causing decay were not identified.

$$PDP = \frac{Number\ of\ Decayed\ Fruits}{Number\ of Total\ Fruits} \times 100\%$$

Shelf life

Shelf life of fruits was evaluated by counting the number of days required to attain fruits remaining still acceptable for marketing as described by Rao et al. (2011). It was decided based on the appearance and spoilage of fruits. When 50% of fruits showed symptoms of shrinkage or spoilage due to pathogens and chilling injury, lot of fruits was considered to have reached end of shelf life.

Statistical analysis

Data were subjected to ANOVA using SAS software version 9.

Table 1. Interaction effect of harvesting stage and storage duration on mean weight loss percentage of sweet pepper fruits under passive refrigeration system.

| Harvesting stage (%) | Weight loss percentage | | | | | Mean |
| | Storage duration (weeks) | | | | | |
	0	1	2	3	4	
0	0.00^n	2.67^k	3.61^{hi}	4.60^{ef}	6.01^b	3.38
25	0.00^n	1.39^m	2.25^l	3.30^{ij}	4.54^{fg}	2.30
50	0.00^n	2.03^l	3.00^j	3.89^h	4.88^{de}	2.70
75	0.00^n	2.28^l	3.30^{ij}	4.27^g	5.47^c	3.06
100	0.00^n	3.28^j	4.23^g	5.16^{cd}	6.50^a	3.83
Mean	0.00	2.33	3.35	4.24	5.48	
$LSD_{(0.05)}$		0.33				
CV (%)		9.29				

Means within a column followed by same letter(s) are not significantly different at 5% LSD test.

Verification of significant differences was done using LSD test at 5% probability level.

RESULTS AND DISCUSSION

Weight loss percentage

The interaction effect of harvesting stage and storage duration on mean weight loss percentage (WLP) of sweet pepper fruits was highly significant (P<0.001); while all other interaction effects were non-significant (P>0.05). At one week of storage, mean WLP of fruits harvested at 0, 25, 50, 75 and 100% colouration stages were 2.67, 1.39, 2.03, 2.28 and 3.28%, respectively; similar trends were observed at other storage times (Table 1). Mean WLP of fruits harvested at full green stage were 0.00, 2.67, 3.61, 4.60 and 6.01 at 0, 1, 2, 3 and 4 weeks of storage, respectively; the same results were apparent at other harvesting stages (Table 1).

The highest and lowest WLP were recorded for combinations of harvested at completely ripened stage and four weeks storage as well as harvested at 25% colouration stage and one week storage under PRS, respectively (Table 1).

Across all storage periods, the WLP of sweet pepper fruits harvested at completely ripened and full green stages were significantly higher than fruits harvested at intermediate stages (Table 1). This is in agreement with the findings of Moneruzzaman et al. (2009) who observed a higher WLP in fruits harvested at early matured stage than intermediate stages. This might be due to poorly developed waxy layer and cuticle on the surface of green pepper fruits as supported by Melaku et al. (2006). The high WLP in completely ripened fruits could be due to changes in permeability of cell membranes, making them more sensitive to the loss of water as confirmed by

Antoniali et al. (2007).

Fruit firmness

The main effects of variety, harvesting stage and storage duration on mean firmness of fruits were highly significant (P<0.001); while all interaction effects were non-significant (P>0.05). The highest fruit firmness of 36.06 N was recorded for variety Telmo-Red whereas the lowest value (30.97N) was recorded for Velez-Yellow variety (Table 2). The mean firmness of fruits harvested at 0, 25, 50, 75 and 100% colouration stages were 38.41, 36.33, 33.60, 31.06 and 28.17 N, respectively. The maximum and minimum fruit firmnesses were recorded at full green and completely ripened harvesting stages, respectively (Table 2). The mean fruit firmness of sweet peppers stored for 0, 1, 2, 3 and 4 weeks under PRS were 35.75, 34.73, 33.35, 32.58 and 31.16 N, respectively. The highest and lowest values were recorded at four weeks and zero week storage periods, respectively (Table 2).

Telmo-Red variety was 14.12% firmer than Velez-Yellow variety (Table 2). This finding is in agreement with results of Lahay et al. (2013) who reported that the value of fruit firmness varied in magnitude between varieties of tomato fruits. The observed variation might be due to genetic or environmental factors as confirmed by Beckles (2012). Ilic et al. (2012) disclosed that the higher pericarp thickness of a variety, the better is the firmness of fruit.

Fruit firmness decreased with increase in harvesting stages (Table 2). The present result is in coherence with the findings of Zhou et al. (2011) who found a decrease in fruit firmness with increasing harvesting stages. The apparent decline in fruit firmness with age might be due to cell wall softening directly influencing the levels of fruit firmness. This is in line with the work of Rao et al. (2011) who found that cell wall softening is due to the activity

Table 2. Effect of variety, harvesting stage and storage duration on mean fruit firmness and total soluble solids under passive refrigeration system.

Variety	Fruit firmness (N)	Total soluble solids (°Brix)
	Mean	Mean
Telmo-Red	36.06[a]	7.22[a]
Velez-Yellow	30.97[b]	6.56[b]
LSD$_{(0.05)}$	0.52	0.10
Harvesting stage (%)	Mean	Mean
0	38.41[a]	5.36[e]
25	36.33[b]	6.40[d]
50	33.60[c]	7.02[c]
75	31.06[d]	7.63[b]
100	28.17[e]	8.03[a]
LSD$_{(0.05)}$	0.82	0.16
Storage duration (Weeks)	Mean	Mean
0	35.75[a]	6.48[e]
1	34.73[b]	6.88[c]
2	33.35[c]	7.35[a]
3	32.58[d]	7.07[b]
4	31.16[e]	6.66[d]
LSD$_{(0.05)}$	0.82	0.16
CV (%)	4.76	4.60

Means within a column followed by the same letter(s) are not significantly different at 5% LSD test.

of softening enzymes such as pectin methylesterase.

The mean fruit firmness progressively decreased with increase in storage time (Table 2). This result is consistence with reports of Lahay et al. (2013) who found a reduction in firmness of fruits during prolonged storage periods. This could be due to high respiration rate and weight loss as supported by Cantwell et al. (2009).

Total soluble solids

The main effects of variety, harvesting stage and storage duration on mean total soluble solids (TSS) were highly significant (P<0.001); while all interaction effects were non-significant (P>0.05). The maximum TSS of 7.22 °Brix was recorded for Telmo-Red variety whereas the lowest (6.56 °Brix) was recorded for Velez-Yellow variety (Table 2). The mean TSS content of fruits harvested at 0, 25, 50, 75 and 100% colouration stages were 5.36, 6.40, 7.02, 7.63 and 8.03 °Brix, respectively. The maximum and minimum TSS contents were recorded at completely ripened and full green harvesting stages, respectively (Table 2). The mean TSS of fruits stored for 0, 1, 2, 3 and 4 weeks under PRS were 6.48, 6.88, 7.35, 7.07 and 6.66 °Brix, respectively. The highest and lowest TSS values were recorded at two weeks and zero week storage periods, respectively (Table 2).

The maximum TSS content was recorded in Telmo-Red variety which showed 0.66 °Brix higher than Velez-Yellow variety (Table 2). This is in agreement with the results of Bernardo et al. (2008) who reported that the value of TSS varied in magnitude between varieties of sweet pepper fruits. The observed TSS variation between varieties might be due to genetic or environmental factors as confirmed by Beckles (2012).

The level of TSS content progressively increased with increase in harvesting stage (Table 2). The Mean TSS in completely ripened fruits was 2.67 °Brix higher than those harvested at full green stage (Table 2). The TSS content in this study is in line with reports of Antoniali ° (2007) who found minimum and maximum TSS values in yellow sweet pepper fruits assessed at full green and completely ripened maturity stages, respectively. The increment in TSS might be due to disassociation of some molecules and structural enzymes in soluble compounds, which directly influence the levels of TSS.

TSS content was increased during the first two weeks storage under PRS followed by a decreasing trend with increase in storage duration (Table 2). This result is in agreement with reports of Rao et al. (2011) who found an increase in TSS as fruits were stored for short period followed by a decreasing trend during prolonged storage periods. The increment in TSS for stored fruits was probably due to increase of respiration and metabolic activity. In this regard, Ali et al. (2011) found that the higher respiration rate increases the synthesis and use of

Table 3. Interaction effect of variety and harvesting stage on mean titratable acidity of sweet pepper fruits stored under passive refrigeration system.

Variety	Titratable acidity (%)					
	Harvesting stage (%)					
	0	25	50	75	100	Mean
Telmo-Red	0.56^c	0.62^b	0.69^a	0.51^d	0.39^g	0.55
Velez-Yellow	0.43^f	0.45^e	0.51^d	0.36^g	0.29^h	0.41
Mean	0.49	0.54	0.60	0.43	0.34	
LSD$_{(0.05)}$			0.03			
CV (%)			7.58			

Means within a column followed by same letter(s) are not significantly different at 5% LSD test.

metabolites result in higher TSS due to the higher change from carbohydrates to sugars.

Titratable acidity

The interaction effect of variety and harvesting stage on mean titratable acidity (TA) was highly significant (P<0.001); while all other interaction effects were non-significant (P>0.05). For Telmo-Red variety, mean TA of fruits harvested at 0, 25, 50, 75 and 100% colouration stages were 0.56, 0.62, 0.69, 0.51 and 0.39%, respectively; while for Velez-Yellow variety, TA of fruits harvested at 0, 25, 50, 75 and 100% colouration stages were 0.43, 0.45, 0.51, 0.36 and 0.29%, respectively (Table 3).

TA values of fruits harvested at full green stage were 0.56 and 0.43% for Telmo-Red and Velez-Yellow varieties, respectively; the same results were apparent at other harvesting stages (Table 3). The highest and lowest TA values were recorded at combinations of Telmo-Red variety and harvested at 50% colouration as well as Velez-Yellow variety and harvested at completely ripened stage, respectively (Table 3).

For both varieties, the TA values of fruits harvested at 50 and 25% colouration stages were significantly higher than fruits harvested at other stages. There was an increasing trend in TA value until fruits attained their half ripening stage and thereafter decreased with increasing harvesting stages for both varieties (Table 3).

The results are in coherence with reports of Anthon et al. (2011) who found that TA of tomato fruits was increased with maturity stages and reached the peak at half ripening stage and thereafter started to decrease. The increment in TA value might be due to the presence of pectin methylesterase enzyme activity; while the reduction in TA of fruits harvested after half ripening stage could be due to high respiration rate and reduction in organic acids as supported by Anthon and Barrette (2012).

Postharvest decay percentage

The three-way interaction effect of variety, harvesting stage and storage duration on mean postharvest decay percentage of fruits under PRS was highly significant (P<0.001). At zero and one week storage periods, all fruits of both varieties were free from any postharvest decay across all harvesting stages. At two weeks of storage, mean PDP of Telmo-Red variety harvested at 0, 25, 50, 75 and 100% colouration stages were 1.63, 0.00, 0.20, 0.90 and 2.33%, respectively; similar trends were observed at three and four weeks under passive refrigeration system (Table 4). Postharvest decay percentages of Telmo-Red fruits harvested at full green stage were 1.63, 4.45 and 5.45 at 2, 3, and 4 weeks of storage, respectively; the same results were apparent at other harvesting stages (Table 4). Similarly, at two weeks of storage, mean postharvest decay percentage of Velez-Yellow variety harvested at 0, 25, 50, 75 and 100% colouration stages were 2.78, 1.16, 1.96, 2.44 and 3.35%, respectively; similar trends were observed at three and four weeks under passive refrigeration system (Table 4).

Postharvest decay percentage of Velez-Yellow sweet pepper fruits harvested at full green stage were 2.78, 5.89 and 7.20% at 2, 3, and 4 weeks, respectively; the same results were apparent at other harvesting stages (Table 4). Starting from two weeks storage period, the highest and lowest postharvest decay percentage were recorded at combinations of Velez-Yellow variety harvested at completely ripened stage and four weeks storage as well as Telmo-Red variety harvested at 25% colouration and two weeks storage under Passive Refrigeration System, respectively (Table 4).

Starting from two weeks of storage, PDP of both varieties harvested at all maturity stages was increased with increasing storage periods (Table 4). Starting from two weeks of storage, fruits of both varieties harvested at completely ripened and full green stages had significantly higher PDP than the other harvesting stages; however it was significantly lower for Telmo-Red variety (Table 4). The present findings are in conformity with reports of Ciccarese et al. (2013) who found that PDP in fruits harvested at completely ripened stage and stored for longer period of time was always higher than fruits harvesting at intermediate stages and stored for less time. Bayoumi (2008) concluded that the higher PDP in late harvesting stage of fruits was due to higher rate of respiration, more skin permeability for water loss and high susceptibility to decay. Moneruzzaman et al. (2009) also determined that fruit PDP increases when fruits are harvested at early matured stage due to poorly developed fruit cuticular wax layer. The increment in PDP during prolonged period of time could be due to the influence of high respiration rate, fruit senescence and enzymatic degradation of fruits' cell wall (Ciccarese et al., 2013).

Table 4. Interaction effect of variety, harvesting stage and storage duration on postharvest decay percentage of sweet pepper fruits stored under passive refrigeration system.

Variety	Harvesting stage (%)	Postharvest decay (%)					
		Storage duration (weeks)					
		0	1	2	3	4	Mean
Telmo-Red	0	0.00[v]	0.00[v]	1.63[rs]	4.45[g]	5.45[e]	2.31
	25	0.00[v]	0.00[v]	0.00[v]	1.39[st]	2.21[op]	0.72
	50	0.00[v]	0.00[v]	0.20[uv]	1.85[qr]	3.23[ij]	1.06
	75	0.00[v]	0.00[v]	0.90[u]	2.07[opq]	3.45[i]	1.28
	100	0.00[v]	0.00[v]	2.33[mo]	4.77[f]	7.30[b]	2.88
	Mean	0	0	1.01	2.91	4.33	
Velez-Yellow	0	0.00[v]	0.00[v]	2.78[kl]	5.89[d]	7.20[b]	3.17
	25	0.00[v]	0.00[v]	1.16[tu]	2.57[lm]	2.94[jk]	1.33
	50	0.00[v]	0.00[v]	1.96[pq]	2.87[k]	3.89[h]	1.74
	75	0.00[v]	0.00[v]	2.44[mn]	3.27[i]	4.45[g]	2.03
	100	0.00[v]	0.00[v]	3.35[i]	6.49[c]	8.38[a]	3.64
	Mean	0.00	0.00	2.34	4.22	5.37	
LSD$_{(0.05)}$				0.29			
CV (%)				8.95			

Means within a column followed by same letter(s) are not significantly different at 5% LSD test.

Table 5. Interaction effect of harvesting stage and storage duration on mean shelf life of sweet pepper fruits stored under passive refrigeration system.

Harvesting stage (%)	Shelf life (days)					
	Storage duration (weeks)					
	0	1	2	3	4	Mean
0	11.17[r]	14.00[no]	19.85[l]	26.32[h]	30.17[de]	20.30
25	14.00[no]	16.17[m]	24.84[i]	31.00[d]	36.00[a]	24.40
50	13.34[p]	15.83[m]	23.31[j]	29.50[ef]	34.00[b]	23.20
75	12.33[q]	14.52[n]	21.50[k]	28.00[g]	33.00[c]	21.87
100	9.67[s]	13.00[pq]	19.00[l]	24.82[i]	29.00[f]	19.10
Mean	12.10	14.70	21.70	27.93	32.43	
LSD$_{(0.05)}$			0.99			
CV (%)			3.97			

Means within a column followed by same letter(s) are not significantly different at 5% LSD test.

Shelf life

The interaction effect of harvesting stage and storage duration on mean overall shelf life (shelf life under PRS plus after being transferred to room temperature) of sweet pepper fruits was highly significant (P<0.001); while all other interaction effects were non-significant (P>0.05). At zero week of storage, mean shelf life of fruits harvested at 0, 25, 50, 75 and 100% colouration were 11.17, 14.00, 13.34, 12.33 and 9.67 days, respectively; similar trends were observed at other storage periods (Table 5). Mean shelf life of fruits harvested at full green

stage were 11.17, 14.00, 19.85, 26.32 and 30.17 days stored for 0, 1, 2, 3 and 4 weeks under PRS, respectively; the same results were apparent at other harvesting stages (Table 5). The maximum and minimum overall shelf lives were recorded at combinations of harvested at 25% colouration stage and four weeks storage under PRS as well as harvested at completely ripened stage and zero week storage under PRS, respectively (Table 5).

Across all storage periods, the shelf life of fruits harvested at 25 and 50% colourations were significantly higher than fruits harvested at full green and late harvesting stages

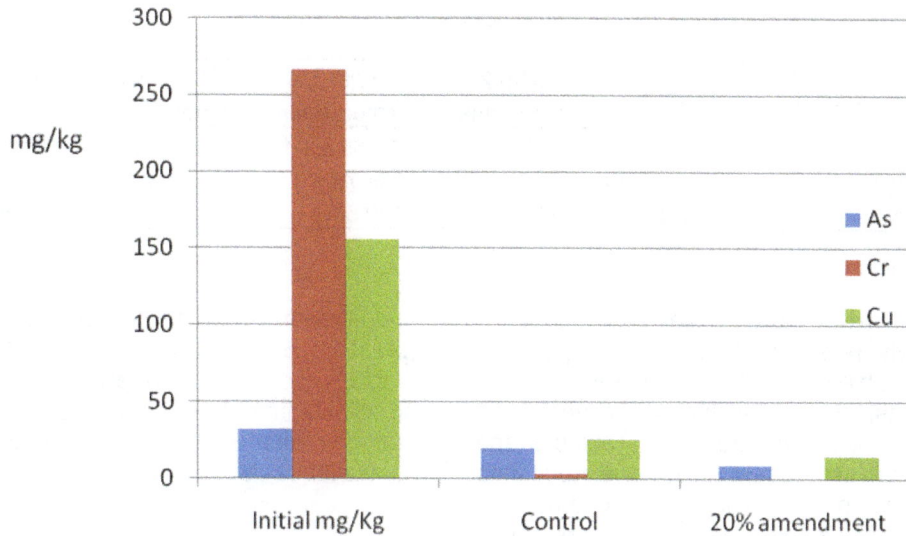

Figure 1. Shows percentage uptake after 20 days of phytoremediation.

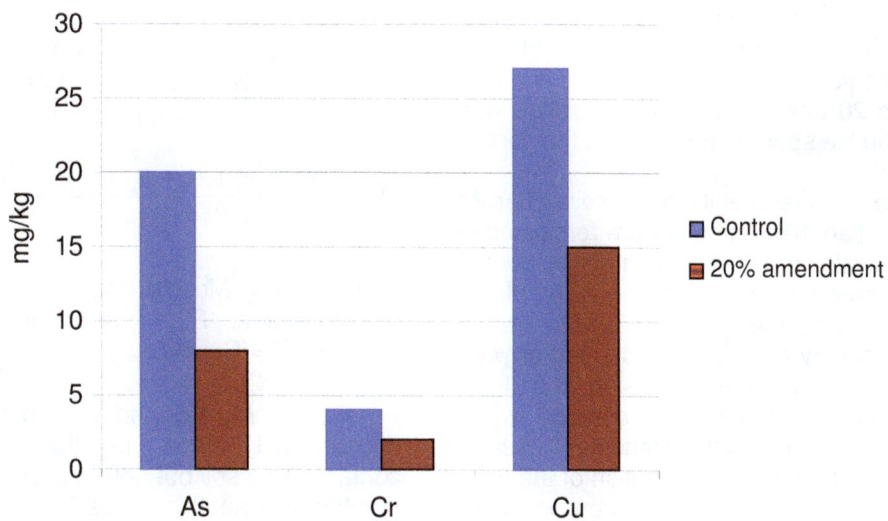

Figure 2. Shows the uptake of the metals by maize plant in both control and soil with 20% amendment.

Equation 2 if calculated). This made it to be highly labile and bioavailable and consequently more dangerous than the other two metals.

Figure 1 compares the percentage uptake of the metals in mg/kg after 20 days of cleanup between the control and soil with 20% amendment. More metals were taken up by plants in the control pots than in the pots with 20% amendment. This results in the plants in the control pots dying before the plants in the pots with amendment.

Figure 2 compares the uptake of the different metals (As, Cr and Cu) after 20 days of phytoremediation in mg/kg between the control and soil with 20% amendment. In both the control pots and in pots with 20%

amendment, copper had the highest uptake. This was followed by arsenic while chromium has the least uptake.

Conclusion

Our studies show that there is a relative advantage in the use of cow dung as soil amendment prior to phyto-remediation of CCA contaminated soil as the plants in soils with amendment out lived those in soil without amendment. Consequently more clean up is expected from living plants than dead plants. Cu and Cr were present in appreciable quantities as organic and residual

Table 9. Total residual metals in soils after 20 days of phytoremediation.

Metals (mg/Kg)	Control	With 2% amendment	With 5% amendment	With 10% amendment	With 20% amendment
Arsenic	25.20 ± 0.00	26.96 ± 1.60	26.65 ± 1.10	26.42 ± 1.20	28.03 ± 1.00
Chromium	252.60 ± 2.40	255.91 ± 3.90	254.78 ± 3.00	254.30 ± 1.30	255.18 ±1.40
Copper	115.30 ± 1.10	120.70 ± 1.00	122.56 ± 1.90	123.80 ± 0.80	126.40 ±1.00

bound. They are thus not bioavailable to plants. They could only be slowly released through decomposition. Apart from arsenic (Table 5) which recorded reductions in the organic fractions, the other metals recorded an increase in the value of organic fractions (Tables 5 and 6). This indicates that the metals must have gone into reactions with organic materials in the amendment to form complexes which are not soluble rendering them unavailable for plant consumption. Bounding of metals is also a method of soil remediation. The slow release through decomposition of these toxic metals to plants also gives the plants a longer lease of life when compared with the control plants. The plants in the control pot experiment were dying before the expiration of the 20 days experimental period (pictures not shown). As a matter of fact, the 20 days experimental duration was adopted based on the life span of the plants in the control pots.

Table 9 shows the residual metals in the soils after 20 days of phytoremediation. More metals were remaining in pots with different levels of amendment than in control pots indicating that more metals were taken up by plants in control pots (no amendment). Plant growth in the control pots were generally retarded with stunted growth, yellowing of leaves, reduced leaf expansion and dying before the expiration of the 20 days duration when compared to the plants in pots with amendment (picture not shown). This is due to heavy consumption of the toxic metals, while those in the pots with amendment were still alive. The increase in the values of pH, CEC and OM especially at 20% amendment level (Table 1) occasioned by the addition of cow dung amendment did more to bound the metals than make them available for plant uptake. The metals bioavailability of soil depends to a large extent on their distribution between solid and solution phase, which in turn is dependent on soil processes like CEC, OM, and pH. The effect of organic matter amendments on heavy metal solubility depend greatly upon the degree of humification of their OM and their effect upon soil pH (Walker et al., 2003). In general, the concentration of an element in the soil solution is believed to depend on the equilibrium between the soil solution and solid phase, with pH playing the decisive role (Lindsay, WL 1979). The soil's ability to immobilize heavy metals increases with rising pH and peaks under mildly alkaline conditions. Heavy metal mobility is related to their immobilization in the solid phase. (Fuller, WH 1979), in discussing the relatively high mobility of heavy metals with regard to pH, considered that in acid soils (pH 4.2 - 6.6), the elements Cd, Ni, and Zn are highly mobile, Cr is moderately mobile, and Cu and Pb practically immobile. Copper is especially tightly held by organic matter occasioned by the addition of amendment. Its availability is low.

Mobility of arsenic, chromium and copper in the CCA contaminated soil

The bioavailability/mobility of metals in soils is assessed on the basis of absolute and relative content of fractions weakly bound to soil components. The relative index of metal mobility was calculated as a "mobility factor" (Cezary and Bal, 2001) using the equation below:

$$M_f = \frac{F_1 + F_2 + F_3}{F_1 + F_2 + F_3 + F_4 + F_5 + F_6} \times \frac{100}{1} \qquad (2)$$

Where: M_f = Mobility factor, F_1 = Soluble form, F_2 = Exchangeable, F_3 = Carbonate, F_4 = Fe-Mn, F_5 = Organic, F_6 = Residual.

F_1, F_2, F_3, F_4, F_5, and F_6 represents the percentage geochemical forms of the metals in the CCA contaminated soil but here corrected to the nearest whole numbers (Table 4). Values from Table 4 when applied to Equation 2 above, assigned mobility factor (M_f) values of 60 for arsenic, 19 for chromium and 8 for copper.

Metal forms bound to carbonate fractions F_3 are relatively less mobile and soluble than exchangeable fractions.

The result shows that arsenic is potentially mobile and biologically available because of its high M_f value of 60. High M_f values are symptoms of relatively high liability and biological availability of heavy metals in soils (Ahumada et al., 1999; Karczewska, 1996). Chromium is relatively mobile with M_f value of 19 while the mobility of copper is low with an M_f value of 8. The high $M_{f.}$ of As may be attributed to the low organic matter of the soil (Rahman et al., 2004). The organic matter of the soil is 2.5%. The use of a modified Tessier et al. sequential extraction procedure by Salbu and Oughton (1998). (six steps) which partitioned the metals As, Cr and Cu among six operationally defined fractions: F_1 (water soluble), F_2 (exchangeable), F_3 (carbonate), F_4 (Fe-Mn), F_5 (organic)

stages (Table 5). The present results are in line with the findings of Dilmacunal et al. (2011) who observed that tomato fruits harvested at breaker stage had a better storability potential under cold storage than the unripe and full red fruits. This could be due to the high weight loss percentage and respiration rate of completely ripened fruits and lack of a well developed fruit cuticular wax layer at full green stage which in turn might have resulted in lower shelf life. Moreover, the increasing trend in overall shelf life of fruits during prolonged storage period might be due to the presence of the new, modern and innovative passive refrigeration system storage equipment. This reality is supported by Shen et al. (2013) who found that refrigeration is used to reduce spoilage and extend the shelf life of fresh fruit by slowing down the metabolism and reducing fruit deterioration.

Conclusion

The postharvest quality and shelf life of sweet pepper fruits was affected by varieties, harvesting stage and storage duration. TSS content was increased while fruit firmness decreased with increasing harvesting stages. Weight loss percentage, postharvest decay and overall shelf life were found to increase; whereas fruit firmness declined correspondingly with increasing storage periods. The present results showed that Telmo-Red variety harvested at 25 and 50% harvesting stages and stored under Passive Refrigeration System storage condition could maintain better postharvest quality and extend their shelf life for more than one month.

REFERENCES

Agonafir Y (1991). Economics of horticultural production in Ethiopia. International symposium on horticultural economics in developing countries. Acta Hortic. 270:15-19.

Ali A, Muhammad M, Sijam K, Siddiqui Y (2011). Effect of chitosan coating on the physicochemical characteristics of Eksotika II papaya (Carica papaya L.) fruit during cold storage. J. Food Chem. 124:620-625.

Anthon E, Barrette M (2012). Pectin Methylesterase activity and other factors affecting pH and titratable acidity in processing tomatoes. J. Food Chem. 132:915-920.

Anthon E, Lestrange M, Barrett M (2011). Changes in pH, acids, sugars and other quality parameters during extended vine holding of ripe processing tomatoes. J. Sci. Food Agric. 93:98-109.

Antoniali S, Paulo M, Ana-Maria M, Rogerio T, Juliana S (2007). Physicochemical characterization of 'zarco hs' yellow bell pepper for different ripeness stages. J. Sci. Food Agric. 64:19-22.

Association of Official Analytical Chemists (AOAC) (2007). Official Methods of Analysis of the Association of Official Analytical Chemists International. In:Horwitz, W. (Ed.), 17th ed., AOAC Press, Arlington, VA, USA.

Bayoumi Y (2008). Improvement of postharvest keeping quality of white

pepper fruits (Capsicum annuum L.) by hydrogen peroxide treatment under storage conditions. Acta Biologica Szegediensis, 52:7-15.

Beckles M (2012). Factors affecting the postharvest soluble solids and sugar content of tomato (Solanum lycopersicum L.) fruit. J. Postharvest Biol. Technol. 63:129-140.

Bernardo A, Martinez S, Alvarez M, Fernandez A, Lopez A (2008). The composition of two Spanish pepper varieties in different ripening stages. J. Food Qual. 31:701-716.

Cantwell M, Nie X, Hong G (2009). Impact of storage conditions on grape tomato quality. ISHS Postharvest Symposium, 6th ed. Antalya, Turkey.

Ciccarese A, Stellacci M, Gentilesco G, Rubino P (2013). Effectiveness of pre- and post-veraison calcium applications to control decay and maintain table grape fruit quality during storage. J. Postharvest Biol. Technol. 75:135-141.

Dilmacunal T, Koyuncu A, Bayindir D (2011). Effects of Several Postharvest Treatments on Shelf Life Quality of Bunch Tomatoes. J. Not Bot. Hortic Agrobo 39(2):209-213.

El-Mougy S, Abdel-Kader M, Aly H (2012). Effect of a new chemical formula on postharvest decay incidence in citrus Fruit. J. Plant Protect. Res. 52(1):156-164.

Ilic S, Trajkovic R, Pavlovic R, Alkalai-Tuvia S, Perzelan Y, Fallik E (2012). Effect of heat treatment and individual shrink packaging on quality and nutritional value of bell pepper stored at suboptimal temperature. Int. J. Food Sci.Technol. 47:83-90.

Lahay M, Devauxa F, Poole M, Seymour B, Causse M (2013). Pericarp tissue microstructure and cell wall polysaccharide chemistry are differently affected in lines of tomato with contrasted firmness. J. Postharvest Bio. Technol. 76:83-90.

Manolopoulou H, Xanthopoulos G, Douros N, Lambrinos G (2010). Modified atmosphere packaging storage of green bell peppers: Quality criteria. J. Bio-Syst. Eng.106:535-543.

Maria S, Zapata P, Castillo S, Guillen F, Martinez-Romero D 2010. Antioxidant and nutritive constituents during sweet pepper development and ripening are enhanced by nitrophenolate treatments. J. Food Chem.118:497-503.

Marin A, Ferreres F, Tomas-Barberan F, Gil M (2004). Characterization and quantitation of antioxidant constituents of sweet pepper (Capsicum annuum L.). J. Agric. Food Chem. 52:3861-3869.

Melaku K, ElkindY, Leikin-Frenkel A, Lurie S, Fallik E (2006). The relationship between water loss, lipid content, membrane integrity and LOX activity in ripe pepper fruit after storage. J. Postharvest Biol. Technol. 42:248-255.

Moneruzzaman M, Hossain S, Sani W, Saifuddin M, Alenazi M (2009). Effect of harvesting and storage conditions on the post harvest quality of tomato (Lycopersicon esculentum Mill) cv. Roma VF. Australian J. Crop Sci. 3(2):113-121.

Nomos (2008). From farms to markets. Providing know-how and finance. International conference on sharing innovative agribusiness solutions. Cairo, Egypt.

Rao R, Gol B, Shah K (2011). Effect of postharvest treatments and storage temperatures on the quality and shelf life of sweet pepper. Sci. Hortic.132:18-26.

Shen Y, Sun Y, Qiao L, Chen J, Liu D, Ye X (2013). Effect of UV-C treatments on phenolic compounds and antioxidant capacity of minimally processed Satsuma mandarin during refrigerated storage. J. Postharvest Biol.Technol. 76:50-57.

Tunde-Akintunde T, Afolabi T, Akintunde B (2005). Influence of drying methods on drying of sweet bell pepper (Capsicum annuum). J. Food Eng. 68:439-442.

Zhou R, Li Y, Yan L, Xie J (2011). Effect of edible coatings on enzymes, cell membrane integrity and cell-wall constituents in relation to brittleness and firmness of Huanghua pears (Pyrus pyrifolia Nakai) during storage. J. Food Chem. 124:569-575.

13

Studies of wine produced from banana (*Musa Sapientum*)

Idise, Okiemute Emmanuel* and Odum, Edward Ikenna

Department of Microbiology, Delta State University, Abraka, Delta State, Nigeria.

Banana, a wonderfully sweet fruit with firm and creamy flesh that come prepackaged in a yellow jacket, available for harvest throughout the year consists mainly of sugars and fibers which make it a source of immediate and slightly prolonged energy. When consumed, reduces depression, anemia, blood pressure, stroke risk, heartburns, ulcers, stress, constipation and diarrhea. It confers protection for eyesight, healthy bones, kidney malfunctions, morning sickness, itching and swelling, improves nerve functions as well as help people trying to give up smoking. Fermentation of banana must for 144 h was carried out using recipes A to D. Recipe A contained a mixture of banana must with natural yeast. A was enhanced with granulated sugar to obtain recipe B. Recipe C contained recipe A augmented with granulated sugar and bakers' yeast while recipe D (control) contained only granulated sugar solution and bakers' yeast. Wine produced had values that ranged from 31.4 ± 0.29 to $33.2 \pm 0.12°C$ for temperature, 3.38 ± 0.017 to 3.54 ± 0.052 for pH, 0.999 ± 0.0085 to 1.02 ± 0.0058 for specific gravity, 0.586 ± 0.018 to 0.71 ± 0.017 for optical gravity, 1.37 ± 0.075 to 1.383 ± 0.152 for percentage (%) alcohol (v/v), 0.271 versus 0.012 to 1.348 ± 0.072 for percentage (%) titratable acidity, 8.2 ± 0.099 to 9.38 ± 0.283 for total aerobic counts and 3.5 ± 0.5 to 4.75 ± 0.1 for R_f. Malo-lactic fermentation after 48 h was evident. Taste testing showed very little differences in wines from recipes A to C. Statistical analyses of tested parameters at 95% confidence level showed no significant differences. The wine from the control was similar to natural palm wine in taste and characteristics. Wine could thus be produced from banana for immediate consumption, within 48 h, using the recipes A to C.

Key words: Banana, flora, fermentation, sugar, wine, flavor, yeast.

INTRODUCTION

Banana (*Musa Sapientum*) is a fruit common in the tropics and is non-seasonal. It is readily available in Nigeria. Due to its high sugar content, it is suitable for the production of wine (Robinson, 2006). Depending upon cultivar and ripeness, the flesh can vary in taste from starchy to sweet and texture from firm to mushy. Both skin and inner part can be eaten raw or cooked. Bananas' flavor is due, amongst other chemicals, to isoamyl acetate which is one of the main constituents of banana oil. Wine is an alcoholic beverage typically made from fermented fruit juice. Any fruit with a good proportion of

sugar may be used for wine production and the resulting wines are normally named after the fruit hence banana, apple, orange, pineapple, strawberries and coconut may be used to produce wine. The type of fruit wine to be produced dictates the fruit and strain of yeast to be involved (Alexander and Charpenter, 2004). Wine production has not been a major market in Nigeria although institutions such as NIFOR (Nigerian Institute for oil palm research) have been involved in production of bottled palm wine using chemical preservatives. Bioaccumulation of chemical preservatives poses potential dangers due to either toxicity or pro-toxicity (Idise and Izuagbe, 1988; Svans, 2008). It is thus pertinent to search for means of producing wines devoid of chemical additives. Banana possesses desirable qualities - high fiber-content which helps restore normal

---
*Corresponding author. E-mail: emmaidise@yahoo.com.

Table 1. Composition of the recipes.

Recipe	Composition
A	1.5 L of fruit slurry + 6.0 L of water.
B	1.5 L of fruit slurry + 6.0 L of sugar solution.
C	1.5 L of fruit slurry + 6.0 L of sugar solution + bakers' yeast.
D	7.5 L of sugar solution + bakers' yeast.

Table 2. Changes in pH with period of fermentation.

Time (h)	A	B	C	D
1	4.3	4.2	4.1	4.0
24	3.4	3.3	3.4	3.4
48	3.3	3.2	3.4	3.5
72	3.4	3.1	3.4	3.4
144	3.3	3.1	3.4	3.3

bowl action, stimulates the production of hemoglobin in the blood, contains potassium and has a low salt content which helps to lower blood pressure as well as control stroke and when consumed along with other fruits and vegetables, banana was observed to be associated with reduced risk of colorectal cancer (Deneo-Pellegrini et al., 1996) and in women, breast cancer (Zhang, 2009) and renal cell carcinoma (Rashidkhani et al., 2005).

According to Uraih and Izuagbe (1990), eating banana as a regular diet can cut the risk of death by stroke as much as 40%. Thus, a wine produced from banana is a worthwhile venture. This study was aimed at small-scale wine production with desirable organoleptic properties from banana for immediate consumption without chemical preservatives.

MATERIALS AND METHODS

Collection of materials

Ripe banana fruits (*M. Sapientum*), sugar and baker's yeast were purchased from Abraka market in Delta State, Nigeria. The fruits were identified at the Botany Department of the Delta State University, Abraka prior to analyses. These were washed with tap water in the laboratory and allowed to air dry.

Preparation of sugar solution

Clean water was boiled for 5 min and allowed to cool. One (1) teacup-full of granulated sugar was dissolved in 1 L of water to obtain the sugar solution.

Preparation of must juice

The method of Uraih (2003) was employed.

Fermentation of orange juice (must)

This was carried out in duplicates according to the method of Uraih (2003) with some modifications (Table 1).

Determination of physico-chemical and microbial parameters

These were carried out in accordance with standard methods reported by Ogunkoye and Olubayo (1977), Kunkee and Amerine (2002), Cowan and Steel (2004) and Fawole and Oso (2008).

Organoleptic evaluation

This was carried out in accordance with the procedure reported by Maragatham and Panneerselvam (2011). The sensory evaluation was done using 8 judge panels after aging for 24 h. Observations recorded for color, clarity, body and taste on a 5 point scale with 5 points for excellent quality and 1 point for bad quality.

Statistical analyses

These were carried out using Microsoft excel 1995 to 2003 at 95% confidence level.

RESULTS AND DISCUSSION

The changes in pH of the banana wines during fermentation are presented in Table 2. It was observed that the pH values reduced with period of fermentation apparently due to the production of acids from the mixed fermentation as well as the microbes in a microbial succession. A malo-lactic fermentation is evident. This result agrees with reports of Robinson (2006) and Okafor (2007). The changes in optical density of the banana wines during fermentation are presented in Figure 1. Increases in values with period of fermentation were

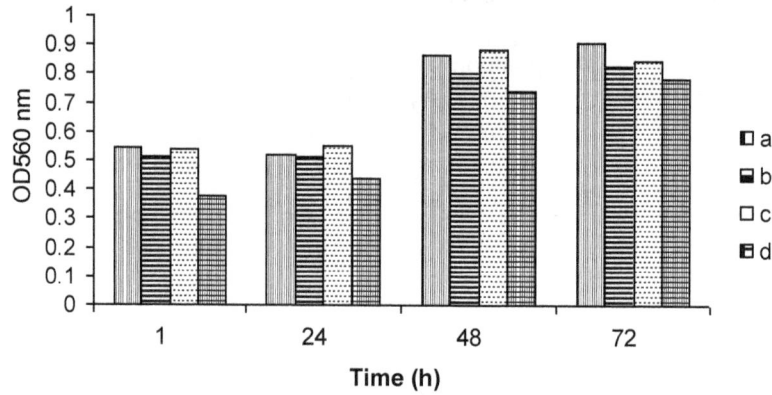

Figure 1. Changes in optical density of banana wine.

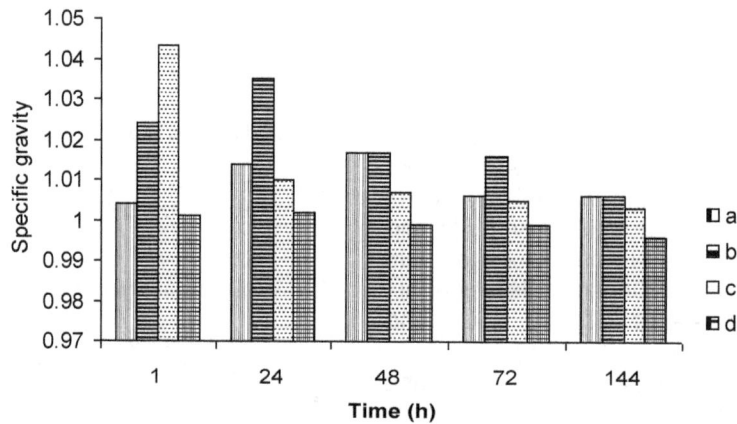

Figure 2. Changes in specific gravity of banana wine.

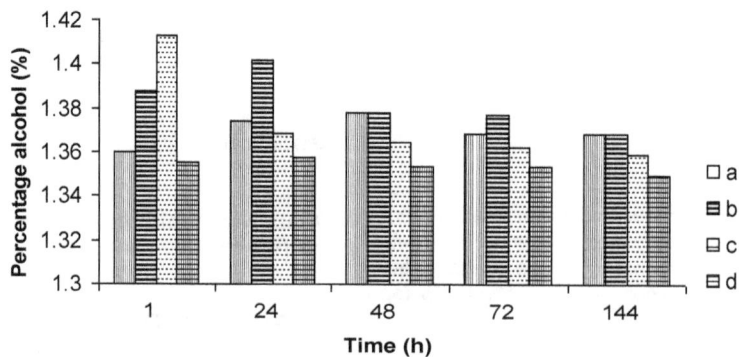

Figure 3. Changes in percentage (%) alcohol of banana wine.

observed apparently due to increasing microbial load with period of fermentation. This result agrees with reports of Amerine and Kunkee (2002) and Okafor (2007). The changes in specific gravity of the banana wines during fermentation are presented in Figure 2. It was observed that values decreased with period of fermentation. This could be due to microbial utilization of nutrients (primarily sugars) in the juice for metabolic activities with the evolution of CO_2 and heat. This result agrees with reports of Uraih (2003) and Okafor (2007). The changes in percentage (%) alcohol (v/v) of the banana wines during fermentation are presented in Figure 3. It was observed

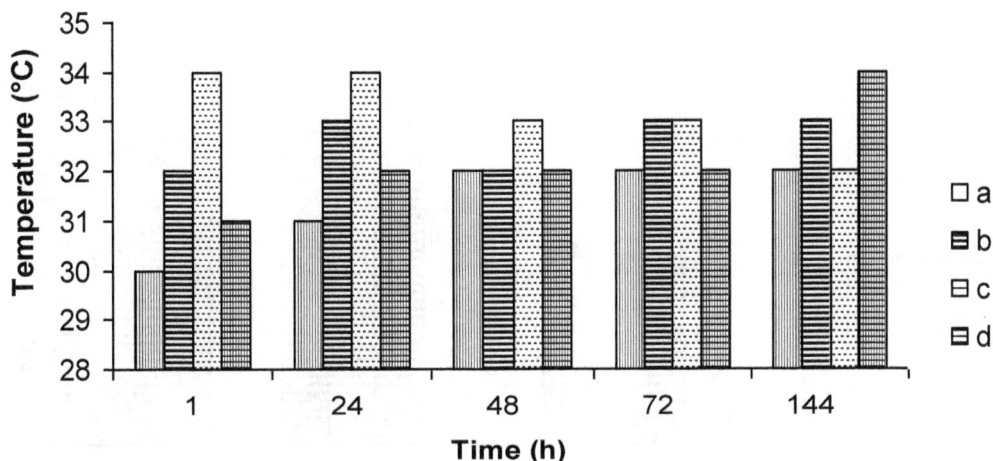

Figure 4. Changes in temperature of banana wine.

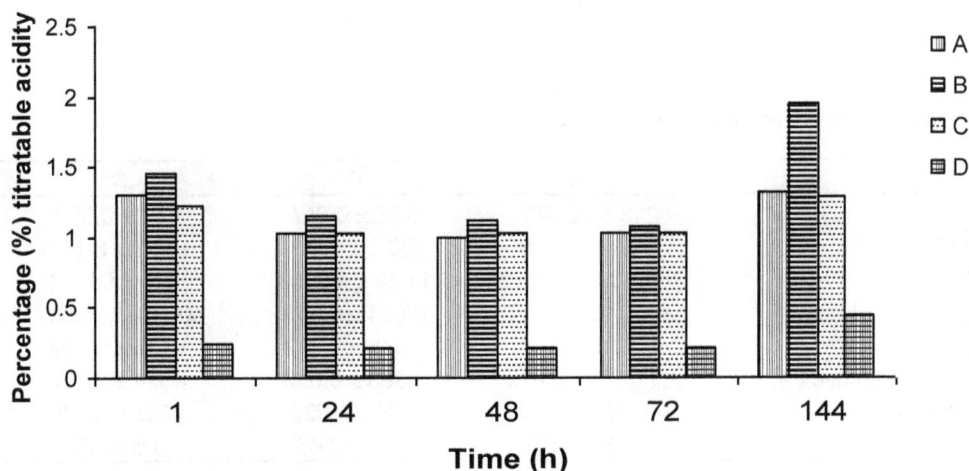

Figure 5. Changes in percentage (%) titratable acidity of banana wine.

that recipe C which was augmented with granulated sugar and bakers' yeast, within 1 h of fermentation had 1.413% compared to 1.360, 1.388 and 1.355% for recipes A, B and D respectively. This could be as a result of mixed fermentation by natural yeast and bakers' yeast. This result agrees with the reports of Wang et al. (2009).

The changes in temperature of the banana wines during fermentation are presented in Figure 4. It was observed that a mean temperature of 32.35°C was recorded from all the recipes. The observed mean temperature could be due to the heat generated during microbial metabolism. This result agrees with the reports of Okafor (2007). The changes in percentage (%) titratable acidity of the banana wines during fermentation are presented in Figure 5. It was observed that the titratable acidity of the recipes decreased up to 48 h of fermentation and thereafter increased with period of fermentation.

fermentation. This could be due to the presence of a malo-lactic fermentation arising from succession of the yeast cells by lactic acid bacteria after 48 h of fermentation. The presence of a malo-lactic fermentation is a desirable phenomenon in wine production due to the attendant buttery flavor. This result agrees with reports of Idise and Izuagbe (1988), Robinson (2006) and Okafor (2007). The changes in microbial load of the banana wines during fermentation are presented in Figure 6. It was observed that recipe C had higher microbial load than other recipes within 1 h of fermentation. This result supports those observed for Figures 4 and 5 and agrees with reports of Uraih (2003), Amerine and Kunkee (2002) and Okafor (2007). The average values of parameters of the various banana wines are presented in Table 3. Recipe B, which was the natural fermentation augmented with sugar produced wine with highest alcohol while

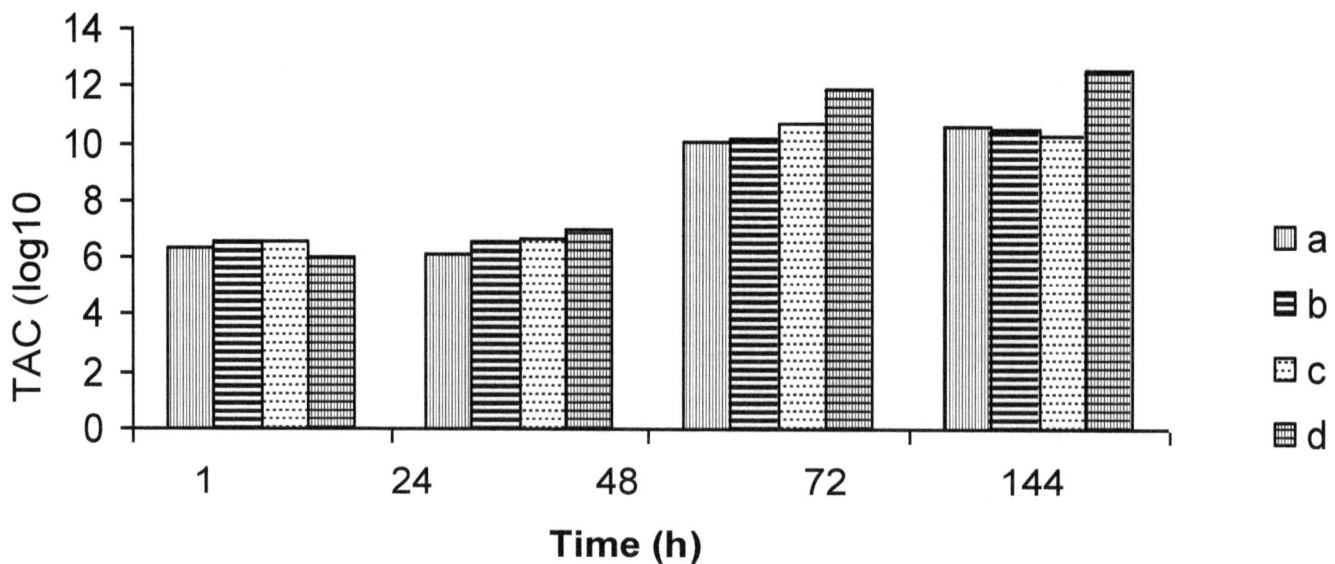

Figure 6. Changes in total aerobic counts of banana wine.

Table 3. Average values of parameters of the various banana wines.

Parameters	A	B	C	D
pH	3.5 ±0.029	3.38 ± 0.017	3.54 ± 0.052	3.52 ± 0.012
Temperature (°C)	31.4 ± 0.29	32.6 ± 0.17	33.2 ± 0.12	32.2 ± 0.35
Specific gravity	1.009 ± 0.0012	1.020 ± 0.0058	1.014 ± 0.0035	0.999 ± 0.0085
Optical density	0.710 ± 0.017	0.664 ± 0.057	0.704 ± 0.008	0.586 ± 0.018
Titratable acidity	1.33 ± 0.05	1.348 ± 0.072	1.115 ± 0.002	0.271 ± 0.012
Alcoholic content percentage (%) (v/v)	1.370 ± 0.075	1.383 ± 0.052	1.374 ± 0.152	1.354 ± 0.014
Microbial load cfu/ml	8.283 ± 0.099	8.20 ± 0.029	8.563 ± 0.126	9.38 ± 0.283
R_f values (cm)	4.75 ± 0.25	3.95 ± 0.65	3.5 ± 0.5	4.1 ± 0.1

Ho accepted as f-cal (0.083649) < f-crit (3.738892).

recipe D, which was sugar solution pitched with baker's yeast produced wine with the lowest percentage (%) alcohol.

The R_f values (cm) at 144 h of fermentation were within the reported values for lactic acid thus supporting the occurrence of a malo-lactic fermentation. Null hypothesis of significant difference was accepted as f-cal (0.83649) was less than f-crit (3.738892). These results agree with the reports of Ogunkoye and Olubayo (1977) and Idise and Izuagbe (1988). The changes in the physical and organoleptic properties of the various banana wines during fermentation are presented in Table 4. It was observed that while wines that received banana fruit must were creamy in color, the wine produced from sugar solution and baker's yeast had similar color and flavor with palm wine. This latter could form the basis for artificial palm wine production either on a small- or medium-scale. These results agree with reports by Idise

and Izuagbe (1988), Uraih (2003) and Okafor (2007). The microcopy of yeast cells from the various recipes after 72 h of fermentation showed no significant differences between the yeast cells of the fermenting broths. It could be inferred that the wild yeast present in the banana wines could be of the same *Saccharomyces* species with the baker's yeast. These results are in agreement with the reports of Idise and Izuagbe (1985), Kunkee and Amerine (2002), Robinson (2006) and Okafor (2007).

CONCLUSION AND RECOMMENDATIONS

There is the possibility of banana wine production using various recipes and the flow chart in our homes for immediate consumption within 48 h without addition of chemical preservatives. There was evidence of Malo-lactic fermentation. The wines produced showed no

Table 4. Physical and organoleptic properties of the various banana wines.

Recipe	Time (h)	Sweetness	Color	Sediments	Frothing
A	1	+	Cream	-	++
	24	-	Dirty cream	+	++
	48	-	Dirty cream	+	+
	72	-	Dirty cream	+	-
	144	-	Cream	+	-
B	1	++	Cream	-	++
	24	+	Dirty cream	+	++
	48	-	Dirty cream	+	+
	72	-	Dirty cream	+	-
	144	-	Cream	+	-
C	1	++	Cream	-	++
	24	+	Dirty cream	+	++
	48	-	Dirty cream	+	+
	72	-	Dirty cream	+	-
	144	-	Cream	+	-
D	1	++	Colorless	-	-
	24	+	White	-	-
	48	-	White	-	-
	72	-	Colorless	+	-
	144	-	Colorless	+	-

appreciable differences in the tested parameters – pH, temperature, optical density, specific gravity, total aerobic counts, percentage (%) alcohol (v/v) and percentage (%) titratable acidity – taste-testing as well as statistically at 95% confidence level. However, there is the need for further research to ascertain the shelf life of the wines.

REFERENCES

Alexander H, Charpenter C (2004). Biochemical Aspect of Stunk and Sluggish Fermentation in Grape Must. J. Ind. Microbiol. Biotechnol., 20: 20-27.

Amerine MA, Kunkee RE (2002). Microbiology of Wine Making. Ann. Rev. Microbiol., 2: 232-258.

Cowan ST, Steel KJ (2004). Manual for the Identification of Medical Bacteria (3rd ed.). Cambridge University Press. London. p. 331.

Idise OE, Izuagbe YS (1988). Microbial and chemical changes in bottled palm wine during storage. Nig. J. Microbiol. 8(1): 175-184

Kunkee RF, Amerine MA (2002). Yeast in Wine Making. In: Rose, H.A and Harrison, J.S. (Edn). The Yeast. Academic Press, London. pp. 5-71.

Maragatham C, Panneerselvam A (2011). Isolation, identification and characterization of wine yeast from rotten papaya fruits for wine production. Adv. Appl. Sci. Res., 2(2): 93-98.

Ogunkoye L, Olubayo O (1977). Basic Organic Practical. 2nd Ed. University of Ife, Ile-Ife printing press. p. 240.

Okafor N (2007). Modern Industrial Microbiology and Biotechnology (1st Edn). Science Publishers, Enfield, New Hampshire. p. 530.

Rashidkhani B, Lindblad P, Wolk A (2005). Fruits, Vegetables and Risk of renal cell carcinoma a prospective study of Swedish women. Int. J. Cancer, 113(3): 451-455.

Robinson J (2006). The Oxford Companion to wine (3rd Edn.), Oxford University Press, USA. p. 840.

Uraih N (2003). Public Health, Food and Industrial Microbiology. (6th Edn.). The Macmillan Press Ltd., London. pp. 196-198.

Uraih N, Izuagbe YS (1990). Public Health, food and industrial Microbiology. University of Benin Press Ltd., Benin-City. p. 373.

Svans P (2008). Preservatives in wine and why we need them. Available at http://ezinearticles.com.

Wang J, Guo L, Zhao G (2009).Whey Alcohol Fermentation with mixed yeast cultures. Int. conf. Bioinforma. Biomed. Eng., 3(11): 1-6.

Zhang CX (2009). Greater vegetable and fruit intake is associated with lower risk of breast cancer among Chinese women. Int. J. Cancer, 124(1): 181-188.

14

Screening of different insect pests of mulberry and other agricultural crops for microsporidian infection

Ifat Bashir[1]*, S. D. Sharma[2] and Shabir A. Bhat[3]

[1]Additional Directorate of Sericulture Development Department, Tulsi Bagh,
Srinagar- 190 001 (J&K), India.
[2]Central Sericultural Research and Training Institute Srirampura Mysore- 570008, India.
[3]Division of Sericulture, Mirgund, Sher-e-Kashmir University of Agricultural Sciences and Technology of Kashmir, Post
Box: 674,GPO Srinagar- 190001, India.

In the present study, different insect pests of mulberry and other agricultural crops were collected from mulberry gardens and agricultural crop fields in and around Mysore, Karnataka, India. The collected insects were screened for microsporidian infection and microsporidian spores were isolated from infected specimens, purified and tentatively designated as NIK- 1Pr, NIK- 1Cc, NIK- 1Cpy, NIK- 1So and NIK- 1Dp. The serological affinity test carried out through monoclonal and polyclonal antibodies, showed negative reaction of these microsporidia which indicated that these are niether *Nosema bombycis* nor Lb_{ms}..

Key words: Agricultural crops, mulberry, pests, microsporidia, monoclonal and polyclonal antibodies.

INTRODUCTION

In the silkworm *Bombyx mori* L, the disease caused by the microsporidian infection is called microsporidiosis and it is commonly known as pebrine. It has been reported long back in silkworm and is caused by an endoparasite, *Nosema bombycis*. The disease has become more complex because in addition to the *N. bombycis* several other species/strains of the microsporidians have been isolated from silkworm (Ananthalakashmi et al., 1994; Bhat and Nataraju, 2004; Selvakumar et al., 2005) and from other insects (Kishore et al., 1994; Kawarabata, 2003). Microsporidia have been found to be the common pathogens infecting insects under natural field conditions (Tanada and Kaya, 1993). Over 100 spp. of microsporidia have been described from insects and these include 40 *Nosema* spp. from different insects (Steinhaus, 1949). Infection due to N. bombycis has also been recorded in the insect orders Diptera (45 species), Lepidoptera (25 species), Ephermeroptera (13 species), Hymenoptera (6 species), Trichoptera (3 species), Coleoptera (2 species), Isoptera (2 species), Plecoptera (2 species) and one species in each of the following orders: Anoplura,

Hemiptera, Odonata, Siphonoptera and Thysanura (Steinhaus, 1949).

Natural infection with *N. bombycis* has been reported in several lepidopteran insects such as *Pieris rapae* (Pieridae), *Spodoptera deparvata* (Noctuidae), *Spodoptera exigua* (Noctuidae), *Spodoptera litura* (Noctuidae) and *Trichoplusia ni* (Noctuidae). The mulberry pyralid, *Diaphania pulverulentalis* (Pyralidae) is also known to harbour *N. bombycis* (Sharma et al., 2003).

The present study has been undertaken with an aim to screen different insect pests of mulberry and some other agricultural crops for microsporidian infection and to see the cross infectivity of microsporidian infection from these insect pests to the economically beneficial insect, the silkworm *Bombyx mori* L.

MATERIALS AND METHODS

Different insect pests were collected from mulberry gardens and agricultural fields in and around Mysore, Karnataka, India by standard insect collection techniques (Donald et al., 1981). The description of these insect pests of mulberry and agricultural crops is presented in Table 1 and Plate 1. The collected insect pests were homogenized individually in 0.6% K_2CO_3 solution. The smear was prepared and observed for the presence of microsporidian spores

---

*Corresponding author.E-mail: ifat_bashir@yahoo.com.

Table 1. Description of the insect pests screened for microsporidian infection.

Insect pest	Common name	Family	Host plants
Sesamia inferens (Walker)	Pink stem borer	Noctuidae	Maize, Rice, Wheat and Sugarcane.
Phytomyza atricornis (Meigen)	Chrysanthemum leaf Miner	Agromyzidae	Cucumber, Lettuce, Pea, Tomato, Beans, Pepper, Onion, Spinach, Celery and Chrysanthemum.
Pieris rapae (Linnaeus)	Cabbage white Butterfly	Pieridae	Broccoli, Cabbage, Cauliflower and Brussels sprouts.
Eupterote mollifera (Walker)	Moringa hairy Caterpillar	Eupterotidae	Mulberry, Drum stick tree, Cardamom and Cashew.
Catopsilia crocale (Cramer)	Common Emigrant	Pieridae	Red gram, Bitter gourd, Sunflower, *Lantana camara* and *Amaltus*.
Eurias hecabe (Linnaeus)	Common grass yellow	Pieridae	Pepper and plants in pea family *viz.,* Indigofera and Yellow pea bush. Also weeds, namely, *Euphorbia geniculata* and *Lantana camara*.
Catopsilia pyranthe (Linnaeus)	Mottled Emigrant	Pieridae	Bittergourd, Red gram and River bean.
Spilosoma obliqua (Walker)	Bihar hairy caterpillar	Arctiidae	Mulberry, Green gram, Soya, Pulses, Sunflower, Jute and Cotton.
Saphygma exigua (Hubner)	Beet armyworm	Noctuidae	Beans, Sugarbeet, Cabbage, Cauliflower, Corn, Tomato, Onion, Turnip and certain weeds , namely, *Parthenium*, *Chenopodium album* and *Amaranthus*.
Colias eurytheme (Boisduval)	Orange sulphur butterfly	Pieridae	Plants in pea family including Alfa alfa and White clover. Also, Milkweeds and Asters.
Diaphania pulverulentalis (Hampson)	Mulberry leaf roller	Pyralidae	Mulberry

at 600 × magnification under Nikon (Type-104) phase contrast microscope. The homogenate was further purified by using percoll. Highly purified microsporidian spores were identified by using monoclonal antibody based Latex agglutination kit (Yakult, Japan) developed for the identification of N. bombycis, Nosema sp. M11 and M12, and polyclonal antibody (Lb$_{ms}$) developed for the identification of Lemerin breed microsporidian. A drop of purified spores of each microsporidia was mixed with an equal amount of monoclonal antibody based spore specific latex agglutination reagent and also the polyclonal antibody on a clean glass slide with glass rod at room temperature and observed under phase-contrast microscope for spore-latex bead agglutination. Five samples were observed in each category. The observation was recorded as agglutination positive (+) for positive affinity and agglutination negative (-) indicating negative affinity of the microsporidian spores isolated from insect pests of mulberry and agricultural crops with that of the respective specific antibodies.

RESULTS AND DISCUSSION

Out of eleven insect pests screened for the microsporidian infection, only five were found infected (Table 2). The microsporidia isolated from these mulberry and agricultural pests were tentatively designated as NIK-1Pr, NIK-1Cc, NIK-1Cpy, NIK-1So and NIK-1Dp wherein NIK represents "National Institute Karnataka" and Pr, Cc, Cpy, So and Dp represent the first letters of the generic and species name of the insect pests, namely, *P. rapae*, *Catopsilia crocale*, *Catopsilia pyranthe*, *Spilosoma obliqua* and *D. pulverulentalis* respectively from which these microsporidia were isolated. Microsporidia have been isolated from different agricultural and mulberry pests, namely, Spodoptera litura, Spodoptera exigua, Helicoverpa armigera, Plutella xylostella, P. rapae Crucivora and Pieris conidia sordida and Spilosoma obliqua (Singh et al., 2008). Several species of microsporidia also have been reported from the spruce budworm, Choristoneura fumiferana (Kees Van Frankenhuyzen et al., 2004).

The results of the affinity test are presented in Table 3. The spores of all the isolated microsporidia did not react positively with the monoclonal antibody based agglutination kit of N. bombycis and Nosema strains,

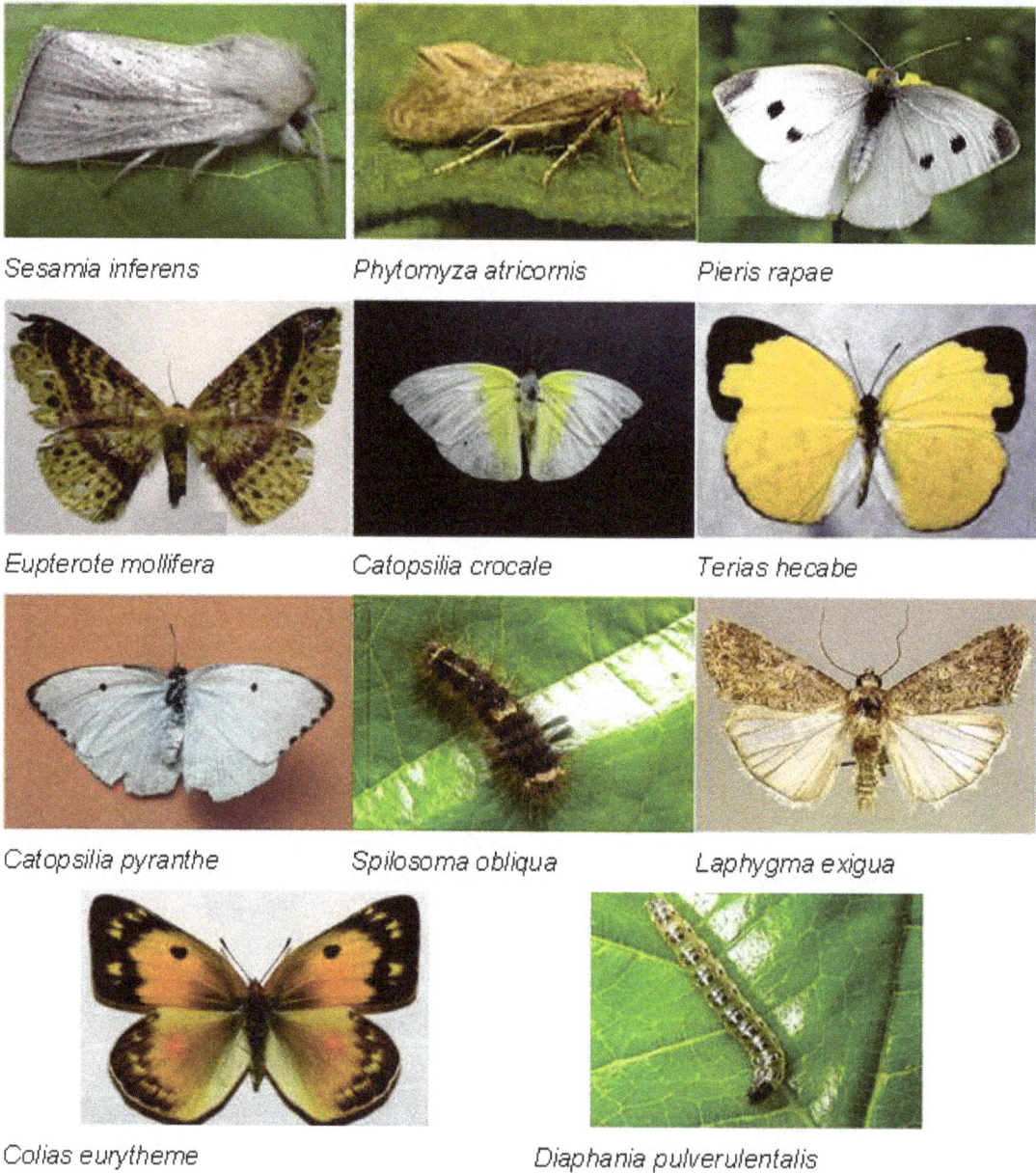

Sesamia inferens	*Phytomyza atricornis*	*Pieris rapae*
Eupterote mollifera	*Catopsilia crocale*	*Terias hecabe*
Catopsilia pyranthe	*Spilosoma obliqua*	*Laphygma exigua*
Colias eurytheme	*Diaphania pulverulentalis*	

Plate 1. Insect pests of mulberry and other agricultural crops.

Table 2. Screening of different insect pests of mulberry and some other agricultural crops for microsporidian infection.

Name of the insect	Place of collection	No. of insects screened	No. of insects infected	Microsp-oridian infection	Infection %
Sesamia inferens (Lepidoptera: Noctuidae)	Gadige Srirangapatna Mallavali Maddur	105	0	-	Nil
Phytomyza atricornis (Diptera: Agromyzidae)	G B Sargur Pandavpura	113	0	-	Nil

ble 2. Contd.

ieris rapae (Lepidoptera: ieridae)	Dharmapura H D Kote Pandavpura C.S.R & T.I, Mysore	90	18	+	20.00
upterote mollifera (Lepidoptera: upterotidae)	Dharmapura Pandavpura Mallavali C.S.R & T.I, Mysore	107	0	-	Nil
atopsilia crocale (Lepidoptera: ieridae)	H D Kote Pandavpura C.S.R & T.I, Mysore	125	23	+	18.40
erias hecabe Lepidoptera: Pieridae	G B Sargur Pandavpura Bogadi C.S.R & T.I, Mysore	155	0	-	Nil
atopsilia pyranthe (Lepidoptera: ieridae	H D Kote Dharmapura C.S.R & T.I, Mysore	75	19	+	25.33
pilosoma obliqua (Lepidoptera: rctiidae)	C.S.R & T.I, Mysore Bogadi G B Sargur H D Kote Maddur	82	21	+	25.60
aphygma exigua (Lepidoptera: octuidae)	Pandavpura Mallavali Dharmapura Bogadi	145	0	-	Nil
olias eurytheme (Lepidoptera: ieridae	H D Kote Dharmapura C.S.R & T.I, Mysore	162	0	-	Nil
iaphania pulverulentalis Lepidoptera: yralidae)	C.S.R & T.I, Mysore Bogadi G B Sargur	88	17	+	19.31

Absence of microsporidian infection; +: presence of microsporidian infection.

namely, M_{11} and M_{12} indicating that the microsporidia isolated from insect pests of mulberry and some other agricultural crops are serologically different from them. The isolated microsporidia also showed a negative reaction towards the polyclonal antibody of Lb_{ms} indicating their serological difference from the Lamerin microsporidian. The screening of different insect pests thus resulted in the isolation of five different microsporidians which are also serologically different from N. bombycis, Nosema spp. M_{11}, M_{12} and Lb_{ms}. The results, thus, indicate that the microsporidians isolated from the insect pests of mulberry and other agricultural crops are different from each other, N. bombycis and also from Lb_{ms}. Such microsporidia thus constitute a potential

Table 3. Serological affinity of the microsporidia isolated from insect pests and their comparison with serological affinity of *Nosema bombycis*.

Microsporidian isolates	Antibodies			
	Nosema bombycis (Monoclonal)	M11 (Monoclonal)	M12 (Monoclonal)	Lbms (Polyclonal)
NIK-1Pr	-	-	-	-
NIK-1Cc	-	-	-	-
NIK-1Cpy	-	-	-	-
NIK-1So	-	-	-	-
NIK-1Dp	-	-	-	-
Nosema bombycis	+	-	-	-

-: Negative reaction; +: positive reaction.

threat of gaining access to silkworm rearing through contaminated mulberry leaf and perpetuate infection despite routine care taken in mother moth examination and sanitation thereby may have an adverse impact on the sericulture industry. Hence, such pests should be kept under check in order to prevent the cross infectivity of microsporidian disease.

REFERENCES

Ananthalakashmi KVV, Fujiwara T, Datta RK (1994). First report on the isolation of three microsporidians (*Nosema spp.*) from the silkworm, *Bombyx mori* L. in India. Indian J. Seric., 33(2): 146-148.

Bhat SA, Nataraju B (2004). Preliminary study on a microsporidian isolate occurring in the Lamerin breed of the silkworm, *Bombyx mori* L. in India. Int. J. Indust. Entomol., 9(2): 265-267.

Donald JB, Dwight MD, Charles AT (1981). Collecting, preserving and studying insects, In "An Introduction to the Study of Insects" CBS College Publishing, Dryden Press, U.S.A. pp. 710-753.

Kawarabata T (2003). Biology of Microsporidians infecting the silkworm, *Bombyx mori*, in Japan. Insect Biotech. Sericol., 72: 1-32.

Kees VF, Peter E, Bob MC, Tim L, Debbie G, Charles V (2004). Occurrence of *Cystosporogenes sp.* (Protozoa, Microsporidia) in a multi species insect production facility and its elimination from a colony of the eastern spruce budworm, *Choristoneura fumiferana* (Clem.) (*Lepidoptera: Tortricidae*). J. Invertebr. Pathol., 87(1): 16-28.

Kishore S, Baig M, Nataraju B, Balavenkatasubbaiah M, Sivaprasad V, Iyengar MNS, Datta RK (1994). Cross infectivity of microsporidians isolated from wild lepidopterous insects to silkworm, *Bombyx mori* L. Indian J. Seric., 33(2): 126-130.

Selvakumar T, Nataraju B, Chandrasekharan K, Sharma SD, Balavenkatasubbaiah M, Sudhakara RP, Thiagarajan V, Dandin SB (2005). Isolation of a new microsporidian sp. (NIK-5hm) forming spores within the haemocytes of silkworm, B.mori L. Int. J. Indust. Entomol., 11(1): 63-66.

Sharma SD, Chandrasekharan K, Nataraju B, Balavenkatasubbaiah M, Selvakumar T, Thiagarajan V, Dandin SB (2003). The cross infectivity between a pathogen of silkworm, *Bombyx mori* L. and mulberry leaf roller, *Diaphania pulverulentalis* (Hampson). Sericologia, 43(2): 203-209.

Singh RN, Daniel AGK, Sindagi SS, Kamble CK (2008). New microsporidia isolated from mulberry insect pest and its cross infectivity to silkworm, *Bombyx mori* L. India, J. Exp. Zool., 11(1): 73-77.

Steinhaus EA (1949). Protozoan infections. In: "Principles of the Insect Pathology", McGraw-Hills Book Company, INC., New York. pp. 592-602.

Tanada Y, Kaya HK (1993). Protozoan infection: Apicomplexa. Microspora, In "Insect Pathology" Academic press, Inc. San. Diego. pp. 414 - 458.

15

Involvement of biotechnology in climate change adaptation and mitigation: Improving agricultural yield and food security

Godliving Y. S. Mtui

Department of Molecular Biology and Biotechnology, University of Dar es Salaam, P. O. Box 35179, Dar es Salaam, Tanzania. E-mail: gmtui@udsm.ac.tz, gmtui@hotmail.com.

In the context of climate change adaptation and mitigation, biotechnology can respond positively towards reducing vulnerability of natural and human systems to climate change effects. This paper reviews different approaches in which both conventional and modern biotechnology can be employed to address climate change adaptation and mitigation for improved crops adaptability, productivity and food security and contributing to the reduction of the greenhouse gases. The current challenges and future perspectives of biotechnology for climate change adaptation and mitigation are highlighted. The negative effects of climate change on agricultural productivity and food security as a result of extreme temperature, drought, salinity and infectious disease vectors include low yield, hunger and malnutrition. Conventional agricultural biotechnology methods such as energy-efficient farming, use of biofertilizers, tissue culture and breeding for adaptive varieties are among feasible options that could positively address the potential negative effects of climate change and thereby contributing to carbon sequestration initiatives. On the other hand, the adoption of modern biotechnology through the use of genetically modified stress-tolerant, energy-efficient and high-yielding transgenic crops also stand to substantially counter the negative effects of climate change. Safe application of biotechnology will greatly complement other on-going measures being taken to improve agricultural productivity and food security. Both conventional and modern agricultural biotechnologies will significantly contribute to the current and future worldwide climate change adaptation and mitigation efforts.

Key words: Adaptation, carbon sequestration, climate change, green biotechnology, marker assisted selection, mitigation.

INTRODUCTION

Climate change is a significant and lasting change in the statistical properties of the climatic system when considered over long periods of time. It can be caused either by the Earth's natural forces, which include solar radiation and continental drift, or human activities (Theodore, 2001). Greenhouse gases are those gaseous constituents of the atmosphere, both natural and anthropogenic, that absorb and emit radiation at specific wavelengths within the spectrum of infrared radiation emitted by the Earth's surface, the atmosphere and clouds (IPCC, 2007). Water vapour (H_2O), carbon dioxide (CO_2), nitrous oxide (N_2O), methane (CH_4) and ozone (O_3) are the primary greenhouse gases in the Earth's atmosphere. Moreover, there are a number of entirely

man-made greenhouse gases in the atmosphere, such as the halocarbons and other chlorine and bromine containing substances. Beside CO_2, N_2O and CH_4, the Kyoto Protocol (http://kyotoprotocol.com) deals with the greenhouse gases such as sulphur hexafluoride (SF_6), hydrofluorocarbons (HFCs) and perfluorocarbons (PFCs).

An increase in the concentration of greenhouse gases leads to increased infrared opacity of the atmosphere, an imbalance that can only be compensated for by an increase in the temperature of the surface-troposphere system. This phenomenon is termed the greenhouse effect (IPCC, 2007).

Adaptation to climate change is a response that seeks to reduce the vulnerability of natural and human systems to climate change effects (IPCC, 2007). Another policy response to climate change is known as climate change mitigation. It refers to human intervention to reduce the sources or decrease intensity of negative climate change effects. Most often, climate change mitigation scenarios involve reductions in the concentrations of greenhouse gases, either by reducing their sources or by increasing their 'sinks'. Examples of mitigation measures include using fossil fuels more efficiently for industrial processes or electricity generation, switching from biomass to renewable energy, improving the insulation of buildings, and expanding forest and other 'sinks' to remove more carbon dioxide from the atmosphere (IPCC, 2007; Sallema and Mtui, 2008). The decline of crops yield, heat stress and ocean acidification are among some of the negative effects of climate change. In order to feed the ever increasing world population, there is a need to double the rate of agricultural production. Biotechnology can contribute positively by mitigating the impact of climate change through green house gas reduction, crops adaptation and increase in yield using less land (Treasury, 2009). This paper seeks to address the contribution of biotechnology to adaptation and mitigation of negative climatic effects.

AGRICULTURAL BIOTECHNOLOGY

Agricultural biotechnology involves the practical application of biological organisms, or their sub-cellular components in agriculture. The techniques currently in use include tissue culture, conventional breeding, molecular marker-assisted breeding and genetic engineering. Tissue culture is the cultivation of plant cells or tissues on specifically formulated nutrient media. Under optimal conditions, a whole plant can be regenerated from a single cell; a rapid and essential tool for mass propagation and production of disease-free plants (Kumar and Naidu, 2006). Advances in breeding help agriculture achieve higher yields and meet the needs of expanding population with limited land and water resources. As a result of improved plant breeding techniques, the productivity gains in worldwide production of primary crops, including maize, wheat, rice and oilseed has increased by 21% percent since 1995, while total land devoted to these crops has increased by only 2% (Treasury, 2009). In molecular assisted breeding, molecular markers (identifiable DNA sequences found at specific location of the genome) are being used. By determining location and likely actions of genes, scientists can quickly and accurately identify plants carrying desirable characteristics, hence conventional breeding can be conducted with greater precision (Mneney et al., 2001; Sharma et al., 2002). Molecular markers can be used in plant breeding to increase the speed and efficiency of the introduction of new genes (marker assisted introgression), understanding of genetic

diversity, taxonomic relationships between plant species and biological processes such as mating systems, pollen or disease dispersal (Johanson and Ives, 2001). Biotechnology enables development of disease diagnostic kits for use in laboratory and field. These kits are able to detect plant diseases early, by testing for the presence of pathogen's deoxyribonucleic acid (DNA) or proteins which are produced by pathogens or plants during infection (Kumar and Naidu, 2006). Conventional agricultural biotechnologies works better when combined with modern biotechnological approaches.

Modern agricultural biotechnology refers to biotechnological techniques for the manipulation of genetic material and the fusion of cells beyond normal breeding barriers. The most obvious example is genetic engineering to create genetically modified organisms (GMOs) through 'transgenic' technology involving the insertion or deletion of genes. In genetic engineering or genetic transformation, the genetic material is modified by artificial means. It involves isolation and cutting of a gene at a precise location by using specific enzymes. Selected DNA fragments can then be transferred into the cells of the target organism. The common practice in genetic engineering is the use of a bacterium *Agrobacterium tumafaciens* as a vector to transfer the genetic trait (Johanson and Ives, 2001). A more recent technology is ballistic impregnation method whereby a DNA is attached to a minute gold or tungsten particle and then 'fired' into the plant tissue (Morris, 2011). Crops may be modified for improved flavour, increased resistance to pests and diseases, or enhanced growth in adverse weather conditions. In recent years, biosafety and genetic engineering projects have been initiated in Africa, with the aim of introducing genetically modified organisms into Africa's agricultural systems. Already, countries like South Africa, Egypt and Burkina Faso have commercialized GMOs while many others have developed the capacity to conduct research and development in modern agricultural biotechnology (Mayet, 2007). 'Green biotechnology' is the term referring to the use of environmentally friendly solutions in agriculture, horticulture, and animal breeding processes (Treasury, 2009).

Recombinant DNA technology has significantly augmented the conventional crop improvement, and has the potential to assist plant breeders to meet the increased food demand predicted for the 21st century. Dramatic progress has been made over the past two decades in manipulating genes from diverse and exotic sources, and inserting them into microorganisms and crops to confer resistance to pests and diseases, tolerance to herbicides, drought, soil salinity and aluminium toxicity, improve post-harvest quality, enhance nutrient uptake and nutritional quality; increase photosynthetic rate, sugar and starch production, increase effectiveness of bio control agents, improve understanding of gene action and metabolic pathways, and production of drugs and vaccines in crops (Sharma et al., 2002 ; Vallad and Goodman, 2004).

BIOTECHNOLOGY FOR CLIMATE CHANGE MITIGATION

Greenhouse gas reduction

Agricultural practices such as deforestation, inorganic fertilizer use and overgrazing currently account for about 25% of green house gases (CO_2, CH_4 and N_2O) emission (Treasury, 2009). Various initiatives under the banner of green biotechnology, may offer solution to decrease green house gases and mitigate climate change by giving farmers opportunities to use less and environmentally friendly energy, carbon sequestration and reduce fertilizer usage (Treasury, 2009).

Use of environmentally friendly fuels

Given the impacts of climate change on agricultural productivity and the role played by agriculture practices in global warming, agricultural techniques must play a crucial role in the fight against climate change. Production of biofuels, both from traditional and GMO crops such as sugarcane, oilseed, rapeseed, and jatropha will help to reduce the adverse effects of CO_2 emission by the transport sector (Sarin et al., 2007; Treasury, 2009). Energy efficient farming will therefore adopt machines that use bioethanol and biodiesel instead of the conventional fossil fuels. Green energy programs through plantations of perennial non edible oil-seed producing plants will help in cleansing the atmosphere and production of biodiesel for direct use in the energy sector, or in blending biofuels with fossil fuels in certain proportions thereby minimizing use of fossil fuels to some extent (Lua et al., 2009; Jain and Sharma, 2010; Lybbert and Summer, 2010).

Less fuel consumptions

Organic farming uses less fuel by the application of compost and mulching techniques which reduce weeds and herbicides spraying due to less ploughing (Maeder et al., 2002). Reduced irrigation would also contribute to reduced fuel usage, thereby reducing the amount of CO_2 release into the atmosphere. Using modern biotechnology such as GMOs and other related technologies facilitate less fuel usage by decreasing necessity and frequency of spraying and reducing tillage or excluding the tillage practice. For example, insect-resistant GM crops reduce fuel usage and CO_2 production by reducing insecticides application.

Reduction of fuel usage due to the application of

biotechnology amounted to savings of about 962 million kg of CO_2 emitted in 2005, while the adoption of reduced tillage or no tillage practices led to a reduction of 40.43 kg/ha or 89.44 kg/ha CO_2 emissions due to less fuel usage respectively (Brookes and Barfoot, 2006, 2008).

Carbon sequestration

The capture or uptake of carbon containing substances, in particular carbon dioxide (CO_2), is often called carbon sequestration. It is commonly used to describe any increase in soil organic carbon content caused by change of land management, with implication that the increased soil carbon storage mitigates climate change (Powlson et al., 2011). Therefore, soil carbon sequestration is an important strategy to mitigate the increase of atmospheric CO_2 concentration. Reducing the amount of conventional tillage is one way of enhancing carbon sequestration. By leaving at least 30% of residue on the soil surface, no-till agriculture reduces loss of CO_2 from agricultural systems and may also play a role in reducing water loss through evaporation, increase soil stability and creation of cooler soil microclimate. Conservation practices that help prevent soil erosion, may also sequester soil carbon and enhance methane (CH_4) consumption (West and Post, 2002; Johnsona et al., 2007). Powlson et al. (2011) have suggested that the climate change benefit of increased soil organic carbon from enhanced crop growth (for example using industrial fertilizers) must be balanced against greenhouse gas emissions emanating from the manufacture and use of such fertilizers.

In modern agricultural practices, genetically modified Round up Ready ^{TM} (herbicide resistant) soybean technology has accounted for up to 95% of no-till area in the United States of America (USA) and Argentina, and led to sequestration of 63,859 million tones of CO_2 (Fawcett and Towery, 2003; Brimner et al., 2004; Kleter et al., 2008). The modified crops reduce the need for tillage or ploughing to allow farmers to adopt 'no till' farming practices. In terms of climate change mitigation, this practice enhances soil quality and retails more carbon in the soil (Brookes and Barfoot, 2008).

Reduced artificial fertilizer use

The dependency on agricultural chemicals to sustain productivity in marginal landscapes has led to a global-scale contamination of the environment with toxins that change the course of biogeochemical cycles (Ogunseitan, 2003). Reduced fertilizer use also means less nitrogen pollution of ground and surface waters. Artificial inorganic nitrogenous fertilizers such as ammonium sulphate, ammonium chloride, ammonium phosphates, sodium nitrate and calcium nitrate are responsible for the formation and release of greenhouse gases (particularly N_2O) from the soil to the atmosphere when they interact with common soil bacteria (Brookes and Barfoot, 2009). To reduce the negative effects of artificial fertilizers, the use of environmentally friendly biotechnology-based fertilizes are being encouraged.

Biofertilizers

Organic farming technologies utilizing bio-based fertilizers (composted humus and animal manure), or crop rotation and intercropping with leguminous plants with nitrogen-fixing abilities are some of the conventional biotechnological options for reducing artificial fertilizer use. In modern biotechnology, the use of mutation or genetic engineering techniques to improve Rhizobium inoculants have resulted to strains with improved nitrogen-fixing characteristics (Zahran, 2001). Biotechnological advances involving the induction of nodular structures on the roots of cereal crops such as rice and wheat offer a bright prospect of non-leguminous plants being enabled to fix nitrogen in the soil (Kennedy and Tchan, 1992; Paau, 2002; Saikia and Jain, 2007; Yan et al., 2008). Another option is the cultivation of GM crops that use nitrogen more efficiently. An example of such crops is the nitrogen-efficient GM canola which not only reduces the amount of nitrogen fertilizer that is lost into the atmosphere or leached into soil and waterways, but it also impacts positively on the economies of farmers through improved profitability (Treasury, 2009). Managing soil nitrogen to match crop needs can reduce N_2O emission and avoid adverse impacts on water quality. Also, manipulating animal diet and manure management can reduce CH_4 and N_2O emission from animal husbandry (Johnsona et al., 2007).

BIOTECHNOLOGY FOR CROP ADAPTATION

Climate change leads in reduced crop yield due to inadequate rainfall, emergence of potential weeds, pests and diseases caused by fungi, bacteria and viruses (Johnsona et al., 2007; Lin et al., 2008). One way of adapting to such calamities is to apply agricultural biotechnologies that counter the effects of such changes by improving crop productivities per unit area of land cultivated.

Biotechnology for increased yield per unit area of land

To satisfy the growing worldwide demand for food crops, two options are available: Either to increase the area under production, or improve productivity on existing farmland (Edgerton, 2009). Given the world's available arable land, and the climate change dynamics, the second option is more feasible. Utilizing organic residues as a source of nutrients for plants, good agronomical practices such as landscape management, crop rotation or mixed farming, and use of traditional and indigenous knowledge on 'non-chemical' pests and diseases control are some of conventional options (Bianchi et al., 2006). Biotechnology and application of advanced techniques in breeding can help agriculture further to achieve higher yields and meet needs of expanding population with limited land and water resources (Treasury, 2009).

Adaptation to biotic stresses

The major aim of agricultural biotechnology is to enhance productivity and maximize productive capacity of diminishing resources. Conventional landscape management practices and breeding initiatives have contributed significantly to crop adaptations through the development of strains that are resistant to biotic stresses such as insects, fungi, bacteria and viruses (Valllad and Goodman, 2004; Bianchi et al., 2006). In modern biotechnology, the ability of a soil bacterium (Baccilus thuringiensis, Bt) gene to be transformed into maize, cotton and other crops to impart internal protection against insects (mainly of the order lepidoptera and diptera) significantly contributes to agricultural pest control strategies. For many farmers, Bt crops are proving to be valuable tools for integrated pest management programs by giving farmers new pest control choices (Zhe and Mithcell, 2011). Transgenic canola (oil seed rape) and soybean have been modified to be resistant to specific herbicides (May et al., 2005; Bonny, 2008). Also, GM cassava, potatoes, bananas and other crops that are resistant to fungi, bacteria and viruses are in development; some have already been commercialised while others are undergoing field trials (Mneney, 2001; Van Camp, 2005). Studies carried out between 2002 and 2005 found out that biotic stress-resistant GM crops account for increases in average yield of 11 to 12% for canola and maize compared to conventional crops (Qaim and Zilberman, 2003; Gomez-Barbero et al., 2008; Brookes and Barfoot, 2008, 2009).

Adaptation to abiotic stresses

Climate change poses an enormous challenge in terms of available agricultural land and fresh water use. Abiotic stresses including salinity, drought, extreme temperatures, chemical toxicity and oxidative stress have negative impacts on agriculture and natural status of the environment. The agricultural sector uses about 70% of the available fresh water and this is likely to increase as temperature rises (Brookes and Barfoot, 2008). Moreover, about 25 million acres of land is lost each year due to salinity caused by unsustainable irrigation techniques (Ruane et al., 2008). It is anticipated that increased salinity of arable land will lead to 30% land loss within 25 years and up to 50% by the year 2050 (Wang et al., 2003; Valliyodan et al., 2006). Therefore, solutions to facilitate crop adaptation to abiotic stressful conditions (drought and salinity) need to be developed. Plant biotechnology programs should give priority to the breeding for drought and salinity tolerance in crops and forests. Conventional approaches to mitigate the effects of drought and salinity stresses involve selection and growing drought resistant crops that can tolerate harsh conditions on marginal lands. Such crops include cassava, millet and sunflower (Manavalan et al., 2009). While mulching to prevent surface water loss has been a common practice for organic farmers; tissue culture and breeding are being used to cross drought tolerant crops with other high yielding species to create a drought tolerant, high yielding hybrids (Apse and Blumwald, 2002; Ruane et al., 2008). However, although adaptation to stress under natural conditions has some ecological advantages, the metabolic and energy costs may overshadow its benefit to agriculture. Therefore, blending traditional and molecular breeding techniques would be most desirable (Wang et al, 2001; Apse and Blumwald, 2002).

Molecular control mechanisms for abiotic stress tolerance are based on activation and regulation of specific stress-related genes. Transgenic plants are engineered based on different stress mechanisms: metabolism, regulatory controls, ion transport, antioxidants and detoxification, late embryogenesis abundance, heat shock processes and heat proteins (Wang et al., 2001, 2003). It has been reported by Zhu (2001) that salt tolerant plants also often tolerate other stresses including chilling, freezing heat and drought. Already, a number of abiotic stress tolerant, high performance GM crop plants have been developed. These include tobacco (Hong et al., 2000); *Arabinopsis thaliana* and *Brasicca napus* (Jaglo et al., 2001); Tomato (Hsieh et al., 2002; Zhang and Blumwald, 2002); rice (Yamanouchi et al., 2002); maize, cotton, wheat and oilseed rape (Yamaguchi and Blumwals, 2005; Brookes and Barfoot, 2006). Plants may also be engineered to reduce the levels of poly (ADP ribose) polymerise, a key stress related enzyme, resulting in plants that are able to survive drought compared to their non-GM counterparts. Field trial results have shown a 44% increase in yield in favour of such GM crop plants (Brookes and Barfoot, 2008). Another technology involving the use of genetic 'switches' (transcription factors and stress genes) from microbial sources is currently under research by the United Kingdom (UK) Agricultural Biotechnology Council (ABC; http://www.abcinformation.org). This technology has been tested and resulted in two-fold increase in productivity for Arabidopsis and 30% yield increase for maize during severe water stress. It has been suggested that comprehensive breeding plan for abiotic stress should include conventional breeding and germplasm selection, elucidation of specific molecular control mechanisms in tolerant and sensitive genotypes, biotechnology-oriented improvement of selection and breeding procedures (functional analysis, marker probes and transformation with specific genes) and improvement and adaptation of current agricultural practices (Wang et al., 2003). With the availability of whole genome sequences of plants, physical maps, genetics and functional genomics tools, integrated approaches using molecular breeding and genetic engineering offer new opportunities for improving stress resistance (Manavalan et al., 2009).

Agroecology and agroforestry

Consequences of global climate change responsible for altering patterns of temperature and precipitation are threatening agriculture in many tropical regions. Agroecological and agroforest management systems, such as shade management in crop systems, may mitigate the effects of extreme temperature and precipitation, thereby reducing the ecological and economic vulnerability of many rural farmers, and improving the agroecological resistance to extreme climate events (Lin et al., 2008). Fungal applications in biotechnology, termed mycobiotechnology, are part of a larger trend toward using living systems to solve environmental problems and restore degraded ecosystems. The sciences of mycoforestry and mycorestoration are part of an emerging field of research and application for regeneration of degraded forest ecosystems (Cheung and Chang, 2009). Mycorestoration attempts to use fungi to help repair or restore ecologically harmed habitats. Whether the habitats have been damaged from human activities or natural disasters, saprophytic and mycorrhizal fungi can help steer the course to recovery. A number of non-legume woody plants such as casuarinas (*Casuartna* sp.) and alders (*Alnus* sp.) can fix nitrogen symbiotically with actinomycete bacteria (*Frankia* sp.), a phenomenon that is beneficial to forestry and agroforesty (Franche et al., 1998). Both endo- and ectomycorrhizal symbiotic fungi together with actinomycetes have been used as inoculants in regeneration of degraded forests (Saikia and Jain, 2007). Therefore, both mycorrhizal fungi and actinorhizal bacteria technologies can be applied with the aim of increasing soil fertility and improving water uptake by plants (Ruane et al., 2008). Afforestation would indirectly contribute to improved agricultural productivity and food security because forests create microclimates that improve rainfall availability. Furthermore, forests act as carbon sinks thereby contributing towards sequestration and concomitant greenhouse reduction effects for climate change mitigation. Consequently, forestry and agroforestry offer the potential to develop

Table 1. Conventional agricultural biotechnologies for climate change adaptation and mitigation.

Measure	Biotechnology	Application	Reference
Climate change mitigation: Reduced artificial fertilize use	No-till practices	Coffee and banana and horticultural farming	West and Post, 2002; Johnsona et al., 2007; Powlson et al., 2011.
	Biofertilizers	Composting and use of animal manure	Treasury, 2009; Powlson et al., 2011.
Carbon sequestration	Agroforestry	Mycorrhizal and actinorrhizal symbiosis	Franche et al., 1998; Zahran, 2001.
		Afforestation (native & exotic trees)	Lin et al., 2008 .
	Biofuels production	Inoculation of nitrogen fixers	Zahran, 2001.
		Biogas from agro wastes	Treasury, 2009.
		Bioethanol from sugarcane	Lybert and Summer, 2010;
		Biodiesel from jatropha, palm oil	Sarin et al., 2007; Lua, 2009; Jain and Sharma, 2010.
Adaptation to climate change: Adaptation to biotic and abiotic stresses	Mulching	Horticlutural practices	Johnsona et al., 2007.
	Tissue culture	Drought tolerant sorghum, millet, sunflower.	Apse and Blumwald, 2002.
	Cross breeding	Drought resistant Pearl millet	Ruane et al., 2008.
	Agroforestry	Shading coffee and banana plantations.	Franche et al., 1998; Saikia and Jain, 2007.
Improved productivity	Increased crop yield per unit area of land	Crop rotation, traditional pesticides.	Edgerton, 2009; Treasury, 2009.

synergies between efforts to mitigate climate change and efforts to help vulnerable populations to adapt to negative consequences of climate change (Verchot et al., 2007). The conventional and modern biotechnological initiatives related to climate change adaptation and mitigation are summarized in Tables 1 and 2.

CHALLENGES AND FUTURE PERSPECTIVES

As the world population is expected to reach 8 billion people by 2028, the demand for food is also expected to increase by 55%. Moreover, out of world's total land area of 13 billion hectares (ha), only 12% is cultivated. In the next 30 years, developing countries will need an additional 120 million hecters for crops (Ruane et al., 2008). Therefore, science and technology should take a lead in spearheading increased agricultural productivity. If we want to feed the world without destroying our resources, science and technology should drive the development of modern agriculture. Genetically modified crop varieties are the most cost effective ways to sustain farming in marginal areas and restore degraded lands to production (Treasury, 2009). Efforts should be made to integrate local and conventional biotechnologies with

modern biotechnology strategies within national policies and legal frameworks in order to increase resilience of local crop varieties against changes in environmental dynamics (Stinger et al., 2009).

Despite the availability of promising research results, many applications of biotechnology have not met their full potential to deliver practical solutions to end-users in developing countries (Ruane et al., 2008). The challenges for the bioenergy sector are concerns about imminent land, water, food and feed conflicts as a result of introduction of large scale plantations of energy crops in limited arable land (Rubin, 2008; Mtui, 2009). In the area of increased soil fertility using biofertilizers, nitrogen fixation research is moving towards genomic studies whereby complete sequences of nitrogen-fixing bacteria are being elucidated (Yan et al., 2008). In forest biotechnology, there is a poor understanding of forest genomics and complex ecosystem processes at landscape scales. It is argued that genomic approaches for monitoring soil microbial communities could become an important tool in understanding the effects of biomass removal for biofuels, or enhancing durable below-ground carbon sequestration (Groover, 2007).

Modern biotechnology has encountered enormous public debates related to risks and benefits of the GMOs

Table 2. Modern agricultural biotechnologies for climate change adaptation and mitigation.

Measure	Biotechnology	Application	Reference
Climate change mitigation:	Engineering herbicide resistance to reduce spraying	GM soy beans GM canola	Fawcett and Towery, 2003; Brimner et al., 2004; Kleter et al., 2008
Less fuel consumption	Engineering insect resistance to reduce spraying	*Bt* maize, cotton, and eggplants	May et al., 2005; Bonny, 2008; Zhe and Mithcell, 2011
Reduced artificial fertilize use	Engineering nitrogen fixation	Genetic improvement of *Rhizobium*; inducing N-fixation to non-legumes	Tchan, 1992; Zahran, 2001; Kennedy and Paau, 2002; Saikia and Jain, 2007; Yan et al., 2008
Carbon sequestration	No-till farming due to Biotechnological advances	Herbicide resistant GM soy beans, canola	Fawcett and Towery, 2003; Kleter et al., 2008
	Green energy	GM energy crops	Lybbert and Summer, 2010
	Nitrogen- efficient GM crops	N-efficient GM canola	Johnsona et al., 2007
Adaptation to climate change:	Molecular marker assisted breeding for stress resistance	Drought resistant maize, wheat hybrids	Wang et al., 2001, 2003
Adaptation to biotic and abiotic stresses	Engineering drought tolerance	GM Arabidopsis , Tobacco, maize, wheat, cotton, soybean	Hong et al., 2000; Jaglo et al., 2001; Yamanouchi et al., 2002; Manavalan et al., 2009
	Engineering salt tolerance	GM tomato, rice	Hsieh et al., 2002; Zhang and Blumwald, 2002
	Engineering heat tolerance	GM Arabidopsis, GM *Brassica* Sp.	Jaglo et al., 2001; Zhu, 2001.
Improved productivity per unit area of land	Increased crop yield per unit area of land	Fungal, bacterial and viral resistant GM cassava, potatoes, bananas, maize, canola.	Mneney, 2001; Van Camp, 2005; Gomez-Barbero et al., 2008

technology in terms of health, environment, socio-economic and ethical issues (Bakshi, 2003). The attitudes and interests of various stakeholder groups supporting or opposing modern biotechnology have led to polarized opinions (Bruinsma et al., 2003; Aerni 2005). There have been opponent activists who dispute the safety of the technology, citing possible risks including: creation of more rigorous pests and pathogens, exacerbating the effects of existing pests, harm to non target species, disruption of biotic communities and loss of species and genetic diversity within species (Snow et al., 2005). Political, socio-economic, cultural and ethical concerns about modern biotechnology are related to the fear of technological "neo-colonialism" in developing countries, intellectual property rights, land ownership, customer choices, negative cultural and religious perceptions, and fear of the unknown (Brink et al., 1998, Makinde et al., 2009). Such public concerns have led to over-regulation of the technology, which threatens to retard its applications (Qaim, 2009). It is suggested that the effects of GMOs should be studied case-by-case, incorporating assessment of potential plant/ecosystem interactions, accessible and relevant indicators and tests

for unforeseen effects (Bruinsma et al., 2003). In order to overcome the challenges currently encountered in development and application of modern biotechnology, governments ought to put in place appropriate biosafety and biotechnology policies and legal frameworks before adopting such technologies (Stringer et al., 2009). Table 3 summarizes major challenges to climate change and agricultural biotechnology, and some proposed solutions.

CONCLUSION

This review shows that safe development and application of plant biotechnology can contribute positively towards climate change adaptation and mitigation through reduction of CO_2 emissions, carbon sequestration, reduced fuel use, adoption of environmentally friendly fuels, and reduced artificial fertilizer use, employing biofuels for improved soil fertility and crop adaptability. These measures are meant to improve agricultural productivity and food security, and at the same time protecting our environment from adverse effects of climate change. There is consensus among scientific

Table 3. Challenges in the climate change and biotechnology debates, and proposed solutions.

Challenge	Proposed solution	Reference
Climate change: Scepticism on the cause of climatic variations: whether it is man-made or natural phenomena.	Arguments should be scientifically-driven; not politically or self-interest driven.	Oreskes, 2004; Doran and Zimmerman, 2009; Anderegg et al., 2011
Carbon/emission trading: an industrialized world issue or the whole world initiative?	Each country in the world has a stake in effecting the reduction of CO_2 emissions.	IPCC, 2007; Barker, 2007
Food security: Overall, the world's food security is not stable.	Science and technology should take a leading role to ensure food sufficiency.	Ruane et al., 2008; Treasury, 2009
Biotic and abiotic stresses threaten food productivity.	Conventional and modern biotechnology interventions are needed to solve the problem.	Gomez-Barbero et al., 2008; Manavalan et al., 2009
Renewable energy: There is imminent land, water, food and feed conflicts in large-scale production of energy crops.	Encourage the use of marginal lands; use second generation sources (agricultural and forest residues) for bioenergy.	Mtui 2007, 2009; Rubin, 2008
Modern biotechnology: Safety concerns on health and environment.	Concerns on side effects of GMOs should be science-based, and should be studied case-by-case.	Bakshi, 2003; Bruinsma et al., 2003; Aerni, 2005; Snow et al., 2005
Socio-economic, cultural and ethical concerns such as IPR issues; loss of traditional crops; fear of the unknown.	National biosafety and biotechnology policies and legal frameworks should guide the technologies.	Treasury, 2009, Qaim, 2009.

community that climate variability is a result of direct and indirect anthropogenic activities. An integrated approach to safe applications of both conventional and modern agricultural biotechnologies will not only contribute to increased yield and food security, but it will also significantly contribute to climate change adaptation and mitigation initiatives.

ACKNOWLEDGEMENTS

The financial support from the Swedish International Development Agency, through the International Science Program of Uppsala University is gratefully acknowledged. The University of Dar es Salaam, Tanzania, and the Department of Biochemistry and Organic Chemistry of Uppsala University are appreciated for logistical support.

REFERENCES

Aerni P (2005). Stakeholder attitudes towards the risk and benefits of genetically modified crops in South Africa. Environ. Sci. Policy, 8: 464-476.

Anderegg WRL, Prall JW, Harold J, Schneider SH (2011). Expert credibility in climate change. Proc. Natl. Acad. Sci. USA. p. 3.

(http://www.pnas.org/cgi/doi/ 10.1073/pcnas.1003187107.

Apse MP, Blumwald E (2002). Engineering salt tolerance in plants. Curr. Op. Biotechnol., 13: 146-150.

Bakshi A (2003). Potential adverse health effects of genetically modified crops. J. Toxicol. Environ. Health, 6(B): 211-226.

Barker T (2007). Mitigation from a cross-sectoral perspective. In: Climate Change 2007: Mitigation. Contribution of Working Group III to the Fourth Assessment Report of the Intergovernmental Panel on Climate Change (B. Metz et al. Eds.)". Cambridge University Press, Cambridge, U.K., and New York, N.Y., U.S.A.

Bianchi FJJA, Booij CJH, Tscharntke T (2006). Sustainable pest regulation in agricultural landscapes: A review on landscape composition, biodiversity and natural pest control. Proc. Royal Soc., 273(B): 1715-1727.

Bonny S (2008). Genetically modified gyphosate-tolerant soybean in USA: Adoption factors, impacts and prospects. A review. Agro. Sustain. Dev., 28: 21-32.

Brimner TA, Gallivan GJ, Stephenson GR (2004). Influence of herbicide-resistant canola on the environmental impact of weed management. Pest Manag. Sci., 61(1): 47-52.

Brink JA, Woodward BR, Da Silva E (1998). Plant Biotechnology: A tool for development in Africa. Electronic J. Biotechnol. Available online, 1(3): 14-15.

Brookes G, Barfoot P (2006). GM Crops: The first ten years – Global socio-economic and environmental impacts in the first ten years of commercial use. J. AgBio. Forum, 9(3): 139-151.

Brookes G, Barfoot P (2008). GM Crops: Global socio-economic and environmental impacts 1996 - 2006. J. AgBio Forum, 11(1): 21-38.

Brookes G, Barfoot P (2009). Global impact of biotech crops: Income and production effects, 1996-2007. J. AgBio Forum, 12(2): 184-208.

Bruinsma M, Kowalchuk GA, van Veen JA (2003). Effects of genetically modified plants on microbial communities and processes in soil. Biol.

Fertil. Soils, 37: 329-337.

Cheung PCK, Chang ST (2009). Overview of mushroom cultivation and utilization as functional foods. Cheung PCK (Ed). John Willey & Sons Inc. (http://onlinelibrary.wiley.com/doi/10 1002/9780470367285.ch1).

Doran PT, Zimmerman MK (2009). Examining the scientific consensus on climate change. Eos. Trans. AGU., 90: 22-23.

Edgerton MD (2009). Increasing crop productivity to meet global needs for feed, food and fuel. Plant Physiol., 149: 7-13.

Fawcett R, Towery D (2003). Conservation tillage and plant biotechnology: How new technologies can improve the environment by reducing the need to plow: CT Information Center, USA. (http://www.ctic.purdue.edu/CTIC/Biotech.html).

Franche C, Laplaze L, Duhoux E, Bogusz D (1998). Actinomycorhizal symbioses: Recent advances in plant molecular and genetic transformation studies. Crit. Rev. Plant Sci., 17(1):1-28.

Gomez-Barbero G, Berbel J, Rodriguez-Cerezo E (2008). BT corn in Spain - the performance of the EU's first GM crop. Nature Biotechnol., 26: 384-386.

Groover AT (2007). Will genomics guide a greener forest biotech? Trends in Plant Sci., 12 (6): 234-238.

Hong Z, Lakkineni K, Zhang K, Verma DPS (2000). Removal of feedback inhibition of delta-pyrroline-5-carboxylate synthase results in increased proline accumulation and protection of plants from osmotic stress. Plant Physiol., 122: 1129-1136.

Hsieh TH, Lee JT, Yang PT, Chiu, LH, Charng YY, Wang YC, Chan MT (2002). Heterogy expression of Arabidopsis C-repeat/dehydration response element binding factor I gene confers elevated tolerance to chilling and oxidative stresses in transgenic tomato. Plant Physiol., 129: 1086-1094.

IPCC (2007). Climate Change 2007. Impacts, adaptation and vulnerability. Working Group II Contribution to the IPCC Fourth Assessment Report. Summary to Policymakers. Available online: (http://www.ipcc.ch).

Jaglo KR, Kleff S, Amunsen KL, Zhang X, Haake V, Zhang JZ, Deits T, Thomashow MF (2001). Components of Arabidopsis C-repeat/dehydration response element binding factor or cold-response pathway are conserved in Brasicca napus and other plant species. Plant Physiol., 127: 910-917.

Jain S, Sharma MP (2010). Prospects of biodiesel from Jatropha in India: A review. Renewable and sustainable Energy Rev., 14(2): 763-771.

Johanson A, Ives CL (2001). An inventory of the agricultural biotechnology for Eastern and Central Africa region. Michigan State University. p. 62.

Johnsona, JMF, Franzluebbersb AJ, Weyersa SL, Reicoskya DC (2007). Agricultural opportunities to mitigate greenhouse gas emissions. Environ. Poll., 150(1): 107-124.

Kennedy IR, Tchan YT (1992). Biological nitrogen fixation in non-leguminous field crops: Recent advances. Plant and Soil, 141: 93-118.

Kleter GA, Harris C, Stephenson G, Unsworth J (2008). Comparison of herbicide regimes and the associated potential environmental effects of glyphosate-resistant crops versus what they replace in Europe. Pest Manage. Sci., 64: 479-488.

Kumar V, Naidu MM (2006). Development in coffee biotechnology – in vitro plant propagation and crop improvement. Plant Cell Tissue Organ Cult., 87: 49-65.

Lin BB, Perfecto I, Vandermeer S (2008). Synergies between agricultural intensification and climate change could create surprising vulnerabilities from crops. BioSci., 58(9): 847-854.

Lua H, Liua Y, Zhoua H, Yanga Y, Chena M, Liang B (2009). Production of biodiesel from Jatropha curcas L. oil. Comp. Chem. Eng., 33 (5): 1091-1096.

Lybbert T, Sumner D (2010). Agricultural technologies for climate change mitigation and adaptation in developing countries: Policy options for innovation and technology diffusion. ICTSD-IPC Platform on Climate Change, ATS Policy Brief 6 (http://ictsd.org/i/publications/77118/).

Maeder P, Filessbach A, Dubois D, Gunst L, Fried P Niggli U (2002). Soil fertility and biodiversity in organic farming. Sci., 296(5573): 1694-1697.

Makinde D, Mumba L, Ambali A (2009). Status of Biotechnology in Africa: Challenges and opportunities. Asian Biotechnol. Rev., 11(3): 1-10.

Manavalan LP, Guttikonda SC, Tran LP, Nguyen HT (2009). Physiological and molecular approached to improve drought resistance in soybean. Plant cell Physiol., 50(7): 1260-1276.

May MJ, Gillian Champion GT, Dewar AM, Qi A, Pidgeon JD (2005). Management of genetically modified herbicide-tolerant sugar beets for spring and autumn environmental benefit. Proc. Biol. Sci., 272(1559): 111-119.

Mayet M (2007). The new green revolution in Africa: Trojan Horse for GMO? A paper presented at a Workshop: "Can Africa feed itself"? – Poverty, Agriculture and Environment – Challenges for Africa. 6-9th June 2007, Oslo, Norway. Center for African Biosafety (www.biosafetyafrica.net).

Mneney EE, Mantel SH, Mark B (2001). Use of random amplified polymorphic DNA markers to reveal genetic diversity within and between populations of cashew (Anacardium occidentale L). J. Hort. Sci. Biotechnol., 77(4): 375-383.

Morris EJ (2011). Modern biotechnology: Potential contribution and challenges for sustainable food production in sub-Saharan Africa. Sustainability, 3: 809-822.

Mtui G (2007). Trends in industrial and environmental biotechnology research in Tanzania. Afr. J. Biotechnol., 6(25): 2860-2867.

Mtui GYS (2009). Recent advances in pretreatment of lignocellulosic wastes and production of value added products. Afr. J. Biotechnol., 8(8): 1398-1415.

Ogunseitan OA (2003). Biotechnology and industrial ecology: New challenges for a changing global environment. Afr. J. Biotechnol., 2(12): 593-601.

Oreskes N (2004). Beyond the ivory tower. The scientific consensus on climate change. Sci., 306: 1686.

Paau AS (2002). Improvement of Rhizobium inoculants by mutation, genetic engineering and formulation. Biotechnol. Adv., 9(2): 173-184.

Powlson DS, Whitmore AP, Goulding KWT (2011). Soil carbon sequestration to mitigate climate change: A critical re-examination to identify the true and false. Eur. J. Soil Sci., 62: 42-55.

Qaim M (2009). The economics of genetically modified crops. Annual Rev. Resour. Econ., 1: 665-693.

Qaim M, Zilberman D (2003). Yield effects of genetically modified crops in developing countries. Sci., 299: 900-902.

Ruane J, Sonnino F, Steduro R, Deane C (2008). Coping with water scarcity in developing countries: What role for agricultural biotechnologies? Land and water Discussion Paper No. 7. Food and Agricultural organization (FAO). p. 33.

Rubin EM (2008). Genomics of cellulosic biofuels. Nature, 454(14). 841-845. doi: 10.1038/nature07190.

Saikia SP, Jain V (2007). Biological nitrogen fixation with non-legumes: An achievable target or a dogma? Curr. Sci., 93(3): 317-322.

Sallema RE, Mtui GYS (2008). Adaptation technologies and legal instruments to address climate change impacts to coastal and marine resources in Tanzania. Afr. J. Environ. Sci. Technol., 2 (9): 239-248.

Sarin R, Sharma M, Sinharay S, Malhotra RK (2007). Jatropha-palm biodiesel blends: An optimum mix for Asia. Fuel, 86(10-11): 1365-1371.

Sharma HC, Crouch JH, Sharma KK, Seetharama N, Hash CT (2002). Applications of biotechnology for crop improvement: Prospects and constraints. Plant Sci., 163(3) 381-395.

Snow AA, Andow DA, Gepts P, Hallerman EM, Power A, Tiedje JM, Wolfenbarger LL (2005). Genetically engineered organisms and the environment: Current status and recommendations. Ecol. Appl., 15(2): 377-404.

Stringer LC, Dyer JC, Reed MS, Dougill AJ, Twyman C, Mkwambisi D (2009). Adaptation to climate change, drought and desertification: Local insights to enhance policy in Southern Africa. Environ. Sci. Policy, 12: 748-765.

Theodore HJ (Ed.) (2001). Climate change 2001: The scientific basis: Contribution of Working Group I to the Third Assessment Report of the Intergovernmental Panel on Climate Change (IPCC). Cambridge, UK: Cambridge University Press. ISBN 0-521-80767-0. http://www.ipcc.ch/ipccreports/tar/wg1/518.htm.

Treasury HM (2009). Green biotechnology and climate change. Euro Bio., p.12. Available online at http://www.docstoc.com/docs/15021072/Green-Biotechnology-and-Climate-Change.

Vallad GE, Goodman RM (2004). System acquired resistance and induced systemic resistance in conventional agriculture. Crop Sci., 44: 1920-1934.

Valliyodan B, Nguyen HT (2006). Understanding regulatory networks and engineering for enhanced drought tolerance in plants. Curr. Opin. Plant Biol., 9(2):189-195.

Van Camp W (2005). Yield enhancing genes: seeds for growth. Curr. Opin. Biotechnol., 16: 147-153.

Verchot LV, Noordwijk MV, Kandj S, Tomich T, Ong C, Albrecht A, Mackensen J, Bantilan C, Anupama KV, Palm C (2007). Climate change: Linking adaptation and mitigation through agroforestry. Mit. Adap. Strat. Glob. Change, 12: 901-918.

Wang W, Vinocur B, Altman A (2003). Plant responses to drought, salinity and extreme temperatures: Towards genetic engineering for stress tolerance. Planta, 218: 1-14.

Wang W, Vinocur B, Shoseyov O, Altman A (2001). Biotechnology of plant osmotic stress tolerance: Physiological and molecular considerations. Acta Hort., 560: 285-292.

West TO, Post, WM (2002). Soil organic carbon sequestration rates by tillage and crop rotation: A global analysis. Soil Sci. Soc. Amer. J., 66: 930-1046.

Yamaguchi T, Blumwals E (2005). Developing salt tolerant crop plants: Challenges and opportunities. Trends in Plant Sci., 10: 615-620.

Yamanouchi U, Yano M, Lin H, Ashikari M, Yamada K (2002). A rice spotted leaf gene Sp17 encodes a heat stress transcription factor protein. Proc. Natl. Acad. Sci. USA, 99: 7530-7535.

Yan Y, Yang J, Dou Y, Chen M, Ping S, Peng J, Lu W, Zhang W, Yao Z, Li H, Liu W, He S, Geng L, Zhang X, Yang F, Yu H, Zhan Y, Li D, Lin Z, Wang Y, Elmerich C, Lin M, Jin Q (2008). Nitrogen fixation island and rhizophere competence traits in the genome of root-associated *Pseudomonas stutzeri* A1501. Proc. Nat. Acad. Sci., 105 (21): 7564-7569.

Zahran HH (2001). Rhizobia from wild legumes: Diversity, taxonomy, ecology, nitrogen fixation and biotechnology. J. Biotechnol., 91: 143-153.

Zhang HX, Blumwald E (2002). Transgenic salt-tolerant tomato plants accumulate salt in foliage but not in fruit. Nature Biotechnol., 19: 765-768.

Zhe D, Mithcell PD (2011). Can conventional crop producers also benefit from *Bt* technology? Agricultural and Applied Association series. Paper No. 103584.

Zhu KJ (2001). Plant salt tolerance. Trends in Plant Sci., 6(2): 66-71.

16

Chromium stress on peroxidase, ascorbate peroxidase and acid invertase in pea (*Pisum sativum* L.) seedling

Surekha and Joginder Singh Duhan[2]*

[1]Department of Botany, Government National Post-Graduate College, Sirsa-125005, India.
[2]Department of Biotechnology, Chaudhary Devi Lal University, Sirsa-125055, India.

In this investigation, chromium (Cr) toxicity on enzymes like peroxidase, ascorbate peroxidase and acid invertase was studied in pea seedling to evaluate the relative tolerance of the different pea varieties. Effect of Cr (0, 1.0, 2.0, 3.0 mM) on different parts of the seedling that is, cotyledon, plumule and radicle were studied separately to have a comparative study of the enzyme activity in these parts of the plants and its varieties. Acid invertase activity in cotyledons of Arkel was not affected significantly by chromium but increased in Rachna and HFP-8712. Chromium decreased acid invertase activity in radicle and plumule. Chromium treatment increased peroxidase activity in all component of seedling and found to be highest in untreated cotyledons of Arkel. Ascorbate peroxidase activity in the radicle and plumule was higher in Rachna. Enzyme activity decreased significantly with the increasing chromium treatment in cotyledons of Arkel while converse was true with regard to HFP-8712. These results indicate that Rachna is more tolerant followed by HFP-8712 and Arkel.

Key words: Chromium toxicity, peroxidase, ascorbate peroxidise, acid invertase, *Pisum sativum*.

INTRODUCTION

Industrialization and technological advancements have led to increase of heavy metals like cadmium (Cd), lead (Pb), mercury (Hg), nickel (Ni), copper (Cu), aluminum (Al), chromium (Cr) and silver (Ag) into the soil environment. Some heavy metals have accumulative effect and some show external toxic effects. The level of protein, nucleic acid and carbohydrates are affected by environmental stresses in growing plant parts due to alteration in the activities of synthetic and hydrolytic enzyme (Dubey, 1997).

At the time of seed germination, the proteins are hydrolyzed and the products are transported to the growing parts of the plant for synthesis of new proteins. Cellular influences like temperature stress (for example, heat shock protein), water supply (for example, desiccation protein), pathogen attack (for example, pathogennesis related (PR) protein), and heavy metal stress (for example, heavy metal stress induced protein) change the cellular protein patterns.

A developmentally and environmentally induced change in the cellular proteins is manifested at qualitative and quantitative levels, for example, increase or decrease in enzymatic activity occurs due to changes in the amount of that particular protein. Chromium (Cr) is the seventh most abundant metal in the earth's crust and an important environmental contaminant released into the environment due to its huge industrial use. Chromium is mainly present in the environment as insoluble Cr (III) and Cr (VI) compounds. These forms differ markedly in their mechanism of crossing the biological membranes. Cr (VI) as chromate, readily permeates through a general

*Corresponding author. E-mail:duhanjs68@gmail.com, duhanjs@rediffmail.com.

Abbreviations: ROS, Reactive oxygen species; **MTS,** metallothioneins; **POX,** peroxidase; **CAT,** catalase; **GPX,** guaiacol peroxidise; **GR,** glutathione reductase; **APX,** ascorbate peroxidise; **SOD,** superoxide dismutase; **Mn-SOD,** Mn-superoxide dismutase.

ion transport system, whereas Cr (III) complexes cannot diffuse through the membrane. The rate of absorption of Cr (VI) in the intestinal track is high as compared to Cr (III) and hence, the hexavalent form of this metal is biologically more toxic (Dubey, 1997). Chronic exposure to the chromium has been reported to cause liver and kidney damage, which are coupled with the appearance of perforations in the nasal septum. It also produces mutagenic and carcinogenic effect on biological systems. Chromium is toxic even at moderately low level. The adverse effect of chromium on plant growth, first noted by Koening (1910), has been documented by numerous workers. It is known to effect seed germination, plant metabolism, minerals nutrition, depress protein and chlorophyll content and to interfere with photosynthetic reaction. These alteration lead to decreased growth and ultimately crop yield coupled with the deterioration in quality of the seeds. Chromium also induces phytotoxic symptoms in plants like morphological changes, proline accumulation and alterations in antioxidant metabolism (Panda et al., 2003).

Heavy metals can induce the generation of reactive oxygen species (ROS) such as super oxide radical (O_2^-), hydrogen peroxide (H_2O_2), hydroxyl radical (OH^-), etc., which cause severe oxidation of the biomolecules like lipids, proteins and nucleic acids (Chaoui et al., 1997; Sumitra and Nayna, 2003). High concentration of these ROS can disrupt the normal physiological and cellular functions. The presence of heavy metal in toxic concentration can result in the formation of ROS, which can be initiated directly or indirectly by heavy metals. To counter the deleterious effects plants have evolved various enzymic and nonenzymic antioxidant systems which can protect the plant from the toxic action of various ROS. These antioxidant activities are induced as a response to adverse and abiotic stresses. ROS formation affects the antioxidant metabolism. Chromium, copper and zinc can induce the activity of various anti-oxidant enzymes like catalase (EC1.11.1.6), super-oxide dismutase (EC1.15.1.1) and glutathione reductase [EC1.6.4.2) (GR)] and also non-enzymes like ascorbate and glutathione (Panda, 2003; Choudhury and Panda, 2004).

Pulses constitute an important source of dietary proteins in human and animal nutrition. Among the pulses, pea has been shown to be a sensitive crop to heavy metal toxicity (Rodriguez et al., 1997). There is a great degree of variability available in pea germplasm which differ in tolerance to stresses, diseases and pest. Varieties used as green vegetables like Arkel, Hisar-Harit etc., are tall, leafy, early flowering and sensitive to water logging and powdery mildews diseases. Those used as pulses like HFP-4, HFP-8712 etc., are dwarf, completely tendriller except the stipules, late flowering and resistant to aforementioned stresses. However, no systematic work has been conducted to decipher the tolerance limit of various cultivars of pea for chromium. So in the light of the foregoing points, the present study was conducted to understand the effect of chromium on peroxidase, ascorbate peroxidase and acid invertase enzymes in pea seedling.

MATERIALS AND METHODS

Seeds

Seeds of uniform size were selected from three different varieties of pea viz: Arkel, Rachna and HFP-8712 differing in their relative tolerance to chromium from Pulses Department, College of Agriculture, Chaudhary Charan Singh Harayana Agricultural University, Hisar, India.

Surface sterilization

Seeds were surface sterilized by treating them with 20% sodium hypochlorite solution for five minutes to which one or two drops of teepol (detergent) also added. The seeds were shaken regularly. After surface sterilization, seeds were washed thoroughly with distilled water.

Germination of seeds and chromium treatment

Surface sterilized seeds were soaked in water. After 48 h of soaking when radicle emerged and acquired a length of approximately 2 mm, these were transferred to Petri plates lined with filter paper these contained 10 ml of a range of $K_2Cr_2O_7$ solution (0, 1.0, 2.0, 3.0 mM Cr (VI) ions). These were than kept in dark at 25±2°C in an incubator. Cotyledons, radicles and plumules were separated after the fifth day of chromium treatment and employed for estimation of different metabolites and associated enzymes.

Extraction and estimation of enzymes

150 mg of fresh weight that is, cotyledons, radicle and plumule were taken separately and washed in chilled distilled water and homogenized separately with a chilled pestle mortar in 5 ml of enzyme extraction buffer. Extraction medium contained 0.1 M phosphate buffer, pH 7.0; 0.25 mM ethylene diamine tetra-acetic acid (EDTA); 2.5 mM cysteine HCl and 2.5% polyvinyl pyrollidone (PVP). The extract was then centrifuged at 10,000 g at 4°C for 20 min. The supernatant was then used for the estimation of enzymes.

Acid invertase

Acivity of acid invertase was measured by estimation of total reducing sugars (glucose and fructose) by dinitrosalicylic acid (DNSA) using the method of Sumner (1935).

1 g of DNSA was dissolved in 20 ml of 2 N NaOH. Added was 50 ml of distilled water and 30 g of sodium potassium tartrate and the volume was made up to to 100 ml by adding distilled water. To a clean test tube, 0.4 ml of 0.2 M acetate buffer (pH 4.8), 0.25 ml of 0.4 M sucrose and 0.35 ml of approximately diluted enzyme extract were added to make a final volume of 1.0 ml. In the control tube, sucrose solution was added only when enzyme had been inactivated by boiling for about 5 min. After 30 min of incubation at 30°C, 1 ml of DNSA reagent was added. The test tubes were kept in a boiling water bath for 10 min and then final volume was made to 5.0 ml and absorbance was recorded at 560 nm. Standard curve was prepared using graded concentration of D-glucose (10- to100 µg/ml) with DNSA reagent. Enzyme activity was expressed in terms

of μg reducing sugars produced mg^{-1} protein.

Peroxidase

Guaiacol + H$_2$O$_2$ $\xrightarrow{\text{Peroxidase}}$ Oxidised guaiacol + 2H$_2$O

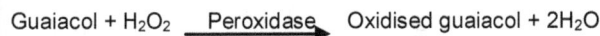

The rate of formation of guaiacol dehydrogenation product is a measure of peroxidase activity and was measured spectrophotometrically at 436 nm.

3 ml (0.1 M) phosphate buffer was pipetted out in test tube and 0.05 ml guaiacol solution added followed by 0.1 ml of enzyme extract. Before assay the temperature was maintained at 25°C. Reaction was started by adding 0.1 ml H$_2$O$_2$, mixed well, placed the cuvette in the spectrophotometer, waited until the absorbance increased by 0.05, stop watch was started and the time required in minutes noted (Δt) to increase the absorbance by 0.1. The enzyme activity was expressed as unit min^{-1} mg^{-1} protein. One unit can be defined as the amount of enzyme which catalyses the conversion of one micromole of hydrogen peroxide per minute at 25°C.

Ascorbate peroxidise

Ascorbate peroxidase activity was measured (Nakano and Asada, 1981) by a modified spectrophotometric method based on the rate of decrease in absorbance of ascorbate at 265 nm during ascorbate oxidation. The assay was performed in 3 ml quartz cuvette containing 0.5 mM ascorbate, 0.1 M phosphate buffer (pH 7.0), 1 mM H$_2$O$_2$. Blank did not contain H$_2$O$_2$. To 0.3 ml of enzyme extract, 0.7 ml of 0.5 mM ascorbic acid was added and reaction was started by adding 0.1 ml H$_2$O$_2$. Decrease in absorbance was recorded at 10 upto 30 sec at 265 nm. The enzyme activity was expressed as unit min^{-1} mg^{-1} protein. One unit can be defined as one micromole ascorbate oxidized min^{-1} (mg of total protein)$^{-1}$.

Statistical analysis

Data analysed as factorial completely randomized design (CRD) using the software "OPSTAT was developed for comparison of treatment (http://hau.ernet.in/link/spas.htm). Critical difference (CD) was calculated at 5% level of significance. One way t-test was applied for significance of the results.

RESULTS

Peroxidase

Maximum peroxidase activity was observed in the untreated cotyledon of Arkel followed by Rachna and HFP-8712 (Figure 1). It increased significantly with increase in chromium treatment in all the tested cultivars. Increase in peroxidase activity was higher in Rachna followed by HFP-8712. Whereas peroxidase activity in untreated radicle was maximum in Rachna followed by Arkel and HFP-8712 (Figure 1). The activity was increased with the increasing dose of chromium treatment.

The maximum increase was observed in Rachna and least in Arkel. The same activity in untreated plumule was found to be comparable in all the tested cultivars (Figure 1). With the increasing dose of chromium treatment, same results were obtained as in case of plumule.

Ascorbate peroxidise

Arkel cotyledons which were not exposed to Cr (VI) showed the maximum activity of ascorbate peroxidase (Figure 2) and the value was significantly less by nearly 250% in HFP-8712. Low chromium treatment (1 mM) enhanced the activity of ascorbate peroxidase except in Rachna where it remained unaffected. Enzyme activity decreased consistently, in Arkel with the increasing dose of treatment, while converse was true with regard to HFP-8712. An increase in enzyme activity was evident by 2.0 mM Cr (VI) treatment in Rachna.

Activity of ascorbate peroxidase enzyme in untreated radicle was found to be maximized in Rachna (Figure 2) while, the activity was nearly identical in other two varieties. Activity of ascorbate peroxidase remained unaffected at lower concentration of 1.0 mM chromium except in Rachna which registered a significant increase at 1.0 and 2.0 mM Cr (VI). Chromium did not affect enzyme activity significantly in other two cultivars.

Plumular ascorbate peroxidase activity of untreated seedling was higher in Rachna followed by HFP-8712 and least in Arkel. The effect of chromium treatment was found to be statistically significant at high concentration (3.0 mM) in comparison to control in all cultivars.

Acid invertase

Activity of acid invertase in the untreated cotyledons was found to be maximam in Arkel followed by Rachna and least in HFP-8712 (Figure 3). Chromium treatment did not affect acid invertase activity significantly in Arkel but increased in Rachna and HFP-8712. The increase in enzyme activity was gradual in Rachna with the increase in substrate Cr (VI) and this gradual increase was evident up to 2.0 mM Cr (VI). However, there was sharp increase (that is, 250%) in activity by 3 mM Cr (VI) as compared to 2 mM treatment in HFP-8712.

Untreated radicle of Rachna showed the maximum activity of acid invertase (Figure 3). This was followed by Arkel and HFP-8712 showed the least activity. The enzyme activity decreased with the increasing dose of chromium treatment in Rachna while, activity remained unaffected by Cr (VI) treatment in Arkel and HFP-8712.

The activity of acid invertase was least in the untreated plumule in Arkel and maximum in Rachna (Figure 3). The activity of this enzyme, in general, decreased with the increasing concentration of chromium except Arkel. Activity of the enzyme remained unaffected by Cr (VI) treatment up to 2.0 mM in HFP-8712 and got enhanced in Arkel at 1.00 mM chromium. One way t- test analysis of results indicates that enzymes activities are significantly correlated with chromium concentrations in almost all the cases (Table 1).

DISCUSSION

Activity of peroxidase in general increased with the

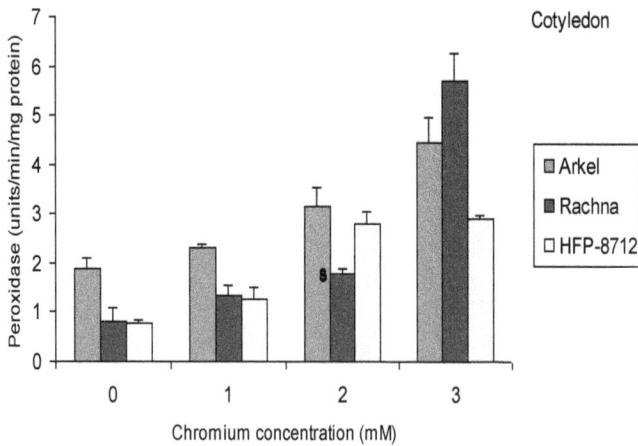

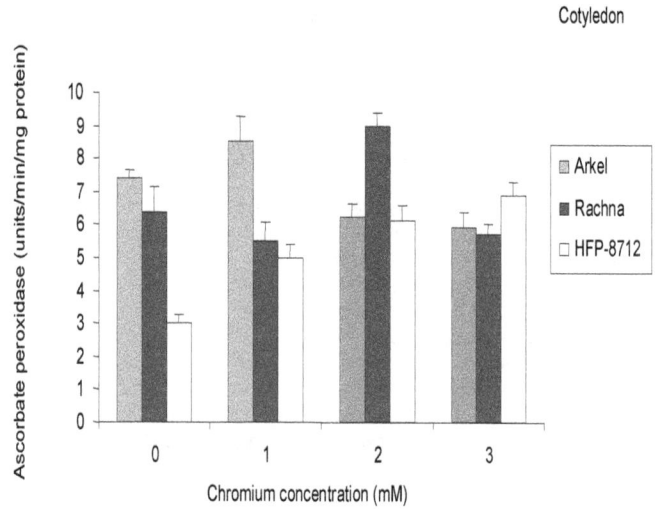

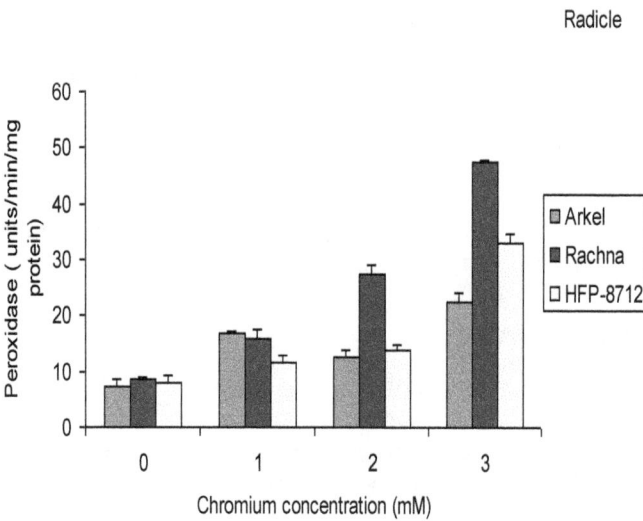

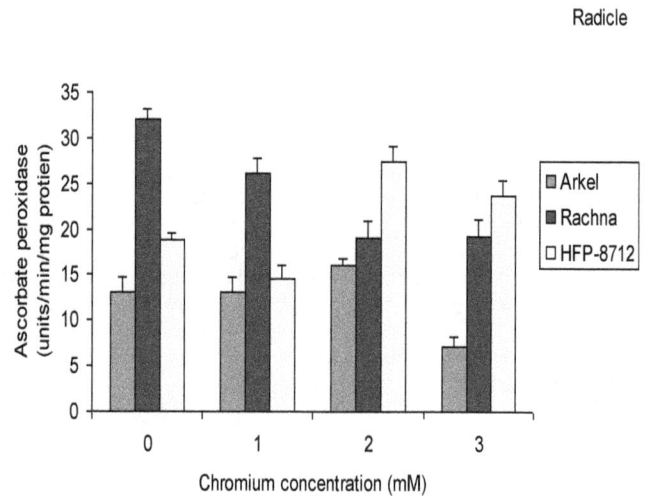

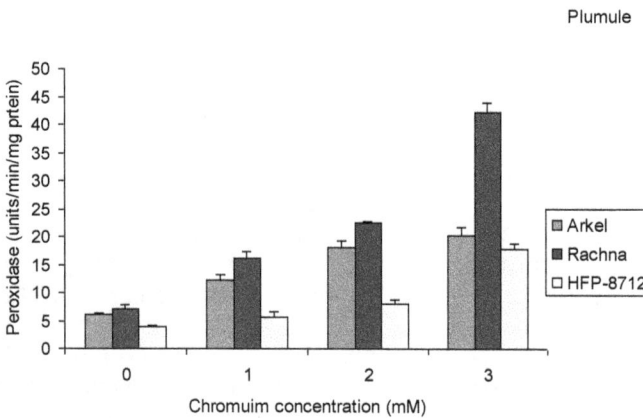

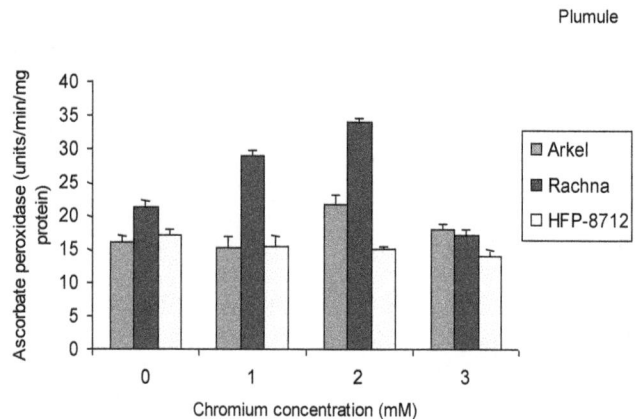

Figure 1. Effect of chromium Cr (VI) on activity of peroxidase in seedling components of pea after five days (Bars on top indicate standard error).

Figure 2. Effect of chromium Cr (VI) on activity of ascorbate peroxidase in seedling components of pea after five days of treatment (Bar on top indicate standard error).

increasing treatment of chromium in cotyledons, radicle and plumule in all the tested varieties. Similar results were reported in cadmium treated pea seedling (Divya, 1999). Pb (II) and Hg (II) treated rice seedling (Mishra

and Choudhari, 1996) and chromium treated radish (Jayakumar et al., 2007). Conversely, Bhattacharjee (1998) reported a gradual decline in activity of peroxidase over untreated control in *Amaranthus*. Seedling under

Cotyledon

Radicle

Plumule

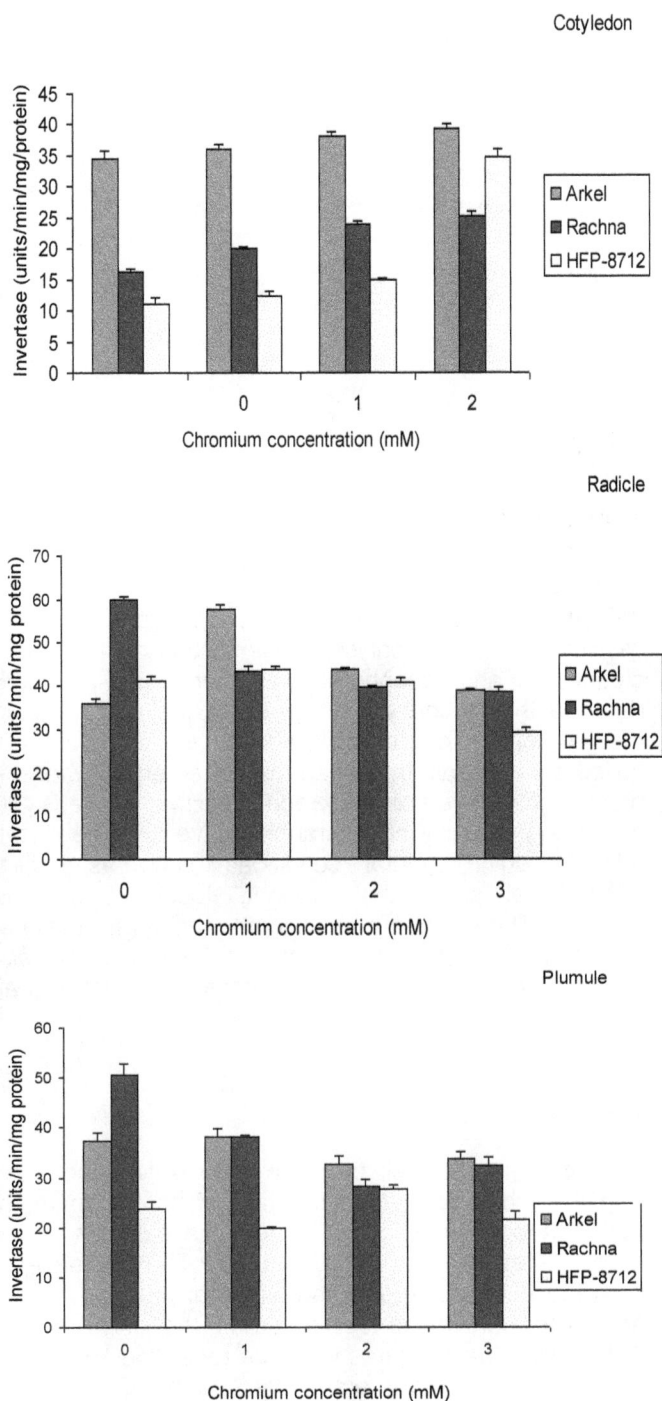

Figure 3. Effect of chromium Cr (VI) on activity of invertase in seedling components of pea after five days of treatment (Bar on top indicate standard error).

hypocotyls elongation in *Phaseolus vulagaris* and showed an increase in the peroxidase activity at both the chromium concentrations (Sumitra and Nayana, 2003).

Panda and Choudhury (2005) found that like copper and iron, chromium is also a redox metal and its redox behaviour exceeds that of other metals like Co, Fe, Zn, Ni

etc. The redox behaviour of a metal has a direct involvement in inducing oxidative stress in plants. Chromium is a redox metal and its redox behaviour exceeds other metals like Co, Fe, Zn, Ni etc. (Sharma and Sharma, 1996) Chromium affects antioxidant metabolism in plants. Antioxidant enzymes like peroxidase (POX), catalase (CAT), guaiacol peroxidase (GPX) glutathione reductase (GR), ascorbate peroxidase (APX) and superoxide dismutase (SOD) are found to be susceptible to chromium resulting in a decline in their catalytic activities. Cell wall-bound peroxidases and Mn-superoxide dismutase (Mn-SOD) coupled together are known to generate hydroxyl radical (OH⁻) from H_2O_2 which may in turn be derived from hydroxycinamic acid in the cell wall (Kukavica et al., 2009).

Peroxidase activity in radish leaves increased with increasing concentration of cobalt from 50 to 250 mg kg^{-1} soil. The peroxidase activity was minimum at 15 mg Co kg^{-1} of soil and highest at 50 mg Co kg^{-1} (Jayakumar et al., 2007). Sharma and Sharma (1996) found that the application of 0.05, 0.5 mM Cr in wheat cultivar cv. UP2003 decreased the activities of both enzyme catalase and peroxidise. Intracellular soluble peroxidases were found to be stimulated by Ni (II) toxicity more in the shoots at a lower concentration than in the roots (Pandolfini et al., 2006). Activity of ascorbate peroxidase increased in the cotyledons of Arkel and HFP-8712 at low level of chromium treatment but it remained unaffected in Rachna. Higher dose of chromium inhibited the activity of ascorbate peroxidase significantly in Arkel. On the other hand, an increase in ascorbate peroxidase activity was evident at 2.0 mM Cr (VI) in Rachna and HFP-8712. Higher dose of chromium (3.0 mM) inhibited the activity of enzyme. Radicle and plumule of Rachna showed the maximum activity of ascorbate peroxidase. Enzyme activity remained unaffected in response to various chromium treatments in plumule of Arkel, but showed a significant decrease in Rachna at 1.0 mM chromium and with a further rise in chromium levels, the activity remained unaffected in Rachna, Plumule of HFP-8712 also showed a decrease in enzyme activity at 1.0 mM chromium than control and thereafter remained unaffected by higher dose of chromium. Activity of asorbate peroxidase remained unaffected at low dose of chromium in case of radicle of Arkel and HFP-8712 and showed an increase in Rachna. But at the highest dose of chromium, radicle of all the tested varieties showed a decrease in enzyme activity. Similar results were reported by Sairam et al. (1998) and they found that abiotic stresses like water stress also increased the antioxidant enzyme like ascorbate peroxidase. Mn^{2+} toxicity resulted in increased activity of ascorbate peroxidase and this increase was more in susceptible genotype than tolerant genotype of bean. However, Divya (1999) reported a decrease in the activity of ascorbate peroxidase with increase in cadmium concentration in radicle and plumule of pea seedling and decrease was prominent in susceptible than the tolerant variety in roots than in shoots. The decline in activity of

Table 1. t-Test statistics of effect of chromium on the activities of the enzymes.

Enzyme	Pea cultivar	Seedling part	Chromium concentration			
			0	1	2	3
Invertase	Arkel	Cotyledon	2.15**	2.37*	2.60*	2.66*
	Rachna	Radicle	2.74*	2.97*	3.19*	3.24*
	HFP-8712	Plumule	2.59*	2.74*	3.25*	3.20*
Peroxidase	Arkel	Cotyledon	2.23**	5.19*	7.57*	6.02*
	Rachna	Radicle	2.97*	3.12*	2.68*	2.83*
	HFP-8712	Plumule	2.73*	2.58*	2.72*	2.58*
Ascorbate peroxidase	Arkel	Cotyledon	2.49*	3.23*	4.04*	6.45*
	Rachna	Radicle	2.40*	2.67*	3.04*	2.70*
	HFP-8712	Plumule	2.88*	2.66*	2.71*	3.78*

**Significant at 1% level of significance; *Significant at 5% level of significance.

this oxidative enzyme has been ascribed to inhibition of enzyme biosynthesis and the denaturation of enzyme proteins (Mohapatra, 1995).

Invertase is an important enzyme of carbohydrate metabolism and hydrolyses non reducing sucrose to reducing sugars like glucose and fructose. Chromium treatment did not affect acid invertase activity significantly in cotyledons of Arkel but increased it in Rachna and HFP-8712. On the other hand, radicle of Rachna showed the maximum activity of acid invertase followed by Arkel while HFP-8712 showed the least activity. The enzyme activity in general, decreased with increasing chromium concentration except in HFP-8712, where it showed an increase at 2.0 mM chromium. Acid invertase activity was least in untreated plumule of Arkel and maximum in Rachna which decreased with increasing concentration of chromium treatment. Dua and Sawhney (1991) also reported a decrease in the invertase activity with the increasing dose of chromium treatment. They found that Cr (VI) ions upto 1.0 mM in the assay mixture did not affect *in vitro* activity of invertase. The metal may be interfering with synthesis of this enzyme. Lowering of the activity of invertase would impair the capacity of cotyledon to generate monosaccharides from sucrose. More importantly, sucrose happens to be the principal form in which sugar are exported. Owing to the deleterious effects of chromium, reduced activity if invertase would restrict the ability of embryonic axis to hydrolyse the incoming sucrose and thus impair its growth. Jha and Dubey (2005) also reported an increase in acid invertase activity in endosperm as well as in embryonic axis under arsenic treatment (25 and 50 µM As_2O_3) in rice seedlings.

Stress condition in general lead to an increased production of toxic reactive oxygen species which is generated in plant cells during metabolic functions especially in chloroplast during photosynthesis. To counteract the hazardous effects of oxygen radical, all aerobic organisms have evolved a complex antioxidative defence mechanism comprising enzymatic constituents as well as free radical scavengers such as ascorbate, glutathione and tocopherol. Karkonen and Fry (2006) reported that ascorbate scavenged H_2O_2 in the culture medium of lignin producing *Picea* cells in spent and boiled spent medium Oxygen toxicity emerges when the production of reactive oxygen species exceeds the quenching capacity of natural protective systems due to adverse environmental conditions, such as chilling (Pinhero et al., 1998), drought, flooding and other stresses. Therefore, the antioxidant mechanism plays an important role not only in plant metal tolerance but also works in any kind of the abiotic stress (Jayakumar et al., 2007).

Conclusion

Acid invertase as well as peroxidase activity increased with the increase in concentration of chromium in the radicle and plumule of the tested pea cultivars except Arkel where it was not affected. The increase in peroxidase activity in Rachna was maximum. Activity of ascorbate peroxidase decreased in the cotyledons of Arkel, while the converse was true regarding HFP-8712. An increase in enzyme activity by 2.00 mM Cr (VI) in the radicle of Rachna was evident. These results indicate that Rachna is more tolerant followed by HFP-8712 and Arkel. The analyses of the results indicate that enzyme activities are significantly correlated with chromium concentrations in almost all the cases.

ACKNOWLEDGEMENT

This work was carried out in the Reproductive Biology Laborartory, Department of Botany, College of Basic Sciences and Humanities, Chaudhary Charan Singh

Haryana Agricultural University, Hisar 125004 (India).

REFERENCES

Bhattacharjee S(1998). Membrane lipid peroxidation, free radical scavengers and ethylene evolution in *Amaranthus* as affected by lead and cadmium. Biol. Plant., 40 (12): 131 - 135.

Chaoui A, Mazhondi S, Ghorbal MHEI, Ferjani E (1997). Cadmium and zinc induction of lipid peroxidation and effects on antioxidants enzymes activities in bean (*Pisum sativum* L.). Plant Sci., 127: 139 - 147.

Choudhury S, Panda SK (2004). Induction of oxidative stress and ultrastructural changes in moss *T. nepalense* (Schwaegr.) growth under Lead (Pb) and Aarsenic (As) Phytotoxicity. Curr. Sci., 87: 342 - 348.

Divya D(1999).Screening of pea cultivars for cadmium toxicity and mechanism of cadmium-calcium interaction. *Ph.D. Thesis*, India: C.C.S. Harayana Agricultural University, Hisar.

Dua A, Sawhney SK (1991). Effect of chromium on activities of hydrolytic enzymes in germinating pea seeds. Environ. Exp. Bot., 31(2): 133 - 139.

Dubey RS (1997). Photosynthesis in plants under stressful conditions. In *Handbook of Photosynthesis* (eds.) Pessarakali, M., New York: Marcel Dekker Inc. pp 857 - 875.

Jayakumar K, Jaleel CA, Vijayarengan P (2007). Changes in growth, biochemical constituents and antioxidant potentials in-radish (*Raphanus sativus* L.) under cobalt stress. Turk. J. Biol., 31: 127 - 136.

Jha AB, Dubey RS (2005). Effect of arsenic on behaviour of enzyme of sugar metabolism in germinating rice seeds. Acta Physiologiae Plantarum, 27(38): 341 - 347.

Karkonen A, Fry SC (2006). Effect of ascorbate and its oxidation products on H_2O_2 production in cell-suspension culture of *Picea abies* and in the absence of cells. J. Exp. Bot., 57(80): 1633 - 44.

Koening P (1910). Studien Uber Die Stimulierienden und Toxischen Wirkungen Der Verscheidenuertigen Chromverbinddungen auf die Pflengen. Lanwrit Jahrb, 39: 775 - 916.

Kukavica M, Vuccinie Z, Maksimovie V, Takahama U, Ovanovie SJ (2009). Generation of hydroxyl radical in isolated pea root cell wall and the role of cell wall bound peroxidase, Mn-SOD and phenolics in their production. Plant Cell Physiol., 50(2): 304 - 307.

Mishra A, Choudhari MA (1996). Possible implications of heavy metals PB (II) and Hg (II) in the free radical-mediated membrane damage in two rice cultivars. Indian J. Plant Physiol., 1: 40 - 43.

Mohapatra S (1995). Chromium toxicity and water stress interaction in green gram *Vigna radiata* L. Wilczek. k 851 during seed germination and seedling growth. M.Phil. Thesis, India: Utkal University, Bhubaneshwar.

Nakano Y, Asada K (1981). Hydrogen peroxide is scavenged by ascorbate specific peroxidise in spinach chloroplasts. Plant Cell Physiol., 22: 867 - 880.

Panda SK (2003). Heavy metal phytotoxicity induces oxidative stress in a moss*Taxithelium* sp. Curr. Sci., 84: 631-663

Panda SK, Choudhary S (2005). Chromium stress in plants. Braz. J. Plant Physiol., 17(1): 95 - 102.

Panda SK, Choudhary I, Khan MH (2003). Heavy metals induce lipid peroxidation and affect antioxidants in wheat leaves. Biol. Plant., 46: 289 - 294.

Pandolfini T Gabbrielli R, Comparini C (2006). Nikel toxicity and peroxidase activity in seedling of *Triticum aestivum*. Plant Cell Environ., 15(6): 719 - 725.

Pinhero G, Reena PG, Yadav RY, Murr DP (1998). Modulation of phospholipase and lipoxigenase activities during chilling: relation to chilling tolerance of maize seedlings. Plant Physiol. Biochem., 36(3): 213 - 224.

Rodriguez EL, Hernandez LE, Bonay P, Ruiz RO (1997). Distribution of cadmium in shoots and root tissues of maize and pea plants: physiological disturbances. J. Exp. Bot., 48: 123 - 128.

Sairam RK, Shukla DS, Saxena DC (1998). Stress induced injury and antioxidant enzymes in relation to drought tolerance in wheat genotypes. Biol. Plant., 40(3): 357 - 364.

Sharma DC, Sharma CP (1996). Chromium uptake and toxicity affect on growth and metabolic activities in wheat, *Triticum aestivum* L. cv. UP2003. Indian J. Exp. Biol., 34: 689 - 91.

Sumitra VC, Nayna GP (2003). Effect of chromium on hypocotyl elongation, wall components and peroxidase activity of *Pisum sativum* seedling. New Zealand J. Horticul., Sci., 31: 115 - 124.

Sumner JB (1935). A more specific reagent for the determination of sugar in urine. J. Biol. Chem., 69: 363.

http://hau.ernet.in/link/spas.htm

17

Influence of preservative solutions on vase life and postharvest characteristics of rose (Rosa hybrid) cut flowers

Hailay Gebremedhin, Bizuayehu Tesfaye, Ali Mohammed and Dargie Tsegay

*Debre Birhan University, College of Agriculture and Natural Resource Science, Department of Plant Science, Debre Birhan, Ethiopia

The experiment was carried out to asses the influence of five preservative solutions (aluminium + ethanol, aluminium + sucrose, ethnol + sucrose, aluminium + ethanol + sucrose and water) and two rose cultivars ('Red Sky' and 'Blizzard'). The scope of the study was to identify the best combination of preservative solutions on rose cultivars. The treatments were arranged in factorial combination in CRD with three replications. Ten (10) cut flowers of each treatment were pre-treated using prepared preservative solution for 24 h in cold room (3 ± 1°C) before storage. Interaction effects of Preservative solutions and cultivars were significant (P < 0.05) on solution uptake on day 16; petal fresh weight on day 4; total soluble solids (TSS) on day 4, 8 and 12 and on vase solution absorbance. Preservative solutions had significant effects on solution uptake on day 1, 4, 8 and 12; TSS on day 1 and 16; petal fresh weight on day 1, 8, 12, and 16. Flower longevity and maximum flower head diameter, relative fresh weight and petal fresh weight loss were significantly (P < 0.05) reduced. Cultivars had significant (P < 0.05) difference on solution uptake and TSS. Aluminium + ethanol + sucrose preservative solution treated cut flowers had shown longest vase life, flower opening, solution uptake, petal fresh weight and TSS on both cultivars; while the values were significantly higher in 'Red Sky' cultivar. The findings provide an alternative for extending the vase life of cut roses and thereby ensure the satisfaction of flower users and sustainability of cut rose flower production.

Key words: Aluminum sulphate, ethanol, preservative solution, quality, rose, sucrose, vase life.

INTRODUCTION

About 20% of fresh flowers lose their quality while passing through the market (harvest, packaging, transportation, and sale) and a large deal of remaining flowers are sold at low quality conditions dissatisfying the consumer (Panhwar, 2006; Asfanani et al., 2008) due to physiological and pathological problems during the postharvest handling. Under normal conditions, cut flowers last only for a few days maintaining their beauty and attractiveness. However, most of the people like to enjoy them in their natural beauty and appearances for a longer period of time having the socioeconomic value of flowers intact (Tsegaw et al., 2011; Zamani et al., 2011). Thus, using appropriate preservatives could help to extend the vase life of the harvested produce for consumer satisfaction and exploitation of the business.

Short vase life of cut flowers is related to wilting, ethylene production and vascular blockage by air and microorganisms (Elgimabi, 2011). Preservative solutions are generally required to supply energy source, reduce microbial build up and vascular blockage, increase water uptake of the stem, and arrest the negative effect of ethylene (Nigussie, 2005). Incorporation of different chemical preservatives to the holding (vase) solution is recommended to prolong the vase life of cut flowers (Ichimura et al., 2006). However, many cut flower growers in Ethiopia rarely put energy source, such as sucrose in the solutions being prepared for post-harvest treatment (Nigussie, 2005).

In addition to this ethylene also adversely affected the longevity and quality of cut flowers; in which STS now widely used commercially to inhibit the acceleration of roses senescence by reducing ethylene related pro-blems. However, since it contains the silver ion which is a potent environmental pollutant and its cost still the agri-cultural use of silver has been criticized.

Thus, alternative techniques for extending the vase life of cut flowers are commercial interest (Serek et al., 1995). Therefore, the objective of the study was to evaluate the effects of different combination of aluminum sulphate, ethanol and sucrose on 'Red Sky' and 'Blizzard' rose cultivars.

MATERIALS AND METHODS

Experimental design, treatments and procedures

The treatments were consisted of five preservative solutions tested on two rose cultivars; arranged in CRD and replicated three times. The flowers were harvested at stage 1 when the buds were tight and the sepals enclosed in the floral bud early in the morning and kept in buckets partially filled with water in upright position (Capdeville et al., 2005). Sorting and grading were done in pr-cooling room.

The preservative solutions were prepared using water and the pH was adjusted to 3.5 to 4.5 with citric acid, except that of aluminum sulphate containing preservative solution which was adjusted to a pH of 3.5, with potassium hydroxide (KOH). Then, immediately after bunches were put in buckets with concentrations of chemical solutions; 0.5 g/L aluminum sulphate, 4% ethanol and 20 g/L sucrose kept in 3 ± 1°C cooling room.

The cut flowers were placed in separate glass jars keeping the bottom of the flower stem; completely immersed in each treatment. Flower stems were cut diagonally using a sharp knife prior to immersing to facilitate absorption of the vase solution. Flowers were kept in the solution for 24 h.

A total of sixty bunches of 10 rose stems were separately soaked in to four litter of water with the respective amount of the combined five preservative solutions. Following 24 h of treatment, the lower most leaves from all flower stems were trimmed off to the height of 15 cm.

Two centimeters of the stem end was given slanted re-cut under water to get stem lengths of 48 cm. Then, the flower stems were taken out of the cold room with all the preservative solutions replaced with ready-made flower food called CHRYSAL 500 ml vase solution at a concentration of 10 g L^{-1} until the completion of the experiment.

Evaluations were made by keeping the flower stems in vase testing room at room temperature with 12 h of photoperiod using cool-white fluorescent lamps. The postharvest physiological characteristics of the flower stems were studied throughout the vase life period.

Data collected

Relative fresh weight (RFW)

Fresh weight of the flowers was determined just before the immersion of the flowers into the solutions and repeated every four days until the vase life of the flowers were terminated. Flowers were taken out of solutions for such a short time as possible (20 to 30 s). The fresh weight of each flower was expressed relative to the initial weight to represent the water status of the flower (Joyce and Jones, 1992).

$$\text{Ralative Fresh Weight} = \frac{\text{Final Weight}}{\text{Initial Weight}} \times 100$$

Solution uptake (S)

Solution uptake was determined by taking four flower stalks and subtracting the volume of water evaporated from a flask of the same volume without cut flower (Chamani et al., 2005).

$$\text{Solution Uptake} = \frac{S(t-1) - St}{\text{Initial Fresh Weight}} \times 100$$

Where, St= Solution weight (g) at time 1, 4, 8, 12 and 16 Days; St-1 = solution weight (g) of the control.

Total soluble solids (TSS)

Tissue sap was extracted from ten petals and TSS was determined using digital Refractrometer (model: RFM 840, Japan) by placing two drops of clear juice on the prism surface and reading was taken as described by Lacey et al. (2001). Data were taken at three days interval and expressed in °Brix.

Solution turbidity of microbial count assessment (VSAbs)

Solution turbidity attributable to microbial growth was assessed at the end of the experiment by measuring absorbance at 400, 500 and 600 nm with a spectrophotometer (Model: JENWAY 6300) and calculating the mean of these values using distilled water as a blank (Knee, 2000).

Petal fresh weight (PFW)

The fresh weight of each flower was expressed relative to the initial weight to represent the water status of the flower (Joyce and Jones, 1992).

Petal dry weight (PDW)

A dry weight of six outer petals was recorded using sensitive balance (Model: SW 1S, Germany) after drying the petals to constant weight in an oven (Model: JM-OD16, Japan) at 70°C.

Maximum flower head diameter (MFHD)

Flower bud diameter was measured daily with Vernier-caliper. The

Table 1. Effect of preservative solutions and cultivars on Solution uptake, RFW and TSS of rose cut flower.

Treatment	Solution uptake (ml/day/g)				RFW (%)					TSS (°Brix)	
	Vase life (days)										
	1	4	8	12	1	4	8	12	16	1	16
PS											
Al+Et	0.43	0.35[a]	0.30[a]	0.24[b]	108.28[a]	104.45[a]	90.18[b]	80.81[b]	72.22[b]	7.17[b]	6.17c
Al+Suc	0.42	0.34[a]	0.30[a]	0.25[b]	108.25[a]	103.85[a]	90.07[b]	79.42[b]	73.05[b]	8.30[a]	7.28[b]
Su+Et	0.43	0.34[a]	0.29[a]	0.24[b]	110.16[a]	107.18[a]	93.99[b]	84.09[b]	73.98[b]	8.70[a]	7.67[b]
Al+Suc+Et	0.46	0.37[a]	0.34[a]	0.29[a]	110.49[a]	109.15[a]	100.69[a]	91.59[a]	81.21[a]	8.73[a]	8.22[a]
Water	0.3	0.28[b]	0.22[b]	0.19[c]	103.37[a]	95.31[b]	83.34[c]	70.18[c]	-	6.72[b]	-
LSD$_{(0.05)}$	ns	0.05	0.04	0.04	ns	6.47	5.94	7.27	5. 36	1.05	0.52
Cultivar											
'Red Sky'	0.46[a]	0.33	0.32[a]	0.26[a]	107.59	103.01	90.94	81.3	76.22	8.15	7.5[a]
'Blizzard'	0.38[b]	0.34	0.26[b]	0.22[b]	108.62	104.97	92.37	81.14	74.01	7.7	7.09[b]
LSD$_{(0.05)}$	0.05	ns	0.03	0.03	ns	ns	ns	ns	ns	ns	0.37
CV$_{(\%)}$	15.11	11.2	14.49	15.24	1	4	8	12	16	11.02	5.79

Means within a column followed by same letter(s) are not significantly different at 5% LSD test. RFW= Relative fresh weight, TSS= total soluble solid, PS= preservative solutions.

MFHD of four cut flowers were recorded using the procedure of Van Doorn et al. (1991).

Flower longevity

Flower longevity was recorded as the number of days on vase until the flowers showed symptoms of bent neck or advanced signs of fading on all petals (Liao et al., 2000).

Statistical analysis

Data were subjected to analysis of variance (ANOVA) using SAS software version 9. 2. Verification of significant differences was done using LSD test at 5% probability level.

RESULT AND DISCUSSION

Relative fresh weight

Preservative solution had highly significant (P < 0.001) effect on RFW of cut flowers at 4, 8, 12 and 16 days after harvesting. At 4, 8 and 12 days after harvesting, RFW of cut flowers treated with Al+Et+Suc, Al+Suc, Al+Et and Et+Suc preservative solutions were significantly higher than those treated with water (Table 1). Starting from eight days after harvesting, cut flowers treated with Al+Et+Suc had significantly higher than treated with other preservative solutions (Table 1). Cultivar had non-significant effect (P > 0.05) on RFW of cut flowers. Interaction effects of preservative solutions and cultivars were non-significant (P > 0.05) on RFW across all days of the vase life.

RFW of cut rose flowers was varied with preservative solutions. RFW was decreased with storage time in all treatments (Table 1). Cut flowers treated with Al+Et+Suc, RFW remained above 100% until day 8; with Al+Suc, Al+Et and Et+Suc remained above 100% till day 4 after harvest (Table 1). Starting from day 4, cut flowers treated with water RFW was decreased sharply (<100%). Similar findings were reported by Tsegaw et al. (2011) who found that RFW of cut flowers treated with HQS were observed to be above 100% until day 9; with other pulsing biocides and preservative solutions it remained above 100% up to day 5 vase life. In line with this, Hajizadeh et al. (2012) reported that RFW of flowers had a decreasing trend during vase life and the lowest value was observed in control at the end of vase life in Rosa hybrid cv. Black magic. The increment in RFW at initial vase life days could be due to the higher solution uptake during the early storage time as supported by Seyf et al. (2012) who found that because of more water absorption, aluminum treated flowers of cut rose 'Boeing' had more RFW than control. The declined RFW during prolonged storage time might be due to high water loss and the declining solution uptake as confirmed by Bayleyegn et al. (2012). In the current study, the best relative fresh weight maintained on cut flowers treated with Al+Suc+Et could be related to reduced microbial load in the vase solution and hence, solution usage.

Solution uptake

Interaction effect of preservative solution and cultivar on

solution uptake of rose cut flowers was significant (p < 0.05) on the 16th day after harvesting. On this vase life day, the highest uptake was recorded on cultivar 'Red Sky' treated with Al+Et+Suc which however, didn't statistically vary from 'Red Sky' treated with Al+Et and Et+Suc as well as the cultivar 'Blizzard'. Preservative solutions had a significant (p < 0.05) effect on solution uptake of cut flowers at 4, 8, and 12 days after harvesting. Solution uptake of the cut flowers treated with all preservative solutions on 4, 8 and 12 days after harvesting were significantly higher than cut flowers kept on control.

However, solution uptakes of the cut flowers in all preservative solutions on 4 and 8 days after harvesting were statistically the same (Table 1). On day 12, solution uptake of cut flowers treated with Al+Et+Suc was significantly higher than those treated with Al+Et, Al+Suc, Et+Suc and water (Table 1). Moreover, Cultivar had a significant (p < 0.01) effect on solution uptake of cut flowers. Mean solution uptakes of cut flowers of cultivar 'Red Sky' on the 1st, 8th and 12th days after harvesting were about 21, 23 and 18%, respectively, higher than on response dates (Table 1).

Solution uptake of cut rose flowers were depends on the type of preservative solutions and the cultivars. Generally, solution uptake decreased with increasing storage time. This could be due to air embolism of cut stem, proliferation of microbes, and plant reaction to wounding as described by Tsegaw et al. (2011). Solution uptake was recorded from cut flowers of 'Red Sky' followed cultivar treated with Al+ Et+Suc and solution uptake was observed in cut flowers of cultivar 'Blizzard' treated with the remaining preservatives (Table 1). On the other hand, the ending vase life of cut flowers treated with water on day 12 could be due to microbial development in the vase solution which might have clogged the xylem tube making the cut flower stems unable to uptake solution from the vase. Pun et al. (2003) reported that even in the flower stem that is removed from the mother plant, certain enzymes are mobilized to the wounded area where chemicals are released in order to try to seal the wound.

Similarly, Knee (2000) reported that the rates of vase solution uptake by Gerbera 'Monarch', Gypsophila 'Crystal' and Matthiola 'Ruby Red' stems were highly variable but generally decreased over time. Cultivar 'Red Sky' showed a higher capacity to absorb solution than the cultivar 'Blizzard' which might be due to better positive response to the preservative solutions than 'Blizzard'. This is similar to the findings of Ichimura et al. (2002) who reported different responses of rose cultivars to chemical compounds caused by genetic variations. Similarly, Nijsse et al. (2001) realized that variability among cultivars as to water uptake may be due to differences in xylem anatomy, which has been shown to greatly influence hydraulic conductivity.

Total soluble solid

Interaction effect of preservative solutions and cultivar on TSS of rose cut flowers was significant (p < 0.05) on day 4, 8 and 12 after harvest. On day 4 of vase life, TSS of cut flowers of cultivar 'Red Sky' treated with Al+Et+Suc significantly higher than the remaining treatments combinations. On day 8, the highest TSS value of cut rose flower was recorded in 'Red Sky' treated with water, however didn't vary from values recorded from same cultivar treated with Al+Et+ Suc and Et+Suc as well as Blizzard treated with Al+Et+Suc preservative solutions. On day 12, Al+Et+Suc treatments in both cultivars recorded significantly higher TSS compared to the remaining preservatives cultivars combinations (Table 2). Preservative solutions had significant (p < 0.001) effect on TSS of cut flowers on the day 1 and 16 after harvest. On day 1 of vase life, TSS of cut flowers treated with Al+Suc, Et+Suc and Al+Et+Suc preservative solutions were significantly higher than those treated with Al+Et and control; while TSS of cut flowers on Al+Suc, Et+Suc and Al+Et+Suc treatments were statistically the same (Table 1). Similarly, TSS of cut flowers treated with Al+Et and water were statistically the same. On day 16, highest TSS were recorded from cut flowers treated with Al+Et+Suc while the lowest TSS on this day was recorded on cut flowers treated with Al+Et but cut flowers treated with Al+Suc and Et+Suc had statistically the same TSS (Table 1). Cultivars had significant (p < 0.05) effect on TSS of cut rose flower petals on day 16. Mean TSS of cut flowers of variety 'Red Sky' on this day were 7.5 °Brix while for cultivar 'Blizzard', TSS of cut flowers were 7.5 and 7.09. But on day one, both cultivars revealed statistically the same TSS of petals (Table 1).

TSS was increased up to eight vase life days and then decreased which confirmed of Elgimabi and Sliai (2013) who reported that sugar content of roses increased at the beginning of the experiment, and then decreased towards the end. Cultivar 'Red Sky' had shown higher TSS value of petals than 'Blizzard' indicating that cultivars could vary in TSS content of cut flowers. In line with these, Tsegaw et al. (2011) reported cultivar 'Red calypso' exhibited the highest TSS value while Akito had the lowest and Viva was found to be intermediate between them. An increase in TSS at the early stage may be due to substitution of the required substrate for respiration by rapid solution uptake whereas the reduction in TSS after the 8th day of vase life may be due to the utilization of the stored food as substrate and inability to substitute it by the low solution uptake as the storage time increased.

Vase solution absorbance (VSAbs)

The interaction effect of preservative solution and cultivar on vase solution absorbance was significant (p < 0.05).

Table 2. Interaction effects of preservative solutions and cultivar on TSS, PFW and vase solution absorbance of rose flowers.

Treatment	Solution uptake (ml/day/g)		TSS (°Brix)						PFW (g)		Vase solution absorbance	
	Day 16		Day 4		Day 8		Day 12		Day 4		day 16	
	'Red Sky'	'Blizzard'	'Red Sky'	'Blizzard'	'Red Sky'	'Blizzard'	'Red Sky'	'Blizzard'	'Red Sky'	'Blizzard'	'Red Sky'	'Blizzard'
Al+Et	0.24^{abc}	0.15^d	8.37^{bc}	7.6^{bcd}	8.47^{bc}	6.6^d	7.73^b	5.87^c	1.53^b	1.47^b	0.050^{de}	0.052^{de}
Al+Suc	0.23^{bc}	0.20^{cd}	8.3^{bc}	8.43^b	9.13^{ab}	8.43^{bc}	7.63^b	7.40^b	1.40^b	1.50^b	0.059^{cd}	0.072^{ab}
Et+Suc	0.28^{ab}	0.16^d	9.4^a	8.17^{bc}	9.3^{ab}	7.6^{cd}	7.90^b	7.63^b	1.53^b	1.50^b	0.068^{bc}	0.065^{bc}
Al+Et+Suc	0.30^a	0.27^{ab}	9.7^a	7.93^{bcd}	9.67^{ab}	9.13^{ab}	9.00^a	8.83^a	1.93^a	1.57^b	0.048^e	0.053^{de}
Water	-	-	7.5^{cd}	7.07^d	7.03^a	7.63^{cd}	6.50^c	6.43^c	1.13^c	1.10^c	0.079^a	0.072^{ab}
LSD$_{(0.05)}$	0.06		0.89		1.11		0.89		0.20		0.009	
CV $_{(\%)}$	15.04		6.37		7.86		7.04		8.07		8.61	

Means within a column followed by same letter(s) are not significantly different at 5% LSD test. TSS= total soluble solid, PFW= petal fresh weight.

Accordingly, the highest (0.079) and (0.048) lowest vase solution absorbance were recorded from cultivar 'Red Sky' treated with water alone and Al+Et +Suc, respectively (Table 2). The significant reduction in vase solution absorbance of cut flowers might be due to the presence of the biocide aluminum sulphate and ethanol as disinfectant. Addition of biocide and disinfectants might have helped in suppressing microbial growth and the clear vase solution obtained in the current study could have made absorption by the cut stems easy.

In conformity with the findings of the current investigation, high absorbance values of vase solution were also reported before in the absence of biocides by Knee (2000). The present results indicated that in all preservative solutions having sucrose did not result in clearer vase solution as compared to the pure water (control); but preservatives containing aluminum sulphate and ethanol together (Al+Et and Al+Et+Suc) had significantly lower vase solution absorbance clearly indicating that sucrose helps for microbial development in the vase and resulted in poor solution uptake by stem. Therefore, the results were convinced that addition of anti microbes decreased solution turbidity which also enhanced solution usage and increased lasting life of the cut flowers.

Petal fresh weight

Interaction effect of preservative solution and cultivar on PFW of rose cut flowers was significant (p > 0.05) on day 4 after harvested. On this particular day, PFW of cut flowers of cultivar 'Red Sky' treated with Al+Et+Suc produced the highest (1.93) while the control in both cultivar recorded the least (1.12 g) on average PFW (Table 3). Preservative solution had a significant (p < 0.05) effect on petal fresh weight of rose cut flowers 1, 4, 8, 12and 16 days after harvest (Appendix 2). However,

PFW of the cut flowers treated with Al+Et, Al+Suc and Suc+Et on day 4, 8 and 16 of vase life were statistically the same (Table 3). The lowest PFW on day 12 was recorded from cut flowers treated with Al+ Suc. Moreover, PFW of the cut flowers treated with Al+Et +Suc on day 4, 8, 12 and 16 were significantly higher than those treated with Al+Et, Al+Suc, Suc+Et and water (Table 3). In the case of Al+Et+Suc, the PFW increased first from day 1 to day 4 then decreased till the end of vase life period. Furthermore, cultivar had a significant effect (p < 0.01) on solution uptake of cut flowers. Cultivar 'Red Sky' had 13.93, 11.66, 12.30 and 8.42% greater petal fresh weight than 'Blizzard' particularly on the 1st, 8th, 12th and 16thdays, respectively (Table 3).

The lowest PFW recorded in Al+Suc indicate that aluminum sulphate is not enough to act as biocide to suppress the microbial unless it is coupled with ethanol. Ethanol is a disinfectant that can enhance water conductance by preventing microbial proliferation. Hence, it could improve effectiveness of aluminum sulphate with the addition of that could be the reason for excellent maintenance of PFW of the cut flowers treated with Al+Et+Suc. These results were also related with the low solution uptake recorded on the current experiment even though it was not significant. While PFW was best maintained in Al+Et+Suc indicated that when ethanol was applied it can act as disinfectant so that enhance solution uptake then maintained PFW.

Several researches shown that the short vase life is related to rapid decline in water uptake and drying of stems (Ichimura et al, 2002; Tsegaw et al., 2011). From Nair and Sharna, (2003) point of view, all preservative solution must essentially contain two components including sugar and germicides. The current findings support this idea. Cognizant of this, van Doorn et al. (1991) reported that flowers placed in water without antimicrobial compounds had a low water potential as a result of vascular

Table 3. PFW and PDW, MFHD and flower longevity (FL) of rose cut flower as affected by different preservative solutions and cultivars.

Treatment	Petal fresh weight (g)				Petal dry weight (g)					MFHD (cm)	FL (days)
	Vase life (days)										
	1	8	12	16	1	4	8	12	16		
PS											
Al+Et	1.52^a	1.23^b	1.07^{bc}	0.72^b	0.18^{ab}	0.19^{ab}	0.19^c	0.17^a	0.15	7.25^b	15.5^b
Al+Suc	1.52^a	1.25^b	0.95^c	0.73^b	0.18^{ab}	0.19^{ab}	0.20^{ab}	0.16^a	0.15	7.46^b	16.0^b
Et+Suc	1.57^a	1.35^b	1.13^b	0.73^b	0.19^a	0.20^a	0.22^a	0.17^a	0.15	8.12^a	16.17^b
Al+Et+Suc	1.68^a	1.53^a	1.28^a	0.85^a	0.18^{ab}	0.19^{ab}	0.21^{ab}	0.16^a	0.15	8.21^a	17.67^a
Water	1.28^b	0.82^c	0.62^d	-	0.18^{ab}	0.18^b	0.16^c	0.14^b	-	6.06^c	12.33^c
LSD$_{(0.05)}$	0.18	0.12	0.12	0.09	0.01	0.02	0.02	0.01	ns	0.63	1.34
Cultivar											
'Red Sky'	1.63^a	1.31^a	1.09^a	0.79^a	0.18	0.18^b	0.19	0.16	0.16^a	7.07^b	16.06^a
'Blizzard'	1.40^b	1.16^b	0.93^b	0.72^b	0.18	0.21^a	0.20	0.16	0.15^b	7.78^a	15.0^b
LSD$_{(0.05)}$	0.11	0.08	0.08	0.06	ns	0.01	ns	ns	0.01	0.40	0.84
CV $_{(\%)}$	9.73	8.618	10.23	10.72	5.97	7.77	7.14	7.05	5.01	7. 02	7.14

Means within a column followed by same letter(s) are not significantly different at 5% LSD test. MFHD= Maximum flower head diameter, FL=Flower longevity, PS= Preservative solutions.

blockage in the lowermost segment of the stem. The reason for best PFW in treatment (Al+Et+Suc) could be due to the main components of preservative solution incorporated.

Petal dry weight

Preservative solution had a significant (p < 0.05) effect on PDW of flower petals throughout the study period. On the 4th and 8th day of vase life, flowers treated with Et+Suc had the highest PDW but not significantly different from Al+Et+Suc and Al+Suc treated flowers. On day 12, cut flowers treated with water had significantly lower PDW compared to those cut flowers treated with preservative solutions. Similarly, on day 16 there was no significant difference recorded among the different preservative solutions (Table 3). Comparing the two rose cultivars, statistically the same PDW were recorded on days 1, 8, and 12. But on day 4, petal dry weights were higher in 'Red Sky' cut flowers whereas on day 16 'Blizzard' had shown significantly higher petal dry weight. In this regard, there was no consistency.

Generally, there was no significant difference recorded on dry mater content of cut flowers treated with Al+Et and tap water. Moreover, in this experiment those cut flowers treated with sucrose containing preservative solution had shown statistically the same petal dry weight in all vase life days and significantly higher on the 8th day after harvest as compared to the control and Al+Et treated flowers. This could be due to the importance of sucrose

for cell expansion and dry mater accumulation as it could help for the endogenous sucrose serve as a substrate of respiration. At 12 and 16 days after harvest PDW of cut flowers treated with sucrose containing preservative solution cut off with those Al+Et which could be due to the effects of respiration. Parallel to this, holding solution containing 8-HQS+Sucrose reduced the respiration rate and physiological loss in weight of spikes of Dendrobium hybrid Sonia-17 (Dineshbabu et al., 2002). This may be due to the solution uptake and accumulated substrate for respiration and decreased due to increment of respiration rate and reduction in substrate for respiration in storage time. In addition, in the current experiment no variation in PDW was found between the two cultivars (Table 3). PDW increased until day 8 after harvest and then decreased till the end of vase life. The rapid decrease in PDW through time could be due to the decreasing solution uptake that compensates the respiration and transpiration.

Maximum flower head diameter

Preservative solutions had significant (p < 0.001) effects on MFHD (Table 3). The largest (8.21 cm) and smallest (6.06 cm) MFHD were registered from cut flowers treated with preservative solution that contained Al+Su+Et and water respectively. MFHD recorded from cut flowers treated with Al+Et+Suc, Al+Et, Al+Suc and Et+Suc preservative solutions were 8.21, 7.25, 7.46 and 8.25 cm, respectively. However, the difference between Al+Et+Suc and Et+Suc was not statistically significant. Cultivar imparted a significant (p < 0.01) difference on MFHD (Table 3). MFHD recorded for cultivar 'Blizzard' and 'Red Sky' was 7.78 and 7.07 cm respectively (Table 3). Interaction effects of preservative solution and cultivars on mean MFHD were non-significant (p > 0.05).

Treatment with Et+Suc had a pronounced effect on flower bud expansion which confirmed with idea of Sarkka (2005) who suggested that carbohydrates are necessary for turgor pressure maintenance and important energy sources facilitating flower opening. In harmony to the present results Ichimura et al. (2002) showed an increased in flower diameter was observed when 20 g of sucrose L^{-1}+200 mg of HQS l^{-1} were used in the pulsing solution, which of course varied among the varieties tested. Al+Et+Suc treated cut flowers was shown better performance in most post harvest characteristics of 'Red Sky' cut flowers than 'Blizzard'. Cultivar 'Blizzard' had better flower diameter indicating that flower diameter could also vary due to the variation in genetic makeup. In confirmation to the current experiment Ichimura et al. (2005) found that an increase in flower head diameter was observed in rose cultivars 'Sonia' and 'Delilah' than other cultivars with identical treatments.

Flower longevity

Preservative solution had significant (p < 0.01) effects on flower longevity of cut flowers (Table 3). Vase life of cut flowers treated with preservative solution Al+Et +Suc, Al+Suc, Et+Suc and Al+Et extended vase life of the cut flowers by 5.33, 3.83, 3.7 and 3.2 days, respectively, as compared to water treated cut flowers (Table 3). Cut flowers treated with Al+Suc, Et +Suc and Al+Et remained with acceptable display life for 16.17, 16 and 15.5 days. Cultivar had a significant effect (p < 0.05) on vase life of cut flowers (Table 3). The number of days where cut flowers of 'Red Sky' and 'Blizzard' remained viable was 16.07 and 15, respectively (Table 3). Interaction effects of preservative solutions and cultivars was non-significant (p > 0.05) effects on flower longevity.

According to Tsegaw et al. (2011) $Al_2(SO_4)_3$, which is a common biocide used in most Ethiopian cut flower growers was not able to extend the vase life of cut flower stems better than the control, treated with tap water. This evidently indicated that combined effect of the chemicals could be the reason for successful vase life extension to 17.67 days of the cut flowers via improving solution uptake, reducing RFW loss, reducing PFW loss, reducing vase and enhancing TSS observed in current study as justified by Hajizadeh et al. (2012) on rose cultivar 'Black magic'. In line with this Wu et al. (1992) reported that ethanol decreases ethylene production and/or sensitivity to ethylene and also act as an antimicrobial compound to prolong vase life of some cut flowers while sucrose can

provide the energy needed to cell processes including maintain the structure and function of mitochondria and the other cellular organelles as reported by Capdeville et al. (2005).The longer vase life which occurred in 'Red Sky' than 'Blizzard' which confirmed by Butt (2005) suggested that variation on vase life could be due to their genetic variability and different responses to chemical compounds. Varieties could also be varying in lasting life due to ethylene production and sensitivity as well as resistance to different disease causing microorganisms (Ichimura et al., 2002).

Conclusion

The best flower longevity, MFHD and lowest vase solution absorbance was maintained due to the treatments of Al+Et+Suc preservative solution and the lowest vase life and MFHD was recorded from cut flowers treated with water. Treatment of the cut flowers using Al+Et, Al+Suc, Suc+Et, and Al+Et+Suc extended the vase life of the cut flowers by 3.2, 3.7, 3.83 and 5.33 days, respectively than control. Generally, it can be concluded that use of Al+Et+Suc preservative solution for flower longevity and maintaining post-harvest characteristics of cut flowers is important for 'Red Sky' and 'Blizzard' cut flowers.

REFERENCES

Asfanani M, Davarynejad G, Tehranifar A (2008). Effects of Pre-harvest Calcium Fertilization on Vase Life of Rose cut Flowers cv. Alexander, Ferdowsi University of Mashhad, Iran.

Bayleyegn A, Tesfaye B, Workneh TS (2012). Effects of pulsing solution, packaging material and passive refrigeration storage system on vase life and quality of cut rose flowers. Afr. J. Biotechnol. 11(16):3800-3809.

Butt SJ (2005). Extending the vase life of roses (rosa hybrid L.) with different preservatives. Int. J. Agric. Biol. http://www.jircas.affrc.go.7(1):97-99.

Capdeville GD, Maffia LA, Finger FL, Batista UG (2005). Pre-harvest calcium sulfate applications affect vase life and severity of gray mold in cut roses. Sci.Hort.103: pp. 329-338.

Chamani AK, Joyce DC, Irvin DE, Zamani ZA, Mostofi Y, Kafi M (2005). Ethylene and anti-ethylene treatment effects on cut 'First Red' rose. J. Appl. Hort. 1:3-7.

Dineshbabu M, Jawaharlal M, Vijayakumar M (2002). Influence of holding solutions on the postharvest life of Dendrobium hybrid Sonia. South Ind. Hort. 50(4-6):451-457.

Elgimabi EL (2011).Vase life Extension of rose cut flowers (Rose hybrida) as influenced by silver nitrate and sucrose pulsing. Am. J. Agric. Biol. Sci.6(1):128-133.

Elgimabi EN, Sliai AM (2013). Effects of Preservative Solutions on Vase Life and Postharvest Qualities of Taif Rose Cut Flowers (Rosa damascene cv. Trigintipetala), Am. Eurasian J. Agric. Environ. Sci. 13(1):72-80.

Hajizadeh HS, Farokhzad A, Chelan GH (2012).Using of preservative solutions to improve postharvest life of Rosa Hybrid cv. Black magic. J. Agric.Technol. 8(5):1801-1810.

Ichimura K, Kawabata Y, Kishimito M, Goto R, Yamada K (2002). Variation with the cultivar in the vase life of cut rose flowers. Bull. Natl. Inst. Flor. Sci. 2:9-20.

Ichimura K, Kishimoto M, Ryo N, Yoshihiko K (2005). Soluble carbohydrates and variation in vase-life of cut rose cultivars 'Delilah' and 'Sonia'. J. Hort. Sci. Biotechnol. 80:280-286.

Ichimura K, Taguch M, Norkoshi R (2006). Extension of the vase life in cut roses by treatment with glucose, isothiazolinonic germicide, citric. JARQ. 40:263-269.

Joyce DC, Jones PN (1992). Water balance of the foliage of cut Geraldton wax flower. J. Postharvest Biol. Technol. 2:31-39.

Knee M (2000). Selection of biocides for use in floral Pulsing. J. Postharvest Biol. Technol. 18:227-234.

Lacey L, McCarthy A, Foord G (2001). Maturity testing of citrus. Farmnote, *Dep. Agri. West. Australia,* 3:1-5.

Nair SA, Singh V, Sharma TV (2003). Effect of chemical preservatives on enhancing vase-life of gerbera flowers. J. Trop. Agric. 41(1,2):56-58.

Nigussie K (2005). Ornamental horticulture: A technical material. Jimma University College of Agriculture and Veternary medicine, Jimma Ethiopia.

Nijsse J, Van der Heijden G, van Ieperen W, Keijzer C, Van Meeteren U (2001). Xylem hydraulic conductivity related to conduit dimensions along chrysanthemum stems. J. Exp. Bot. 52:319-327.

Panhwar F (2006). Postharvest technology of fruits and vegetables. *ECO Services International,* Hyderabad Sindh, Pakistan.

Pun UK, Ichimura K (2003). Role of sugars in senescence and biosynthesis of ethylene in cut flowers. J. ARQ, 4:219-224.

Sarkka L (2005). Yield quality and vase life of cut roses in year round greenhouse production. Academic Dissertation, University of Helsinki, Finland. p. 64.

Serek M, Tamari G, Sisler EC, Borochov A (1995). Inhibition of ethylene-induced cellular senescence symptoms by 1-methylcyclopropene, a new inhibitor of ethylene action. Physiol. Plant 94:229-232.

Seyf M, Khalighi A, Mostofi Y, Naderi R (2012). Study on the effect of aluminum sulfate treatment on postharvest life of the cut rose 'Boeing' (*Rosa hybrid* cv. Boeing). J. Hortic. For. Biotechnol. 16(3):128-132.

Tsegaw T, Tilahun S, Humphries G (2011). Influence of pulsing biocides and preservative solution treatment on the vase life of cut rose (Rosa hybrid L.) varieties. J. Appl. Sci. Technol. 2(2):1-18.

Van Doorn WG, De Witte Y (1991). Effect of bacterial suspensions on vascular occlusion in stems of cut rose flowers. J. Appl. Bact. 71:119-123.

Wu MJ, Lorenzo Z, Saltveit ME, Reid MS (1992). Alcohols and carnation senescence. Hort Sci. 27:136-138.

Zamani S, Kazemi M, Aran M (2011). Postharvest life of cut rose flowers as affected by salicylic acid and glutamin. World Appl. Sci. J. 12(9):1621-1624.

18

Effect of humic acid application on accumulation of mineral nutrition and pungency in garlic (*Allium sativum* L.)

Manas Denre[1, 4] , Soumya Ghanti[2] and Kheyali Sarkar[3]

[1]Department of Agricultural Biochemistry, Bidhan Chandra Krishi Viswavidyalaya, Mohanpur, Nadia-741252, West Bengal, India.
[2]Department of Spices and Plantation Crops, Bidhan Chandra Krishi Viswavidyalaya, Mohanpur, Nadia-741252, West Bengal, India.
[3]Department of Botany, Raniganj Girls' College, Raniganj, Burdwan-713347, West Bengal, India.
[4]Department of Soil Science and Agricultural Chemistry, Birsa Agricultural University, Kanke, Ranchi-834006, Jharkhand, India.

Humic acid promote the conservation of mineral nutritions and as well as stimulate the pungency usually being more prominent in the cloves of garlic bulb. The effect of humic acid application on accumulation of mineral nutritions and pungency in garlic (*Allium sativum* L.) cv. 'Gangajali' was studied. Here, we observed that the maximum concentration of Ca, Fe and S were shown when plants were treated with 400 ppm humic acid. While, in the case of Mg, P and Zn content, the maximum values were observed by application of 200 ppm humic acid. The maximum concentration of K, Cu, Mn were observed when plants were treated with 300 ppm humic acid. Regarding, pungency, content was determined as pyruvic acid development significantly increased with increase in concentration of humic acid applications. Our results also showed significant positive correlations between Mg and P, Mg and Zn, P and Zn, Cu and PAD, and S and PAD, respectively. Based on average values and ANOVA of overall variables, the highest result was observed by application of 300 ppm of humic acid followed by 400 and 200 ppm of humic acid, which may be the proper value addition in garlic bulb by enhancing the mineral nutritions and pyruvic acid development that needs to be studied in the future.

Key words: *Allium sativum* L., humic acid, mineral nutritions, pungency.

INTRODUCTION

Currently, the major challenges of plant scientists and agronomists are to enhance crop yields in more resource, efficient and environmentally friendly cropping systems. One of the potential systems involved is creation of innovative means for plant nutrition and growth promotion. The urgency to emphasize the importance of humic substances (HS) and their value as fertilizer ingredients has never been more important than at present, as the content of organic matter in agricultural soils has reached drastically low levels (Loveland and Webb, 2003). The value of HS in soil fertility relates to the many functions these complex organic compounds perform. It is well established that HS improve the physical, chemical and biological properties of soil and favourably influence plant growth (Nardi et al., 2002). Although seed treatment and foliar application of HS is increasingly used in agricultural practice, the mechanism of possible growth promoting effect is usually attributed to hormone-like impact, activation of photosynthesis and improved nutrient uptake (Chen and Aviad, 1990; Fernandez et al., 1996; Kulikova et al., 2005). Humic acids (HA) are characterized as a heterogeneous natural resource, ranging in color from yellow to black, having high molecular weight, and resistance to decay. Humic acid, as a commercial product contains 44-58% C, 42-46% O, 6-8% H and 0.5-4% N, as well as many other elements (Larcher, 2003; Lee and Bartlette, 1976). It improves soil fertility and increases the availability of nutrient elements by holding them on mineral surfaces. The humic substances are mostly used to remove or decrease the negative effects of chemical fertilizers from the soil and have a major effect on plant growth, as shown by many scientists (Linchan, 1978; Ghabbour and Davies, 2001; Pal and Sengupta, 1985).

As per literature survey many researchers reported that the humic substances stimulated root development and enhanced nitrogen, K^+, Cu^{2+} and Mn^{2+} content (Bidegain et al., 2000) in ryegrass. According to Adani et al. (1998), commercial humic acid affected tomato root fresh and dry weights of tomato as well as iron content, depending on the source of the humic acid. The two concentrations (20 and 50 mg/L) of humic acid, resourced from fertilizer, caused iron to increase to 113 and 123%, whereas humic substance derived from leonardite increased iron content to 135 and 161% in tomato roots. Fernández-Escobar et al. (1999) found that application of HA stimulated chlorophyll content and accumulation of K, B, Mg, Ca and Fe in leaves of olive trees. The foliar application of humic substances becomes effective in promoting uptake and accumulation of nutrients in leaves of olive trees (Fernandez et al., 1996). The foliar application of humic substances exerted positive effect on nutrient status of Thuja orientalis L. as reported by Zaghloul et al. (2009). The humic acid application can also greatly improve plant growth and nutrient uptake as reported by Dursun et al. (2002) and Paksoy et al. (2010).

Often called the "stinking rose," garlic may be known for its odor as much as its flavor, but it is actually odorless until its cells are ruptured by being "bruised, cut or crushed" (Simon et al., 1984; Tuckar et al., 2000; Woodward, 1996). Garlic's scent comes primarily from sulfur compounds. When a garlic clove is cut, alliin, an "odorless, sulfur-containing amino acid derivative" (Small, 1997) reacts with the enzyme alliinase to form allicin and other sulfur compounds (Koch et al., 1996; Tuckar et al.,

2000; Woodward, 1996). Allicin breaks down into diallyl disulfide, which is largely responsible for garlic's odor (Koch et al., 1996; Tuckar et al., 2000). In addition to scent, allicin is also responsible for many of garlic's health benefits including its antioxidant, anti-microbial, cholesterol-lowering and blood-thinning properties (Blumenthal, 2000) and is likely to play a role in garlic's anti-cancer effects (Koch et al., 1996).

The goal of the present study was to evaluate the effect of foliar application of commercially produced humic acid on accumulation of mineral nutritions and pungency in cloves obtained from bulb of garlic (Allium sativum L.) grown in the field experiment. The research findings are based on the key parameters necessary for evaluation of mineral nutrients (Ca, Fe, Mg, P, K, Zn, Cu, Mn and S) and pungency (PAD) quality as victual food and hoped to obtain information for patients and researchers.

MATERIALS AND METHODS

Field experiment

Sandy loam soil was plowed twice and 50 MT•ha⁻¹ of well-rotted cow manure incorporated. Synthetic fertilizer at 40 N:60 P:40 K kg•ha⁻¹ was applied as preplant to the soil. Nitrogen was from urea, phosphate was from single superphosphate, and potash was from muriate of potash. Garlic cloves obtained from bulbs (weighing about 35 g each) of cv. Gangajali was planted 3 cm deep in furrows with 15-cm spacing between rows and 10 cm between plants in plots that were 1.5 × 1.5 m². The experiment was established in the last week of October 2012 at the Research Farm, Bidhan Chandra Krishi Viswavidyalaya, Mohanpur, Nadia, and West Bengal, India. Additional nitrogen at 40 kg•ha⁻¹ was applied 30 days after planting. The experiment consisting of five treatments including control (no humic acid applied) were arranged in a randomized complete block design with three replications of each treatment. The detail treatments are summarized in Table 1.

Because garlic is shallow-rooted, supplementary irrigation was required and nine irrigation events providing approximately 5 cm of water each at 15 day intervals were applied, with the first immediately after planting. There were four hand weedings within 9 weeks of planting. The insecticide malathion at 1 ml•L⁻¹ (Rallis India Ltd., Mumbai, Maharashtra, India) was applied to control thrips and the fungicide Dithane M-45 at 2.5 g•L⁻¹ (Indofil Industries Ltd., Andheri, Maharashtra, India) was applied to control purple blotch disease caused by Alternaria porri (Ellis) cif. Three applications of both pesticides were started 30 days after planting and at 15 day interval. After harvesting, ten bulbs were collected from each treatment. Fresh cloves, separated from bulbs, were washed, dried with a soft tissue, peeled, and finely chopped before analysis of mineral nutritions and pungency (PAD).

Preparation of plant samples

Digestion of plant samples

Wet digestion by A.O.A.C. (1970) was used.

Procedure:

1. 1.0 g of ground material was weighed into a 250 ml conical flask.

Table 1. Preparation of humic acid solution for spray on garlic (*Allium cepa* L.) plant.

Standard stock solution (ml)	Diluted with distilled water (ml)	Solution made (ppm)
20	1000	100
40	1000	200
60	1000	300
80	1000	400

Extraction solution: In a 500 ml volumetric flask with 200 ml of distilled water, was added 80g NaOH, 8 ml ethanol and brought to volume 500 ml with distilled water. Standard stock solution (5000 ppm): Weighted out 1.075 g of humic acid and diluted to 200 ml with extraction solution and shaken for 1 h. The source of humic acid was granular, peat, brown coal (Maharashtra Chemicals and Fertilizers, Nageshwar Nagar, Malegoan, Pune-413115 and Maharashtra, India). The spraying was done three times with sticker starting from 25 days after planting and subsequent ones at an interval of 15 days during vegetative stage.

2. 4 ml of $HClO_4$, 25 ml of concentrated HNO_3 and 2 ml of concentrated H_2SO_4 were added to the sample in the conical flask.
3. The content were mixed and heated on a hot plate.
4. The heating continued until dense white fumes appeared.
5. 2 ml of concentrated HNO_3 was added and heated for a minute.
6. It was allowed to cool and 40 ml of distilled water was added and boiled for half a minute on a hot plate.
7. It was cooled and filtered with Whatman No. 42 filter paper into a 100 ml Pyrex volumetric flask and made up to the mark with distilled water.
8. The solution was preserved for the determination of mineral nutritions.

Amount of Cu, Fe, Mn and Zn were determined with an atomic absorption spectrophotometer (model 2380, Perkin-Elmer, Shelton, Conn.) and potassium content was analyzed with a flame photometer (model 1020, Chemito, Mumbai, India). Calcium and Mg were determined by titration using eriochrome black T and calcon indicators (Jackson, 1973). Phosphorus was determined calorimetrically by the phospho-vanado molybdate yellow color method (Jackson, 1973). Sulfur was determined by turbidimetry using the method of Butters et al. (1959). Pungency of garlic bulbs was determined as pyruvic acid (Anthon and Barrett, 2003; Schwimmer and Weston, 1961). Pyruvic acid concentration was determined with 2, 4-dinitrophenylhydrazine using the method of Schwimmer and Weston (1961).

Statistical analysis

Data were analyzed statistically by using Daniel's XL Toolbox 6.52 software for analysis of variance.

RESULTS AND DISCUSSIONS

Calcium (Ca)

In our present study (Table 2), calcium is known to show remarkable variation in its effects among treatments. In garlic, calcium content significantly increased positively with increase of concentration of humic acid applications as compared to the control. The increase was ~1.36 (100 ppm), ~1.88 (200 ppm), ~2.30 (300 ppm) and ~2.77 (400 ppm) fold, respectively. Our results are in agreement with that of Akinci et al. (2009), they also reported that the humic acid applications increased calcium concentration

in broad been roots, and same was reported in tomato by David et al. (1994).

Iron (Fe)

The iron content (Table 2), in response to humic acid applications did show significantly increased effect in all treatments except in 100 ppm of humic acid only as compared to the control, which (HA_1) was also increased over the control, though not significantly. Our results support that of Akinci et al. (2009), who found that the Fe^{3+} increased in humic acid treated broad bean roots as compared to the control. In tomato plants grown in green house conditions, applying humic acid increased the Fe^{3+} content in its roots (David et al., 1994). The maximum value was observed by application of 400 ppm of humic acid (~2.13 fold).

Magnesium (Mg)

Increase in the concentration of magnesium of maize fodder in response to humic acid application was reported by Daur and Bakhashwain (2013). Our results also showed that (Table 2) the magnesium concentration significantly increased in all treatments except 400 ppm of humic acid only as compared to the control treatment, in which (HA_4) also increased over the control, though not significantly. The highest magnesium concentration was observed by application of 200 ppm (~3.10 fold) followed by 100 ppm (~2.33 fold) of humic acid.

Phosphorus (P)

Phosphorus is a major mineral nutrient which is essential to all plant life mostly in terrestrial plants. It also activates crucial enzymatic reactions and contributes to the osmotic pressure of the vacuole, which helps to maintain structural rigidity. In the present study (Table 2), the concentration of phosphorus, with significantly positive

Table 2. Effect of humic acid applications on accumulation of mineral nutrient (mg.100^{-1}g) and pungency (mmol.100^{-1}g) in garlic (*Allium sativum* L.).

Treatment	Ca	Fe	Mg	P	K	Zn	Cu	Mn	S	PAD
HA$_0$ (control)	177.09^{n}	1.69	27.56	160.00	400.77	1.11	0.33	1.69	0.68	4.39
HA$_1$ (100 ppm)	241.76 ±9.23	1.97 ±0.18	69.00 ±3.55	233.59 ±1.61	679.06 ±25.96	1.46 ±0.27	0.37 ±0.07	1.95 ±0.04	0.87 ±0.06	5.77 ±2.19
HA$_2$ (200 ppm)	333.00 ±14.33	3.07 ±0.16	91.67 ±3.18	309.11 ±3.44	933.09 ±43.92	1.60 ±0.11	0.44 ±0.11	2.22 ±0.15	1.00 ±0.07	7.96 ±0.68
HA$_3$ (300 ppm)	407.95 ±13.21	3.05 ±0.05	53.33 ±3.23	153.79 ±3.30	1179.11 ±69.88	1.25 ±0.04	0.52 ±0.03	2.29 ±0.08	1.20 ±0.1	8.60 ±1.43
HA$_4$ (400 ppm)	489.99 ±12.00	3.60 ±0.15	33.05 ±1.95	141.06 ±1.46	1013.23 ±13.12	1.18 ±0.04	0.49 ±0.03	2.00 ±0.15	1.56 ±0.1	10.03 ±1.04

Data are mean ± standard deviation values (*n*=3).

influences were seen in a limited range of humic acid application from 0.00 to 200 ppm. While, 300 and 400 ppm of humic acid applications did not show negative effect on concentration of phosphorus as compared to the control. However, Abdel-Rezzak and El-Sharkawy (2013) reported that the humic acid, significantly increased in concentration of phosphorus in garlic cloves during 2008/2009.

Potassium (K)

As per literature survey, many researchers reported that the humic substances provoked a better efficiency of plant water uptake and improved the potassium concentration (Delfine et al., 2005; Morard et al., 2011; Daur and Bakhashwain, 2013). However, humic acid signifi-cantly increased in the potassium concentration in cucumber at 20 and 40 ppm of humic acid appli-cations as compared to the control (Mohsen Kazemi, 2013).

Our results also revealed that (Table 2) the humic acid applications exerted significantly positive influence on concentration of potassium content as compared to the control. The highest concentration was observed by application of 300 (~2.53 fold) followed by 400 (~2.94 fold) and 200

ppm (~2.33 fold) of humic acid, respectively. While, according to Samson and Visser (1989) humic acid induced increase in permeability of bio-membranes for electrolytes accounting for increased uptake of potassium.

Zinc (Zn)

The beneficial effect of humic acid in soil might have prevented the formation of insoluble complexes of Zn and facilitating their uptake by plants (Tenshia and Singaram, 1992). In our present experiment, with respect to Table 2, it was shown that the concentration of zinc significantly increased in 200 ppm (~1.44 fold) of humic acid application only, while remaining treatments that is, 100, 300 and 400 ppm of humic acid also increased, apparently, though not significantly. However Akinci et al. (2009) reported that the zinc content decreased in humic acid treated plants. On the other hand, Zn^{2+} with decrease in broad bean root may be related with the Fe^{3+} causing the absorption of Zn^{2+} and its toxicity (Olsen, 1972).

Copper (Cu)

In the present study, application of humic acid

through different treatments could produce no significant differences in the content of copper (Table 2). Therefore, no significant effects could be observed by application of humic acid on the content of copper. However, copper content in *Vicia faba* L. treated with HA decreased by 27% but did differ significantly from controls (Akinci et al., 2009).

Eyheraguibel et al. (2008) also found that the Cu^{2+} increased significantly in HA treated maize plant roots by 14% as compared to control. According to Mackowiak et al. (2001), in wheat plants grown with HEDTA, Cu^{2+} cannot freely enter its root since HEDTA can make a stronger bond with Cu^{2+} as compared to humic acid Cu^{2+} bonds. David et al. (1994) stated that in tomato plants grown under low nutrient media, addition of humic acid causes increase of Cu^{2+} in its roots while Cu^{2+} concentration increased in tomato stems, under high nutrient treatment.

Manganese (Mn)

In the present experiment, with respect to Table 2, it is shown that garlic : manganese concentration exerted significantly positive effects in 200 (~1.31 fold) and 300 ppm (~1.35 fold) of humic acid applications, while, other applications of humic

Table 3. Pearson's correlation matrix of all variables.

	Ca	Fe	Mg	P	K	Zn	Cu	Mn	S
Ca									
Fe	0.964*								
Mg	-0.068	0.104							
P	-0.268	-0.057	0.933*						
K	0.887*	0.881*	0.252	-0.041					
Zn	-0.071	0.095	0.984*	0.950*	0.192				
Cu	0.932*	0.907*	0.073	-0.204	0.981*	0.011			
Mn	0.629	0.696	0.598	0.316	0.905*	0.512	0.821		
S	0.981*	0.917*	-0.184	-0.351	0.793	-0.158	0.851	0.482	
PAD	0.990*	0.988*	0.063	-0.131	0.907*	0.059	0.932*	0.695	0.955*

*Significant at 5%, Student's t-test.

acid like 100 and 400 ppm, did not show any significant effects over the control. The result also seems to be related to the antagonistic effect of Ca^{2+} on Mn^{2+} uptake (Bozcuk, 2000).

Sulfur (S)

Sulfur is an essential component of important metabolic and structural compounds in plants (Marschner, 1995). Garlic is known as a S-demanding crop, as it is a component of secondary compounds, that is, allicin, cycloallicin and thiopropanol, which not only control the taste, pungency and medicinal properties of garlic, but also are important for resistance against pests and diseases (Schnug, 1993; Brown and Morra, 1997; Raina and Jaggi, 2008). Our present study shows that the sulfur content (Table 2), positively increased with increased concentration of humic acid applications, which significantly increased in 200 (~1.47 fold) 300 (~1.76 fold) and 400 ppm (~2.29 fold) humic acid applications, respectively as compared to the control.

Pyruvic acid development (PAD)

A common assessment of pungency is made by measuring pyruvate, formed as a stable primary compound from the enzymatic decomposition of flavor precursors and formed in a mole-for-mole relationship with the flavor precursors. We indicated that, concentration of pyruvic acid development (Table 2) had positive increment among all the treatments, which significantly increased in 300 (~1.96 fold) and 400 ppm (~2.28 fold) humic acid applications, respectively as compared to the control.

Correlation among variables

There are correlations between pairs of variables (Table 3). Most of the mineral nutrient like Ca had significant positive correlation with Fe, K, Cu, S and PAD. There are also positive significant correlations of Fe with K, Cu, S and PAD. Here also significant positive correlations between Mg with P, Mg with Zn, P with Zn, Cu with PAD and S with PAD were seen, respectively. There are significant positive correlations of K with Cu, Mn and PAD.

These relationships indicate that improving the primary (P and K) and secondary nutrients (Ca, Mg and S) to enhance micronutrients (Fe, Zn, Cu and Mn) concentration in garlic (*Allium sativum* L.) bulbs could accompany improvement of quality as well as improve pungency (PAD).

Conclusions

In the present study, remarkable variable effects were seen on accumulation of mineral nutritions and pungency content in response to humic acid application in clove of garlic (*A.sativum* L.) bulb. Based on average values and ANOVA results, the highest result was observed by application of 300 followed by 400 and 200 ppm humic acid, which may be the proper value addition in cloves of garlic bulb by enhancing the mineral nutritions and pyruvic acid development that needs to be studied in the future.

Conflict of Interests

The author(s) have not declared any conflict of interests.

ACKNOWLEDGEMENTS

The authors are grateful to the department of Agricultural Biochemistry, Bidhan Chandra Krishi Viswavidyalaya, Mohanpur, Nadia-741252, West Bengal, and India for supporting to carry out the research work.

REFERENCES

Abdel-Rezzak HS, El-Sharkawy GA (2013). Effect of biofertilizer and humic acid applications on growth, yield, quality and storability of two garlic (Allium sativum L.) cultivars. Asn. J. Crop Sci. 5(1):48-64.

Adani F, Genevini P, Zaccheo P, Zocchi G (1998). The effect of commercial humic acid on tomato plant growth and mineral nutrition. J. Pl. Nutr. 21:561-575.

Akinci S, Buyukkeskin T, Eroglu A, Erdogan BE (2009). The Effect of Humic Acid on Nutrient Composition in Broad Bean (Vicia faba L.) Roots. Not. Sci. Biol. 1(1):81-87.

Anthon GE, Barrett DM (2003). Modified method for the determination of pyruvic acid with dinitrophenylhydrazine in the assessment of onion pungency. J. Sci. Food Agric. 83:1210-1213.

AOAC (1970). Official Methods of Analysis. Association of Official Agricultural Chemists, Washington, D.C.

Bidegain RA, Kaemmerer M, Guiresse M, Hafidi M, Rey F, Morard P, Revel JC (2000). Effects of humic substances from composted or chemically decomposed poplar sawdust on mineral nutrition of ryegrass. J. Agric. Sci. 134:259-267.

Blumenthal M (2000). Herbal medicine: expanded Commission E monographs. Newton, MA: Integrative Medicine Communications (HSA Library).

Bozcuk S (2000). Bitki fizyolojisi, Hacettepe Üniversitesi, Fen Edebiyat Fakültesi, Ankara, Türkiye 3. Baskı, Ankara.

Brown PD, Morra MJ (1997). Control of soil-born plant pests using glucosinolate containing plants. Adv. Agron. 61:161-231.

Butters B, Chenery EM (1959). A rapid method for the determination of total sulfur in soils and plants. Analyst. 84:239-245.

Chen Y, Aviad T (1990). Effects of humic substances on plant growth. In Humic Substances in Soil and Crop Sciences, eds. MacCarthy P, Clapp CE, Malcolm RL, Bloom PR. Wisconsin (USA): ASA and SSSA, Madison. pp. 161-186.

Daur I, Bakhashwain AA (2013). Effect of humic acid on growth and quality of maize fodder production. Pak. J. Bot. 45(S1):21-25.

David PP, Nelson PV, Sanders DC (1994). A humic acid improves growth of tomato seedling in solution culture. J. Pl. Nutr. 17:173-184.

Delfine S, Tognetti R, Desiderio E, Alvino A (2005). Effect of foliar application of N and humic acids on growth and yield of durum wheat. Agron. Sustain. Dev. 25(2):183-191.

Dursun A, Güvenc I, Turan M (2002). Effects of different levels of humic acid on seedling growth and macro- and micro-nutrient contents of tomato and eggplant. ACTA Agrobotanica. 56:81-88.

Eyheraguibel B, Silvestre J, Morard P (2008). Effects of humic substances derived from organic waste enhancement on the growth and mineral nutrition of maize. Bioresource Technol. 99:4206-4212.

Fernandez RE, Benlock M, Barranco D, Duenas A, Ganan JAG (1996). Response of olive trees to foliar application of humic substances extracted from leonardite. Sci. Hortic. 66:191-200.

Fernández-Escobar R, Benlloch M, Barranco D, Dueñas A, Gutérrez Gañán JA (1999). Response of olive trees to foliar application of humic substances extracted from leonardite. Sci. Hortic. 66(3-4):191-200.

Ghabbour EA, Davies G (2001). Humic substances: Structures, models and functions, Royal Society of Chemistry, England.

Jackson ML (1973). Soil Chemical Analysis. Prentice Hall of India Pvt. Ltd., New Delhi.

Kazemi M (2013). Effect of foliar application of humic acid and potassium nitrate on cucumber growth Bull. Environ. Pharmacol. Life Sci. 2(11):03-06

Koch HP, Lawson LD (1996). Garlic: the science and therapeutic application of Allium sativum L. and related species. 2nd ed. Baltimore, MD: Williams & Wilkins.

Kulikova NA, Stepanova EV, Koroleva OV (2005). Mitigating activity of humic substances direct influence on biota, Use of humic substances to remediate polluted environments: From theory to practice, Perminova, I.V.; Hatfield, K. and Hertkorn, N.; Springer, Netherlands, pp. 285-310.

Larcher W (2003). Physiological Plant Ecology: Ecophysiology and stres physiology of functional groups, 4th. Edition, Springer, New York.

J. 65:1744-1750.

Lee YS, Bartlett RJ (1976). Stimulation of plant growth by humic substances, Soil Sci. Soc. Am. J. 40:876-879.

Linchan DJ (1978). Humic acid and nutrient uptake by plants. Plant Soil 50:663-670.

Loveland P, Webb J (2003). Is there a critical level of organic matter in the agricultural soils of temperate regions: A review. Soil Till. Res. 70:1-18.

Mackowiak CL, Grossl PR, Bugbee BG (2001). Beneficial effects of humic acid on micronutrient availability to wheat, Soil Sci. Soc. Amer.

Marschner H (1995). Mineral Nutrition in Higher Plants. London: Academic Press. p. 889

Morard P, Eyheraguibel B, Morard M, Silvestre J (2011). Direct effects of humic-like substance on growth, water, and mineral nutrition of various species. J. Plant Nutr. 34(1):46-59.

Nardi S, Pizzeghello D, Muscolo A, Vianello A (2002). Physiological effects of humic substances on higher plants. Soil Biol. Biochem. 34:1527-1536.

Olsen SR (1972). Micronutrient interactions, in Micronutrients in Agriculture, Mortvedt, J. J., Giordano, P. M., and Lindsay, W. L., Eds., Soil Science Society of America, Madison, WI, pp. 243-264.

Paksoy M, Turkmen O, Dursun A (2010). Effects of potassium and humic acid on emergence, growth and nutrient contents of okra (Abelmoschus esculentus L.) seedling under saline soil conditions. Afr. J. Biotechnol. 9(33):5343-5346.

Pal S, Sengupta MB (1985). Nature and properties of humic acid prepared from different sources and its effects on nutrient availability. Plant and Soil. 88:91-95.

Raina SK, Jaggi RC (2008). Effects of sulphur in presence and absence of farmyard manure on onion (Allium cepa) under onion-maize (Zea mays) cropping sequence. Ind. J. Agric. Sci. 78:659-62.

Samson G, Visser SA (1989). Surface active effects of humic acids on potato cell membrane properties. Soil Biol. Biochem. 21:343-347.

Schnug E (1993). Physiological functions and environmental relevance of sulphur containing secondary metabolites. In: De Kok, L. (Ed.). Sulphur Nutrition and Assimilation in Higher Plants (pp. 179-190). The Hague: SPB Acadamic Publishing.

Schwimmer S, Weston WJ (1961). Enzymatic development of pyruvic acid in onion as a measure of pungency. J. Agric. Food Chem. 9:301-304.

Simon JE, Chadwick AF, Craker LE (1984). Herbs: an indexed bibliography 1971-1980 - the scientific literature on selected herbs, and aromatic and medicinal plants of the temperate zone. Archon Books. (HSA Library).

Small E (1997). Culinary herbs. Ottawa: NRC Research Press. (HSA Library).

Tucker AO, De-Baggio T (2000). The big book of herbs: a comprehensive illustrated reference to herbs of flavor and fragrance. Loveland, CO: Interweave Press. (HSA Library)

Woodward P (1996). Garlic and friends: the history, growth and use of edible Alliums. South Melbourne, Victoria: Hyland House.

Zaghloul SM, El-Quesni EMF, Mazhar AAM (2009). Influence of potassium humate on growth and chemical constituents of Thuja orientalis L. seedlings. Ozean J. Appl. Sci. 2:73-78.

19

Anthology of historical development and some research progress glimpses on phytochemical antioxidants phenomenon

Daramola, B.

Department of Food Technology, Federal Polytechnic, PMB 5351, Ado-Ekiti, Ekiti State, Nigeria.

The inevitability of applications of antioxidants in protection of human and preservation of dormant living systems such as food, drugs, cosmetics and other allied chemicals against internal and external stresses have made antioxidants an area of active research world over. Study impact of antioxidant research has advanced from topic level to subject level as revealed by the volume of antioxidants research publications. Each cardinal research interest is engaged in scientific exploration with view to gain mechanistic understanding and consequently raise the bar of knowledge in order to maximise exploitation of antioxidants benefits. The cardinal research interest is so diverse and the volume of publications is so enormous and profusely dispersed. Therefore, it is academically worthwhile to pool some of the research developments into a single piece which could offer accessibility to array of study briefs that appeared in many journals which could motivate readership to seek further knowledge on specific area of antioxidant research interest. In this review, glimpses of developments on antioxidant research that transverse research cardinal perspectives such as phytochemical antioxidant genesis, highlights mechanism of action. Modern methods of extraction and evaluation techniques, quantitative structure-activity relationship (QSAR) and rational design strategy for antioxidants were reviewed. The research future of antioxidants of phytochemical origin was projected. These academic collections should motivate readership to seek further knowledge for product research and development of antioxidants of phytochemical origin and natural product analogues.

Key words: Antioxidants, phytochemicals, cardinal research glimpse, lead references.

INTRODUCTION

All organisms or substance whether living or non-living are vulnerable to oxidative process with several consequences. For instance, in a living thing oxidative process result to a number of oxygenated radicals which are cytotoxic. Consequently, this leads to a spectrum of disease condition such as cancer, cognitive dysfunctions, coronary heart disease and many more (Finkel and Holbrook, 2000; Steinmetz and Potter, 1991) in human beings. In food, oxidative radicals lead to loss of nutritional and sensory quality and consequently loss of economic value (Giese, 1996). This undesirable oxidation phenomenon could be prevented using antioxidants.

In term of origin, antioxidant can be natural or synthetic. Synthetic antioxidant are effective in inhibiting peroxidation especially in non-edible products, such as petroleum based chemicals, but are surrounded with league of limitations largely based on health risk concern. However, natural antioxidants are safe and renewable among other advantages hence preferred to synthetic antioxidants for application in foods, drugs and cosmetics. Recalling that oxidative stress occurs in all living systems, nature endowed the systems with a means of preventing lipid peroxidation. The activity of substances that prevent oxidation is antioxidation and the group of the substances is called antioxidants. In plants, this group of substances that prevent oxidative damaged have genealogical linkage to plant chemicals called phytochemicals or secondary metabolites.

Frontier studies have been conducted on the application of antioxidants with view to gain knowledge and exploit the preservation and protection endowment of antioxidants.

This review reports a survey on major classes of frontier researches of antioxidants scattered in many scholarly journals largely from the perspective of phytochemicals or analogues. This review on phytochemical antioxidant research status should update readership on present knowledge and motivate reader to seek further information for phytochemical antioxidant research and product development.

Phytochemical evolution and defence arguments

Phytochemicals also called nutraceuticals, phytochemicals, phytonutrients and sometimes referred to as functional foods possess antioxidants activity, some modify the immune system and others alter enzymes that metabolize drugs in our system. However, this review limits its purview to antioxidants. As implied by the name, phytochemicals are the chemicals produced by plants. These plant chemicals are biologically active but are not considered essential or priority nutrients such as proteins, carbohydrates, fat, minerals and vitamins. Therefore, it mainly contributes health maintenance and therapeutic properties of food to its consumers. That is, play a role of secondary and tertiary functions of food. In the beginning, phytochemicals were first known to be extradites and as such thought to be waste product. No sooner than later it became clear that phytochemical are arsenal of defence mechanism. The following relates the genesis of phytochemicals. When plants first evolved, there was little free oxygen in the atmosphere, as oxygen level increased as a result of plant metabolism (plants take in carbon dioxide and give off oxygen) their environment became polluted, and production of highly reactive oxygen which are cytotoxic follow afterwards. In order to combat the adverse

effect of the reactive species, plant cell mutates to synthesis chemicals referred to as plant chemicals (Figure 1) that can neutralize or absorb the toxic radicals. In addition, the plants are prone to environmental stress such as heat and radiation and biological attack notably bacteria and viruses and pests.

The following evidences signalled that phytochemicals are strictly for protection and defence purpose. First, phytochemicals are localized at the peripheral surfaces, such as bark of plant stem because it is vulnerable to attack because it exposes directly to attacking agents. However, the trunk cortex at the central of the stem, covered by the bark has low amount and concentration of phytochemicals because it is covered by the stem therefore protected from biological and environmental attacks.

Second, flower and immature leaves contain high amount of phytochemicals because they are struc-turally weak, therefore their presence will afford defence option for the vulnerable plant part. However, it is noted that as the plant leaves and flower grow and mature and structurally strong, the phytochemical content of the named plant parts proportionally decrease. Thirdly, similar explanation holds for root parts and seeds (plant young in embryo). Fourth, plants that survive in the desert and hot regions are known to be rich in phytochemicals. The basis for this is that such desert surviving plants have an efficient mechanism of mopping off radiation (sun) generated radicals that are cytotoxic to the plant.

Fifth, when any part of plant is injured, it quickly respond by secreting extrudates to heal the cut as well as offering protection against probably invading micro and macro organisms.

Ultraviolet (UV) screen

The energy of UV light reaching the earth is sufficient to induce photochemical degradation of many plant components; however, nature equipped terrestrial plants with capability of evolution of barriers to absorb this UV radiation by increasing accumulation of plant chemicals to avert damage. It is apparent that flavonoids such as flavones and flavonols are responsible for UV screen because they are prominent in plant parts such as flower and leaves (Harborne, 1980). Also, phytochemicals such as flavonoids are often concentrated in or around epidermal tissues, where their screening potential will be greatest (Ibrahim et al., 1987; Schmelzer et al., 1988).

Pharmacology of phytochemicals

The aim of the review in this section is not designed to treat pharmacological principles of phytochemicals, but to allude to the relationship between disease condition and

$$CO_2 + H_2O$$

Respiration   Photosynthesis

O_2 O_2

Polysaccharides Monosaccharides
glycosides   → Shikimic acid

Pyruvic acid

Peptide

Acetic acid
(acetyl CoA) 2^0 metabolites
                                                                              intermediate
                                                                              (Prephenic acid)

2^0 metabolite intermediates   Aliphatic
(mevalonic acid,   amino acids   Nitrogeneous
dimethylallyl   source (NH_3)
pyrophosphate)   Alkaloids

                                    Matonic acid

                                                        Aromatic amino
                                                        acids

                                                              denitrification

                        Polylcetides

Terpenoids
Steroids   Cinnamic
                                                                              acids

Fatty acids   Flavonoids,
Fat   other aromatics   Coumarins

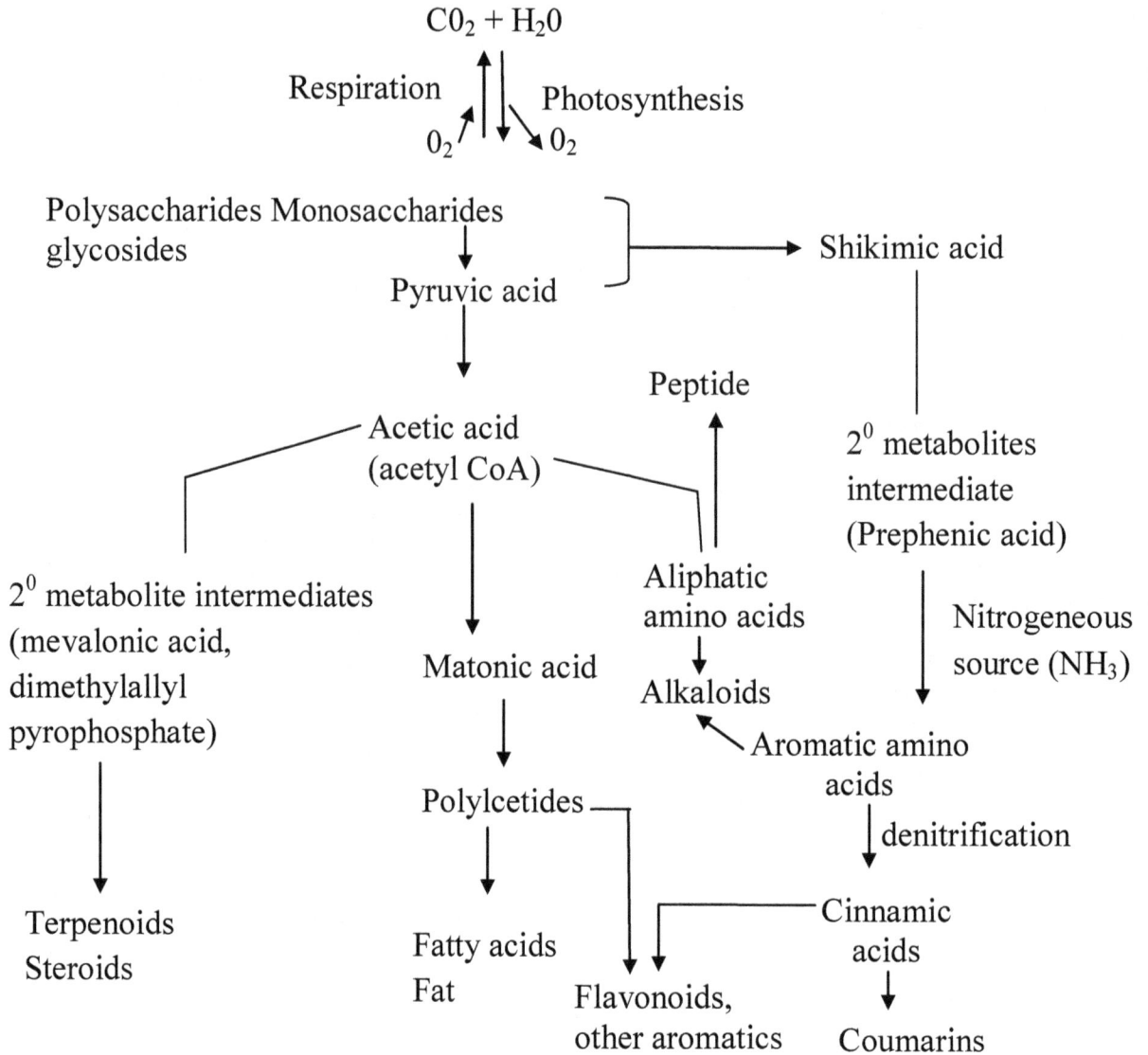

Figure 1. Notable streams of secondary metabolism adapted for academic use from: Essential Inorganic and Organic Pharmaceutical Chemistry. Olaniyi et al., 1998 Shaneson C.I Limited.

antioxidant- pharmacology activities of phytochemicals. For thorough understanding of the mechanism process readers are urge to seek detail information in professional texts.

Gastric ulcer

Simply, the aetiology of gastric ulcer involves increase effect of stress hormones which lead to increased glandular secretion which denatures proteins in plasma membranes and catalyses the hydrolysis of polysaccharide moieties of proteoglycans in the protective mucous coat covering the luminal surface of the stomach and the upper intestine to a perilous extent during prolong stress. Consequently, making the lumen surfaces

to be weak and vulnerable to injury described as gastric ulcer. Phytochemicals such as flavonoids and glycosides have been reported to protect against gastric disorders such as cancer. This activity is accomplished by ability to transfer acyl group to hydroxyl group of cyclooxygenase (Kumar et al., 2011).

Inflammation

Inflammation is the integrated response of many defence systems of the body to the invasion of a foreign body. Inflammation involves action of the complement systems, blood coagulation, humoral and cellular immunity, cytokines, tissue hormones, angiogenesis and repair processes. It is produces free radicals (Miller, 1996).

Phytochemicals such as flavonoids have been found to be prominent inhibitors of cyclooxygenase (COX) and Lipooxygenase (LOX) that affects inflammation. The activity of flavonoids such as quercetin, apigenin, tea catechin in the inhibition of COX and inducible nitric oxide synthase was related to antioxidant activity (Kumar et al., 2011).

Cancerous conditions

Cancerous condition is abnormal growth condition resulting from disturbance in growth metabolism. Cancer cells manifest in uncontrolled proliferation, differentiation, loss of functions, invasiveness and metastasis that differentiate it from normal cells. Cancer undergoes the stage of initial development, and progression by modulation of cellular proliferation, differentiation, apoptosis, angiogenesis and metastasis (Rang et al., 2007). Phytochemicals such as flavonoids have been shown to be highly effective scavengers of most types of oxidizing molecules, notably singlet oxygen and other free radicals that are probably involved in DNA damage and tumour promotion. This mechanism of therapeutic action expresses antioxidative action.

Antimicrobial activity

Phytochemicals of various classes have been used extensively since pre-historic times for treatment of various diseases. Propolis has been used, referred in old testament for its healing properties. Crude and fractionated extracts of tropical seed of bitter kola (*Garcinia kola*) had been reported to exhibit antimicrobial activities against some micro-organisms notably *Candida albicans, Esherichia coli, Salmonella enteric* that are important in food spoilage and intoxification (Daramola and Adegoke, 2007). Flavonoids and alkaloids are the dominant bio-active components identified in the fractional flavonoids isolated from T*ermanalia ballerica* possess antifungal activity against *C. albicans*. And some glycosylated flavonones are effective against *Aspergillus flavus*. A summary of antibacterial, antimicrobial and antiviral activities of flavonoids a class of phytochemical is tabulated and presented (Kumar et al., 2011; Cushnie and Lamb, 2005).

Treatment of thrombosis

Platelet aggregation progressively contributes to atherosclerosis and acute platelet thrombus formation. Activated platelets adhering to vascular endothelium generate lipid peroxides and oxygen free radicals which inhibit endothelial function of prostacylin and nitric oxide (Middleton et al., 2000).

Etiology and treatment of cardiovascular diseases

Cardiovascular diseases (CVS) are today the principal cause of death in both developing and developed countries. CVS diseases include atherosclerosis, coronary heart disease, arterial hypertension and heart failure. The major reason behind CVS Diseases is oxidative stress. Oxidative stress is a condition of imbalance endogenous oxidants and reactive oxygen/-nitrogen species (RONS) with predominance of reactive species. Products of oxidative stress modify low density lipoprotein particles and subsequent induction of inflammation (Kumar et al., 2011).

Endothelial dysfunction associated with increased AMI platelet aggregation. Common consequences of AMI are heart failure and arrhythmias because patients with heart failure and arterial hypertension have been diagnosed with increased production of reactive oxygen species (ROS) (Mladenka et al., 2010). Studies revealed that long-term administration of flavonoids can decrease the incidence of cardiovascular disease and their conesquences, since all the disorders can be mitigated by flavonoids. Flavonoids are the most studied phytochemicals in relation to antioxidant activity. All these revealed the capability of antioxidant in management of various diseases conditions.

Antioxidants phenomenon

Although, metabolic process channel the provision of energy for vital cell activities in a living system, however, this process leads to the unavoidable production of oxygen derived free radicals (Mccord, 1994) and harmful toxins such as tobacco smoke and indiscriminate burning of materials such as tyre and ageing related diseases that have been confirmed to be causative agents for myriad of diseases notably cancer, rheumatoid arthritis, heart attack, stroke and Alzheimers disease and others. In addition, free radicals and other oxidants are known to cause oxidative damage to lipids, proteins and nucleic acids. These oxidants are important factors in the development of a number of diseases as itemised above (Ames et al., 1993). Ordinarily, there is a balance between antioxidants and oxidants. When the equilibrium between oxidants and antioxidants defence systems is impaired in favour of the oxidants, the condition is known as oxidative stress (Halliwell and Gutteridge, 1999). Abundant evidences exist that oxidative stress triggers many undesirable processes at cellular, tissue and organism levels, consequently playing a major role in pathogenesis of many human diseases named above and others such as ischemia, atheroscherosis, chronic renal failure and many more. These undesirable conesquences of oxidative stress accounts for the justification for application of exogenous antioxidants with view to abort or prevent undesired chemical damage caused by oxidative stress (Augustin et al., 1997)

Some aspect of biological organelle as targets of endogeneous radicals

The basis of the spectrum of diseases is stemmed from susceptibility of biological molecules to radical attack. For example susceptible lipid molecules present in the biological membrane are most prone to free radical attack (Roy et al., 2013). In addition, DNA and protein-like macro molecules also constitute vulnerable targets for free radical attack. Free radical mutates the DNA and RNA by pairing with electrons in the DNA chains leading to cellular electronic imbalance (Evans and Cooke, 2004). Ageing is often characterized by the accumulation of mitochondrial DNA mutations as well as improper clearance of reactive oxygen species produced by the respiratory chain resulting in early aging. More importantly, when transport proteins (protein critical for rapid homeostatic mechanism) are affected by free radicals, or when inherent antioxidant defences are overwhelmed, toxics occurrence ensues (Salvi et al., 2001). Such occurrences hand-in spectrum of chronic pathological conditions as well as other known fatal degenerative diseases. In terms of electronic transport chain, free radicals are produced inevitably during cellular metabolism such as by electron leakage from the electron transport chain and redox enzymes as well as by some lymphocytes while defending the human system against foreign organism (St Pierre, 2002).

Antioxidants

Antioxidants simply means against oxidation. Their physiological effects have been harnessed for management of public health. Going by the definition of oxidation and reduction for antioxidants then it can be claimed that the mechanism of therapeutic and pharmacological actions of phytochemicals illustrated here-above is in accord with at least one of the oxidoreduction definition of antioxidants. Hence all the pharmacological exhibition of phytochemicals expresses one form of antioxidants or another. The broad spectrum of biological activities within the group and the multiplicity of actions displayed by certain individual members make the flavonoids group one of the most intriguing classes of biologically active compounds and thus these are often termed 'bioflavonoids' (Singla et al., 2001). Flavonoids occur in practically all parts of plants including fruits, vegetables, nuts, seeds, leaves flowers and bark (Middleton, 1984). Phytochemicals are very important because some symptoms originally thought to be due to vitamin C deficiency such as bruising due to capillary fragility were found in early studies to be relieved by crude vitamin C extract but not by purified vitamin C.

Bioflavonoids were found to be essential components in correcting this bruising tendency and improving the permeability and integrity of the capillary lining. These bioflavonoids include hesperidin, citrin, rutin, flavones, flavonols, catechin and quercetin (Singla et al., 2001).

Also, the antioxidative properties have been employed in preservation of lipid food systems thereby circumventing undesirable changes such as objectionable odour and flavour, rancidity and bleaching of fatty food colours, consequently prolong the shelf-life of the food (Giese, 1996).

Antioxidants in food

One of the major causes of loss of quality in foods is liquid peroxidation which leads to quality deterioration, rancidity, discoloration and loss of nutrients such as vitamins (Nawar, 1996; Hidalgo et al., 1998). The deteriorative process of oxidation occurs naturally in all foods, not just those with high fat content (Giese, 1996). This makes the addition of antioxidants useful in most fat-containing foods.

Although, oxidative damage to foods can be prevented or delayed using improvements in food processing and preparation, refrigeration and packaging but they are much more expensive in comparison to the cost of adding antioxidants. In terms of origin, antioxidants can be synthetic or natural; though synthetic antioxidants are effective in preventing lipid peroxidation but their activity is surrounded by league of limitations that are centrally linked to health risk and poor process carry-through. However, exploitation of natural antioxidants especially from plant sources has greatly increased in recent years. The development on application of antioxidants from natural sources is favoured by a number of factors notably: (1) safety, since they are part of food man has been eating for thousands of year. (2) effectiveness since they survive processing operations as found in institutional food preparations (3) Their use is not guided by regulatory rules (4) Their source is renewable (Daramola et al., 2009).

Han-Seung et al. (2004) listed in their report several factors such as light, relative humidity, temperature, availability of oxygen and some metals that affect the production of lipid oxidation products. For example, lipid oxidation is likely the most common mechanism of oxygen uptake in fried foods such as potato chips. Also, lipid oxidation in meat and meat products is one of the major causes of spoilage and deterioration of organoleptic properties leading to off-flavour development, colour degradation and nutritive loss (Genot et al., 1997). This undesirable occurrence can be inhibited by the use of antioxidants.

Nature of antioxidant action

As the name implies antioxidants could function by any of

Table 1. Definition of oxidation and reduction.

Oxidation	Reduction
Addition of oxygen	Removal of oxygen
Addition of electro negative element (s) or ion	Addition of electronegative elements or ions
Removal of hydrogen	Addition of hydrogen
Removal of electro positive elements	Addition of electronegative elements or ions
Loss of electron(s)	Gain of electron
Increase in oxidation	Decrease in oxidation number

reductive action process presented in Table 1. However, the principal natures of antioxidant action are nomenclaturally designated as:

Reducing agents: Reducing agents function by transfers of hydrogen atom. Such compounds include ascorbic acid, erythorbic acid, ascorbyl palmitate and sulphites.

Chelating agents: Although some scientific opinion holds that chelating agents are not true antioxidant but are often used with antioxidative compounds. This is because chelating agents grab and hold or complex with pro-oxidative metal ions such as iron and copper. Examples of chelating agents are citric acid and its salt, phosphates and the salts of ethylene diamine tetraacetate (EDTA). However, considering the universal definition of antioxidant in Table 1, reducing agents are functionally antioxidants. Generally, the mode of antioxidant action can be oxygen scavenger, radical scavenger and capability to repair damaged molecules. This is customarily expressed by enzymic antioxidants

Natural antioxidant - plant phenolics functional groups

Virtually all phytochemicals would exhibit antioxidative properties. A treaty on comprehensive list that include: simple phenolics, tannins, coumarins, anthraquinones, xanthones, chromones, flavonoids, anthocyanins saponins, alkaloids, and steroids and respective glycosides can be found in pharmacognosy text such as Trease and Evans (2002) and natural products texts. However, this review shall center on phenolics and derivatives with reference to flavonoids. Phenolics are virtually ubiquitous to all plant bio-constituents therefore, it is logical to think that they play a critical role with respect to the survival of plants. As already stated phenolics are important in playing defence role in plants, more importantly as an antioxidant. This section reviews fundamental chemical properties of phenolics that accounts for their anti-oxidative properties.

The common feature of phenolics is the presence of a hydroxyl-substituted benzene ring within their structure. However, some non-hydroxylated precursors or derivatives eg cinnamic acid (3-phenyl propenric acid), are sometimes tagged 'honourary phenolics' although these do not exhibit all the characteristics of true phenol-

lics (Parr and Bolwell, 2000). The interaction of the hydroxyl groups of phenolics with the λ-electrons of the benzene ring gives the molecules special properties, most notably the ability to generate free radicals, where the radical is stabilized by delocalization. By this formation, the relatively long lived radicals are able to modify radical-mediated oxidation processes. Phenolics which possess two ortho-positioned hydroxyl groups are very good antioxidants. Many phenolics chelate metal ions, but tight binding requires vicinal hydroxyl groups such as those present in the B-ring of quercetin and on caffeic acid (Morei et al., 1993). This metal-binding capacity is relevant to one aspect of phenolic antioxidant activity since free transition metals ions are pro-oxidant because they are profoundly present in biological systems. Also, they produce free radicals easily in the presence of hydrogen peroxide. Besides, phenolic hydroxyl groups, increase the potential of electronic delocalization. More importantly phenolic groups are easily ionized, thus serve as weak acids, which ultimately influence the chemical reactivity of total phenolics (Parr and Bolwell, 2000). Others such as phenolics are good hydrogen donor in the formation of hydrogen bonds. Some polymeric phenolics carry large numbers of such donor groups, with the result that complexes formed with other molecules are very stable and tend to precipitate out. This is the basis for tanning abilities of tannins (hydrolysable tannins; for example, esters of garlic acid and the condensed tannins; for example, flavan-3-ol polymers).

Mechanism of oxidation: Autoxidation

As reported by Giese (1996), oxidation occurs in three steps as explained below:

First initiation step: Fat free radicals are formed when hydrogen atoms are lost from the fatty acid group. The resultant fat free radicals react with oxygen to form peroxyl free radicals. The peroxyl free radicals act as strong initiators or catalysts for further oxidation by extracting hydrogen from another molecule triggering propagation.

Second propagation step: The earlier formed peroxyl radicals remove a hydrogen atom from a lipid to form a relatively stable hydroperoxide and a new unstable fatty

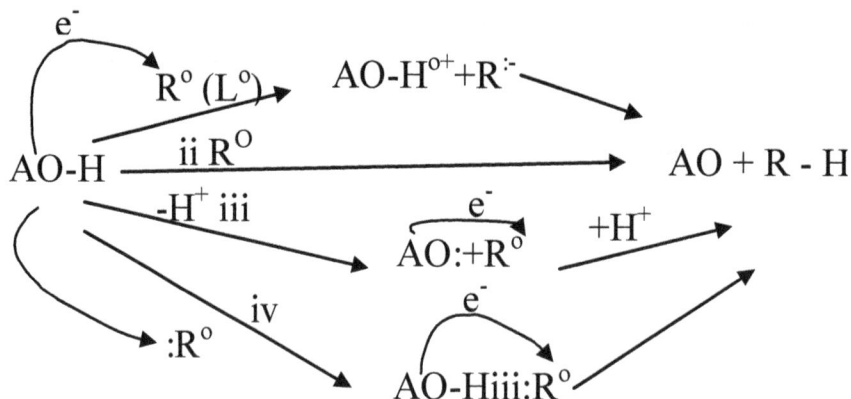

Figure 2. Mechanism of radical scavenging by an antioxidant.

radical. The unstable fatty radical will then react with oxygen to form another new reactive peroxyl radical.

Third, termination step: The final step in autoxidation involves the split of hydro peroxides to form smaller short chain organic compounds such as aldehydes, ketones, alcohols and acids which are responsible for the off-odours, off-flavour characteristics of rancid fats, oils and their products. It is important to state that autoxidative process is ended when two unstable radicals react. Besides, the termination step can also be accomplished when a fatty radical reacts with a stable antioxidant radical. The mechanism of autoxidation and antioxidant action has been structurally represented in the work of Dorko and Edwards (1993).

Mechanism of antioxidant action

According to the mode of action, food antioxidants can be classified as free radical terminators, chelators of metal ions or as oxygen scavengers that react with oxygen in a closed system (Dziezak, 1986). Free radical terminators also known as primary antioxidants react with higher energy lipid radicals to convert them to thermodyna-mically more stable product. They are believed to contribute hydrogen or electron from the phenolic hydro-xyl groups. These effects may either inhibit the initiation or propagation step (Giese, 1996) as illustrated in the equations below. An antioxidant, AH apparently reacts with radical produced during autioxidation according to the scheme (Dugan, 1985):

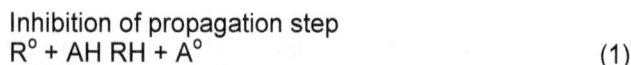

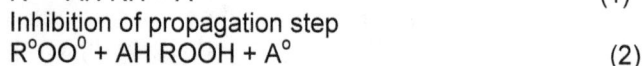

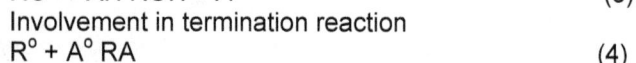

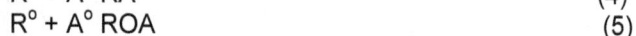

Inhibition of propagation step
$R^{\circ} + AH\ RH + A^{\circ}$ (1)
Inhibition of propagation step
$R^{\circ}OO^{\circ} + AH\ ROOH + A^{\circ}$ (2)
$RO^{\circ} + AH\ ROH + A^{\circ}$ (3)
Involvement in termination reaction
$R^{\circ} + A^{\circ}\ RA$ (4)
$R^{\circ} + A^{\circ}\ ROA$ (5)

The antioxidant free radicals formed in (1), (2) and (3) are stable and low energy free radicals that do not start a chain propagation process but rather enter some termi-nation reaction with lipid radical to form lipid - antioxidant complex.

Generalised pathways of radical scavenging DA-2 by antioxidant

The generalized pathways depicted in Figure 2 according to Evans et al. (1992), Mukai et al. (1992) and Van Acker et al. (1996) explains mechanism of antioxidant action in four different mode designated as follows: (i) electron transfer from antioxidant to active radical produces a cation radical and an anion. The electron transfer is succeeded by proton transfer from the cation radical to the anion. (ii) Direct hydrogen atom transfer between the antioxidant and the active radical (iii) Deprotonation of the antioxidant followed by electron transfer from the resulting anion to the active radical. This is immediately followed by protonation of the anion derived from the active radical and (iv) proton-coupled electron-transfer for phenolic antioxidants as a fourth pathway distinguished by some DA-3 author notably Mayer et al. (2002), DiLabio and Johnson (2007) and Tishchenko et al. (2008).

Extraction and analysis of plant phenolics

All plants are endowed with phenolic compounds and plant foods and medicinal plants are rich sources of phenolics that can act as antioxidants that can prevent heart diseases (Jin et al., 2010; Wijngaam et al., 2009), reduce inflammation (Mohammad et al., 2012), lowers the incidence of cancers and diabetes. The protection arrogated to the consumption of food plant products such as fruits, vegetables and legumes is essentially asso-ciated with the presence of phenolic compounds.

Therefore, there is need for their isolation prior to characterisation. The objective of this section is to review current methods of extracting natural product of phenolic origin that are known to exhibit antioxidant activity from plant materials.

Sample preparation

The fundamental factors for consideration during preparation of plant samples are: nature of sample matrix, chemical properties of the phenolics, with respect to polarity, concentration, number of aromatic rings and hydroxyl groups (Roberts et al., 2013). Consequently, no single extraction procedure is suitable for the extraction of phenolics from all plant materials. Other factors for consideration include particles since, temperature and all forms of pretreatment to enhance the extraction of phenolic compounds. Such pre-treatment include removal of fat especially when necessary to remove lipid from fat - containing samples as accomplish by Weidner et al. (2012) prior to extraction of phenolics from ground seeds of grapes.

Solvent extraction is the most common technique employed for the extraction of phenolics. However, notable parameters influencing the yield of phenolics include nature or chemical property of the solvent, extraction time, temperature, solvent to sample ratio, number of repeat extraction of sample. As well as nature of bioactive or phenolic compound to be isolated. The commonest solvents used are: water, acetone, ethyl acetate diethyl ether, chloroform, alcohols (methanol, ethanol, propanol). A comprehensive review on accom-plishments with respect to extraction process and factors affecting phenolic extraction can be found in Roberts et al. (2013). However, it is imperative to state that solvent modification do greatly influence extraction of phenolic compounds such that solvent modification could be by acid, alkaline or sulphated water.

Modern extraction techniques for phenolics

Although, there are merits such as simplicity, cheap apparatus and high extraction rate, the convectional procedures of Soxhlet, tested reflux extraction procedure is still used in many research and institutional centres especially in developing countries. It has some draw backs, notably (1) long extraction time, (2) the need to use large volumes of hazardous organic solvents, which constitute environmental pollutants, and health hazards to workers (3) interference with and degradation of targeted components due to both internal and external factors such as light, air, high temperature (Santana et al., 2009; Altuner et al., 2012). The flaws associated with Soxhlet solvent extraction method necessitate the evolve-ment of new extraction techniques outlined herein: Ultra-

sound-assisted extraction (UAE), microwave assisted extraction (MAE), ultrasound-microwave assisted extraction, supercritical fluid extraction (SFE), sub-critical water extraction (SCWE) and high hydrostatic pressure processing. These methods are characterized by short extraction times, decrease release of toxic pollutants as a result of reduction in the amount of organic solvent used. Summary of the novel extraction techniques for phenolic constituents and lead references are presented in Table 2.

ROS and methods of assessment of antioxidant activity

Since it is ROS that are the most important substrates for target by antioxidants to scavenged, summary of ROS that are relevant to the food matrix and ROS that could be found in vivo is shown in Table 3. There many methods for the assessment of antioxidative potentials of samples. Notable methods (Table 4) outlined herein are limited to physical and chemical methods.

Improvement of antioxidant activity

There are two broad types of strategies to be employed for the designing of novel antioxidant. They are: (1) Modification of the existing antioxidant to meet specific requirement or demand. (ii) Molecular construction/-synthesis of antioxidants based on theoretical/data. This is often referred to as de novo design (Zhang, 2005). The efficacy of both strategies defends on antioxidant structural requirements obtained from qualitative SARS and QSARS of antioxidants.

Modification of existing antioxidants

Activities of antioxidants are governed by many factors and antioxidative properties requirement are diverse. Therefore there are needs to improve existing ones and design new ones with superior activity to existing ones. In this section, highlights of modification of antioxidant with view to improve activity are presented. The molecular structure of antioxidant could be altered with view to enhance its activity.

Qualitative SARS for phenolic antioxidants and analogues

Of all the natural antioxidants, flavonoids and its analogues have the highest frequency of study hence used for illustration herein. The essence of structure activity relationship study is to define dominant structural factors that influence activity of a molecule. Bors et al.

Table 2. Some novel extraction techniques for the extraction of phenolic compounds.

Name	Operation Principles	Examples of plant extraction	Lead Ref Samples
Ultrasound- assisted extractors	Application of ultra sonic radiation (waves) that create cavitational bubbles around sample tissue to disrupt cell wall thereby releasing content.	- *Potentilla altrosanguinea* - Pinus radiate	Toma et al., 2001 Vinatoru, 2001 Kalpana et al., 2008
Microwave assisted extracted	Microwaves are non-longing radiation, inducing molecular motion in materials resulting in sample heating, the stem generated swells and rupture the cells thereby releasing their active components	- *Androgatus paniculata* - Green tea polylends	Wang et al., 2010 Vasu et al., 2010
Ultrasound/microwave assisted extraction	The coupling of ultrasonic and microwave to extract bioactive constituents. The principle is the simultaneous exertion of the two methods explained above. The synsigism of the technique lend reduction of extraction time, consumption of lower volume of solvents and comparative high yield.	-*Spatholobus suberectus* - Burdocth leaves	Lou et al., 2010 Xian et al., 2011
Super critical fluid Extraction	The transformation of a solvent to a fluid at particular temperature and pressure marks its critical points. Such fluid is termed super critical fluid. It has penetration power thus efficient for extraction of bioactive components	- Sweet basil - *Momordica charantia*	Leal et al., 2008 Shan et al., 2012
Subcritical water extraction	Also called superheated water, pressurized water or hot liquid water extraction. It is simple, high extract quality, low extraction time. Water becomes subcritical when its liquid form is preserved at 100-347°C and 10-60 bar. It extracts essentially polar compounds.	- *Morinda citrifolia* - Green tea	Pongnaravane et al 2006 Etoh et al., 2010
High Hydrostatic pressure extraction (HHPE)	This method is non-thermal but super-high hydraulic pressure (1000-8000 bar). HHPE involves creation of huge pressure difference between the cell membrane interior and exterior consequently allows solvent to penetrate into the cells leakage of cell components (bioactive substances)	- *Maclura pomifera* - Cashew apples	Altuner et al., 2012 Queiroz et al., 2010
Pulse electric field	Also a non-thermal technique with low energy, that is effectual in cell membrane breakdown and efficient mass transfer.	- Straw berry juice - Apple juice	Odriozola et al., 2008 Turk et al., 2010
Accelerated solvent extraction	An automated solvent technique that operates under nitrogen, high pressure and temperature. these condition lend high solvent penetration and dislodge of bioactive constituent		Wibisono et al., 200 Richier et al., 1996

Table 3. Relevant ROS for examining potential antioxidants.

In vivo	Food matrix
O_2 (Superoxide radical)	O_2
Singlet O_2	Singlet O_2
H_2O_2	H_2O_2
Lipid peroxides	Lipid peroxides
HOCl*	-
RO (alkoxy radicals)[a]	RO
RO_2 (Peroxyl radical$_2$)[a]	R O_2
NO (Nitric oxide) NO_2 (nitrogen dioxide)	NO, NO_2
ONOO (Peroxynitrite)	(Nitrite preservation)
OH (hydroxyl radical)	OH

*HOCl is produced by activated phagocytes in the human body. Many bleaches and disfectants contain its sodium salt (NaOCl), so it is possible that food constituents might sometimes come into contact with this molecule. [a]Radicals formed by the breakdown of lipid hydroperoxides, either thermally (as in heated oils/fats) or catalysed by transitional metal ions (both in foods and *in vivo*). Source: Aruoma et al., 1997.

Table 4. Notable methods of assessment of antioxidant activity

Method/ instrument	Principal oxidant/ Reagent	Antioxidant activity unit	References
Electron spin resonance spectroscopy	Methyl linoleate	Measure rate of oxygen depletion	Skibsted et al., 2001
Free-radical scavenging activity UV-Spectro photometer 515 nm	DPPH 2, 2 di-phenyl -1- picrylhydrazyl	2 DPPH radial scavenging activity	Brand-Williams et al., 1995
Free-radical scavenging activity UV-Spectro photometer 532 nm	Deoxyribose model	% Hydroxyl radical scavenging activity	Halliwell et al., 1987
Ferric Reducing antioxidant power 500 nm (FRAP)	Ferric thiocyanate method	% oil-acid peroxidation	Osawa and Namiki, 1981
Total phenolic content/spatrophatium	Folin Ciocalteau reagent	Total phenolic content	Taga et al, 1984
Total phenolic content/spectrophotometer 470 nm	β-carotene linoleic acid bleaching method	Bleaching/double bond oxidation	Taga et al, 1984
fluorescence	ORAC method	Peroxyl radical scavenging activity	Cao and prior, 1995; Ou et al., 2001
Copper chelating capacity 200-600 nm	$CuCl_2$		Afanasen et al., 1989
ABTS* radical cation 658nm, 734 nm	MnO_2 ABTS spectro photometer	ABTS radical cation scavenging activity	Re et al., 1999
Superoxide anion radical scavenging activity 550nm	Nitroblue tetrazolium salt (NBT)	Anion scavenging activity	Kuda et al., 2005
Spectrophotomer 515 nm	1, 3 Diethy1-2-thiobarbituric acid method	% Lipid peroxidation	Furuta et al., 1997, Suda et al., 1994
Conjugated diene mtd spectrophotometer 234 nm	Linoleic acid-emulsion		Lingnert et al., 1979
Total antioxidant capacity method	Oxygen radical absorbance capacity		Cao et al, 1996

Ferric reducing antioxidant power = FRAP; oxygen radical absorbance capacity = ORAC.

(1990) indicated three structural factors being the most crucial for flavonoids antioxidant activity namely; i) an ortho-dihydroxy (catechol) structure in the B ring; ii) a 2, 3-double bond in conjugation with a 4-oxo function (1, 4, pyrone moiety) in the C ring; iii) the additional presence of both 3 and 5 hydroxyl group. These structural factors could be manipulated to improve the antioxidant activity of flavonoids. For example it has been proposed and confirmed that a five - membered analog of α - tocopherol is more active than the six - member analogue because the formal is more planer than the latter and consequently, enables λ-type lone pairs to exert its full stabilizing effect on the radical. This lay the foundation for the designing and improvement of a novel antioxidant 2,3-dihydro -5- hydroxy-2,2- dipentyl 4,6 ditertbutyl benzofuran. The major improvements as reviewed by Zhang (2005) are: i) reduction of OH BDE and prohibition of the free radical of BO - 653 (Figure 3) from attacking other biological targets due to substitution of two O - tert butyl moiety, ii)

Improved cellular mobility of BO - 653 within and between membranes and lipoproteins, and iii) the opened- 7 - position, which facilitates the addition of peroxy radical to the phenoxy radical of BO - 653.

Rational design strategy for antioxidants

The most important features of an excellent radical-scavenging antioxidants are: (a) the

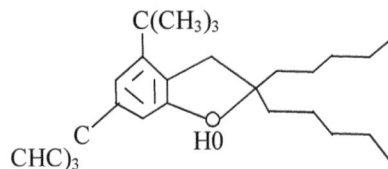

Figure 3. Structures of BO - 653.

X(O,S,N,C)- H BDE or IP should be appropriate. Low BDE and IP are beneficial to enhance the direct radical-scavenging activity in non-polar or polar solvents. However, in polar solvents, possible proton dissociation should be considered because anions are more active than neutral counterparts to donate on electron and some electron-withdrawing groups become electron donating in anion forms; for examole, - COOH, CHCOOH (b) the solubility should be suitable in the applied environments. For example, hydrophobic antioxidants tend to exhibit better activity in an emulsion system, while hydrophilic antioxidants are more effective in bulk lipids, often observed as 'polar paradox'. (c) The toxicity of anti-oxidant and their metabolites, including antioxidant derived radicals should be as low as possible.

De novo antioxidant design

This implies either the assembling of the good features of two or more antioxidants into one molecule or to find new structures by computer aided methodologies. Some examples as illustrated by Zhang (2005) are explained herein: By combining the essential moiety of α-tocopherol and uric acid into one molecule a new antioxidant lead structure; hydroxyphenyl-urea was proposed. Most of which their derivatives exhibit 10 times higher antioxidant activity than α-tocopherol or uric acid. The enhanced radical scavenging activity of hydroxyphenyl-urea deri-vatives were attributed to the fact that the odd electron can be better stabilized by the P-Ome group and the urea moiety.

Similarly, combining the aromatic moiety of structure of α-tocopherol and dione moiety of lycopene, Palloza et al. as reported by Zhang (2005) designed a new antioxidant tagged FeAOX-6 which was a better antioxidant than α-tocopherol and lycopene, alone or in combination. In addition, a planar catechin analogue was designed and synthesized with view to enhance radical scavenging activity and reduce the pro-oxidant toxicity of catechin. More examples and instructive details can be found in the report of Zhang (2005).

FABRICATION OF ANTIOXIDANTS USING QSAR

Since un-denied facts exist that there is need for exoge-nous antioxidants, research has gathered a library of in-formation with respect to activity and other properties of

antioxidant. The available information has revealed that no single antioxidant is adequate to address all oxidative stress conditions. Secondly, existing antioxidants application is associated with one form of limitation or the other.

Consequently, there is need for designing an anti-oxidant with an improved potency and functional speci-ficity (St Piere, 2002). This feat would be accom-plished by the advancement accomplished in quantum mecha-nical treatment of atoms and progress made in appli-cation of computer information technologies in che-mistry. Therefore, antioxidants are now being fabricated with view to carry all the potentials needed to prevent, cure or at least manage disease conditions associated with all radicals.

The first step in accomplishing this ambition is by design of antioxidant using quantitative structure-activity relationship (QSAR). The QSAR technique mathema-tically correlates the biological activity of the molecules with their various structural features that impart a distinct variation in the different physicochemical properties of the molecules. Therefore, the QSAR technique provides an easy, non-destructive and economical route for identify-cation and designing of novel antioxidants prior to synthesis and assessment. Descriptors could be used for either homogenous or heterogeneous groups. All the descriptors used have correlation with antioxidant activity. The fundamental descriptors used for QSAR study is presented in Table 5.

FUTURE RESEARCH DIRECTION ON PHYTOCHEMICAL ANTIOXIDANT

Since the application of antioxidants is inevitable for maintenance of human health and preservation of foods and non-food products, its demand shall continue to increase and research would need to address the following among others: while extensive research work had been accomplished on primary antioxidant func-tionality, there are sparse studies on secondary and tertiary functionalities of antioxidants. Consequently, secondary and tertiary functionalities antioxidants should be designed and fabricated for treatment of spectrum of disease conditions implicated with oxygenated radicals. In addition, there would be adoption of green extraction protocols in obtaining antioxidants of natural origin by application of methods such as plant milking technology (Chemat et al., 2012).

Similarly, enhancement of anti-oxidant metabolites accumulation by manipulation of factors such as environ-mental and cultural as demon-strated by Karaaslan et al. (2013) should be prioritised in phytochemical antioxidant research.

CONCLUSION

Since the functionality of antioxidants in the prevention or

Table 5. Some Types of QSAR Descriptors

Model, Number	Descriptor	Type	Unit
Semi-empirical descriptors			
1.	Homo energy (HOMO)	Electronic	eV
2.	LUMO energy (LUMO)	Electronic	eV
3.	Energy gap (HOMO-LUMO)	Electronic	eV
4.	Electronic energy (EE)	Electronic	Kcal/mol
5.	Polarizability (P)	Electronic	$\hat{O}^{03}$
6.	Energy of heat of formation (HP)	Thermodynamic	Kcal/mol
7.	Total energy (TE)	Thermodynamic	Kcal/mol
8.	Binding energy (BE)	Thermodynamic	
9.	Hydration energy (HE)	Thermodynamic	
10.	Log P	Thermodynamic	
11.	Refractivity	Thermodynamic	A^{03}
Dragon 3D descriptor			
1.	Randic molecular profiles		
2.	Geometrical descriptors		
3.	RDF descriptors		
4.	3D-MORSE descriptors		
5.	WHIM descriptors		
6.	GETAWAY descriptors		Bo-2

Sources: OM and KIM (2008).

mitigation against degenerative diseases and shelf life extension of oxidizable foods and drugs have been established, efforts have been concerted to engage in frontier research for maximum exploitation of protection and preservation potentials inherent in antioxidants of phytochemical origin. This review pooled up-to-date research briefs on antioxidants of phytochemical origin that are scattered in many journals and articles into one piece. The future of research on phytochemical anti-oxidants was projected. This paper should offer anti-oxidant status information to readership with view to stimulate readership to seek further information for research and development of improved antioxidant

Conflict of Interests

The author(s) have not declared any conflict of interests.

REFERENCES

Afanasen IB, Dorozhko AI, Brodskii AV Kostyuk VA, Potapovitch AI (1989). Chelating and free radical scavenging mechanisms of inhibitory action of rutin and quercetin in lipid peroxidation. Biochem. Pharmacol. 38:1763-1769.

Altuner EM, Islek C, Ceter T, Alpas H (2012). High hydrostatic pressure extraction of phenolic compounds from *Maclura pomifera* fruits. Afr. J. Biotechnol. 11:930-937.

Ames BN, Shigenaga MK, Hagen TM (1993). Oxidants, antioxidants and the degenerative diseases of aging. Proc. Natl. Acad. Sci. USA 90:7915-7922.

Aruoma OI, Spencer JPE, Warren D, Jenner P, Butler J, Halliwell B (1997). Characterization of food antioxidants, illustrated using commercial garlic and ginger preparations. Food Chem. 60(2):149-156.

Augustin W, Wiswedel I, Noack H, Reinheckel Th, Reichelt O (1997). Role of endogenous and exogenous antioxidants in the defence against functional damage and lipid peroxidation in rat liver mitochondria. Mol. Cell. Biochem. 174:1-2, 199-205.

Bors W, Heller W, Michel C (1990). Flavonoids as antioxidants: determination of radical-scavenging efficiencies. Methods Enzymol. 186:343-355.

Brand-Williams W, Cuvelier MF, Berset C (1995). Use of a free radical method to evaluate antioxidant activity. Food Sci. Technol. 28:25-30.

Cao G, Wang G, Prior R (1996). Total antioxidant capacity of fruits. J. Agric. Food Chem. 44:701-705.

Cao G, Prior RL (1999). The measurement of oxygen radical absorbance capacity in biological samples. Meth. Enzymol. 299:50-62.

Chemat F, Vian MA, Cravotto G (2012). Green extraction of natural products: concept and principles. Int. J. Mol. Sci. 13:8615-8627.

Cushnie TPT, Lamb AJ (2005). Antimicrobial activity of flavonoids. Int. J. Antimicrob. Agents 26:343-356.

Daramola B, Adegoke GO (2011). Bitter Kola (*Garcinia kola*) seeds and health management potential. In V.R. Preedy, R.R. Watson V.B. Patel, (Editors). Nuts and Seeds in Health and disease prevention (1st edition) pp213-220 London, Vurlington, San diego: Academic press (imprint of Elsevier).

Daramola B, Adegoke GO (2007). Nutritional composition and antimicrobial activity of fractionated extracts of *Garcinia kola* Heckel Pakistan J. Sci. Ind. Res. 50(2):104-108.

Daramola B, Adegoke GO, Osanyinlusi SA (2009). Fractionation and assessment of antioxidant activities of *Garcinia kola* seed. J. Food Agric. Environ. 7(1):27-30.

Dilabio GA, Johnson ER (2007). Lone pair δ and δ' δ interactions play an important role in proton-coupled electron transfer reactions. Journal of the American Chemical Society 129(19):6199-6203.

Dorko CL, Edward MK (1993). Antioxidants used in foods. Presented at the Inst of Technologists. Short course: Ingredient Technology. Chicago July 9-10.

Dugan LE Roy (1985). Lipids in food chemistry part I Fennema OR ed Marcel Dekker, New York pp. 139-189.

Etoh H, Ohtaki N, Kato H, Kulkarni A, Morita A (2010). Sub-critical water extraction of residual green tea to produce a roasted green -like extract, Biosci. Biotechnol. Biochem. 74:858-860.

Evans MD, Cooke M (2004). Factors contributing to the outcome of oxidative damage to nucleic acids. Bioassays 26:533-542.

Finkel T, Holbrook NJ (2000). Oxidant, oxidative stress and the biology of aging. Nature 408:239-247.

Furuta S, Nishiba Y, Suda I (1997). Fluorometric assay for screening antioxidative activity of vegetables. J. Food Sci. 62:526-528.

Genot C, Kansci G, Meynier A, Gandemer G (1997). The antioxidant activity of carnosine and its consequences on the volatile profiles of liposomes during iron/ascorbate induced phospholipid oxidation. Food Chem. 60(2):165-175.

Giese J (1996). Antioxidants: Tools for preventing lipid oxidation. Food Technol. 50(1):73-81.

Halliwell B, Guteridge JMC (1999). Oxygen toxicity, transition metals and diseases. In: Free Radicals in Biology and Medicine 2nd ed. Japan Scientific Societies Press Tokyo, Japan.

Halliwell B, Gutteridge MC, Arouma OL (1987). The deoxyribose method: a simple test tube assay for determination of rate constants for reactions of hydroxyl radicals. Anal. Biochem. 165:215-219.

Han-Seung S, Youn Suk L, Jong-Koo H, Myunghoon L, Giacin JR (2004). Effectiveness of antioxidant-impregnated film in retarding lipid peroxidation. J. Sci. Food Agric. 84:993-1000.

Harborne JB (1980). Plant phenolics. In Encyclopedia of Plant Physiology, Vol 8, Secondary Plant Products. Ed by Bell EA and Charlwood BV Springer, Berlin pp. 329-402.

Hidalgo FJ, Ahmad I, Alaiz M, Zamora R (1998). Effect of oxidized lipid/amino acid reaction products on the antioxidative activity of common antioxidants. J. Agric. Food Chem. 46:3768-3771.

Ibrahim RK, Deluca V, Khouri H, Latchinian L, Brisson L, Charest PM (1987). Enzymology and compartmentation of polymethoxylated flavonol glucosides in Chrysosplenium americanum. Phytochem. 26:1237-1245.

Jin D, Mumper RJ (2010). Plant Phenolics: extraction, analysis and their antioxidant and anticancer properties review. Molecules 15:7313-7352.

Kalpana K, Kapil S, Harsh PS, Bikram S (2008). Effects of extraction methods on phenolic contents and antioxidant activity in aerial parts of Potentialla atrosanguinea Lodd. And quantification of its phenolic constituents by RP-HPLC. J. Agric. Food Chem. 56:10129-10134.

Karaaslan M, Ozden M, Vardin H, Yilmaz FM (2013). Optimisation of phenolic compound biosynthesis in grape (Bogazkere cv.) callus culture. Afr. J. Biotechnol. 12(25):3922-3933.

Kuda T, Tsunakawa M, Goto H, Araki Y (2005). Antioxidant properties of four edible algae harvested in the Noto Peninsula, Japan. J. Food Composition Analysis 18:625-633.

Kumar B, Sandhar HK, Prasher S, Tiwari P, Salhan M, Sharma P (2011). A review of phytochemistry and pharmacology of flavonoids. Int. Pharm. Sci. 1(1):25-40.

Leal PF, Maia NB, Carmello QAC, Catharino RR, Eberlin MN, Meireles MAA (2008). Sweet basil (Ocimum basilicum) extracts obtained by supercritical fluid extraction (SFE): Global yields, chemical composition, antioxidant activity and estimation of the cost of manufacturing. Food Bioprocess Technol. 1:326-338.

Lingnert H, Valientin K, Eriksson CE (1979). Measurement of antioxidative effect in model system. J. Food Process Preserve. 3:87-103.

Lou ZX, Wang HX, Zhu S, Zhang M, Gao Y, Ma CY, Wang ZP (2010). Improved extraction and identification by ultra performance liquid chromatography random mass spectrometry of phenolic compounds in burdock leaves. J. Chromatogr. A 1217:2441-2446.

Mayer JM, Hrovat DA, Thomas J.L, Borden WT (2002). Proton-coupled electron transfer versus hydrogen atom transfer in benzyl/toluene, methoxy/methanol and phenoxyl/phenol self-exchange reactions. J. Am. Chem. Soc. 124:11142-11147.

McCord JM (1994). Free radicals and prooxidants in health and nutrition. Food Technol. 48(5):106-110.

Middleto EJ (1984). The flavonoids. Trends Pharmacol. Sci. 8:335-338.

Middleton EJR, Kandaswami C, Theoharides TC (2000). The effects of plant flavonoids on mammalian cells: implications for inflammation, heart disease and cancer. Pharmacol. Rev. 52:673-751.

Miller AL (1996). Antioxidant flavonoids: Structure, function and clinical usage. Altern. Med. Rev. 1:103-111.

Mladenka P, Zatloukalova L, Filipsky T, Hrdina R (2010). Cardiovascular effects of flavonoids are not caused only by antioxidant activity. Free Radic. Biol. Med. 49:963-975.

Mohanlal S, Parvathy R, Shalini V, Mohanan R, Helen A, Jayalekshmy A (2012). Chemical indices, antioxidant activity and anti-inflammatory effect of extracts of the medicinal rice 'Njavara' and staple varieties. J. Food Biochem. 36:1-12.

Nawar WW (1996). Lipids in Food Chemistry 3rd ed Fennema O.R Ed Dekker New York pp. 225-319.

Odriozola - Serrano I, Soliva Fortuny R, Martin-Belloso O (2008). Phenolic acids, flavonoids, vitamin C and antioxidant capacity of strawberry juices processed by high-intensity pulsed electric fields or heat treatment. Eur. Food Res. Technol. 228:239-248.

Olaniyi AA, Ayim JSK, Ogundaini AO, Olugbade TA (1998). Essential Inorganic and Organic Pharmaceutical Chemistry. Shaneson C.I Ltd pp. 516.

Osawa T, Namiki M (1981). A novel type of antioxidant isolated from leaf wax of Eucalyptus leaves. J. Agric. Food Chem. 45:735-739.

Ou B, Hampsch-Woodill M, Prior RL (2001). Development and validation of an improvedoxygen radical absorbance capacity assay using fluorescein as the fluorescent probe. J. Agric. Food Chem. 49:4619-4626.

Pongnaravane B, Goto M, Sasaki M, Anekpankul T, Pavasant P, Shotipruk A (2006). Extraction of anthraquinones from roots of Morinda citrifolia by pressurized hot water: Antioxidant activity of extracts. J. Super Crit. Fluids 37:390-396.

Queiroz C, Moreira FF, Lavinas FC, Lopes MLM, Fialho E, Valente-Mesquita VL (2010). Effect of high hydrostatic pressure on phenolic compounds, ascorbic acid and antioxidant activity in cashew apple juice high pressure. Res. 30:507-513.

Rang, HP, Dale MM, Ritter JM, Flower RJ (2007). Rand and Dale's Pharmacology. Seventh Edition, Churchill Livingstone.

Re R, Pellegrini N, Proteggente A, Pannala A Yang M and Rice Evans C (1999). Antioxidant Activity: applying an improved ABTS radical cation decolorization assay. Free Radic. Biol. Med. 26:1231-1237.

Richter BE, Jones BA, Ezzell JL, Porter NL, Avdalovic N, Pohl C (1996). Accelerated solvent extraction. A technique for sample preparation. Ann. Chem. 68:1033-1039.

Roberts TH, Khoddami A, Wilkes MA (2013). Techniques for analysis of plant phenoliccompounds. Mol. 18:2328-2375.

Roy K, Mitra I, Saha A (2013). Predictive modelling of antioxidant coumarin derivatives using multiple Approaches: descriptor-based QSAR, 3D-pharmacophore mapping and HQSAR. Scientia Pharma Ceutica. 81:57-80

Salvi A, Carrupt PA, Tillement JP, Testa B (2001). Structural damage to proteins caused by free radicals: assessment, protection by antioxidants and influence of protein binding. Biochem. Pharmacol. 61:1237-1242.

Santana CM, Ferrera ZS, Torres PME, Santana RJJ (2009). Methodologies for the extraction of phenolic compounds from environmental samples: New approaches. Mol. 14:298-320.

Schmelzer E, Jahnen W, Hahlbrock K (1988). In situ hybridization of light-induced chalcone synthase in RNA, chalcone synthase, and flavonoid end products in epidermal cells of parsley leaves. Proc Natl. Acad. Sci. USA 85:2989-2993.

Shan B, Xie JH, Zhu JH , Peng Y (2012). Ethanol modified superficial carbondioxide extraction of flavoroids from Momordica charantia L and its antioxidant activity. Food Bioprod. Process 90:579-587.

Singla AK, Garg A, Gargs, Zaneveld LTD (2001). Chemistry and pharmacology of the citrus bioflavonoids hesperidin. Phytother. Res. 15:655-669.

Skibsted LH, Pedulli GF, Pedrielli P (2001). Antioxidant mechanism of flavonoids. Solvent effect on rate constant for chain breaking reaction of quercetin and epicatechin in antioxidation of methyl linoleate. J. Agric. Food Chem. 49:3034-3040.

Steinmetz KA, Potter JD (1991). Vegetables, fruits and cancer. II

Mechanisms. Cancer Causes, Contr. 2:427-442.

St. Pierre J (2002). Topology of superoxide production from different sites in the mitochondrial electron transport chain. J. Biol. Chem. 277:44784-44790.

Suda I, Furuta S, Nishiba Y (1994). Fluorometric determination of a 1, 3-diethyl-2-thiobarbituric and malondialdehyde adduct as an index of lipid peroxidation in plant materials. Biosci. Biotechnol. Biochem. 58:14-17.

Taga MS, Miller EE, Prath DE (1984). Chia seeds as a source of natural lipid antioxidants. J. Am. Oil Chem. Soc. 61:928-931.

Tishchenko O, Truhlar DG, Ceulemans A, Nguyen MT (2008). A unified perspective on the hydrogen atom transfer and proton-coupled electron transfer mechanisms in terms of topographic features of the ground and excited potential energy between phenol and radicals. J. Am. Chem. Soc. 139:7000-7010.

Toma M, Vinatoru M, Paniwnyk L, Mason T (2001). Investigation of the effects of ultrasound on vegetal tissues during solvent extraction. Ultrason. Sonochem. 8:137-142.

Turk MF, Baron A, Eugene V (2010). Effect of pulsed electric fields treatment and mash size on extraction and composition of apple juice. J. Agric. Food Chem. 58:9611-9616.

Vasu S, Palaniyappan V, Badami S (2010). A novel micro-assisted extraction for the isolation of andrographolide from *Andrographis paniculata* and its *in vitro* antioxidant activity. J Nat. Prod. 24:1560-1567.

Vinatoru M (2001). An overview of the ultrasonically assisted extraction of bioactive principles from herbs. Ultrason. Sonochem. 8:303-313.

Wang L, Qin P, Hu Y (2010). Study on the microwave assisted extraction of polyphenols from tea. Front. Chem. Eng. Chin. 4:307-313.

Weidner S, Powalka A, Karamac M, Amarowicz R (2012). Extracts of phenolic compounds from seeds of three wild grape vines : comparison of their antioxidant activities and the content of phenolic compounds. Int. J. Mol. Sci. 13:3444-3457.

Wibisono R, Zhang J, Saleh Z, Stevenson DE, Joyce NI (2009). Optimization of accelerated solvent extraction for screening of the health benefits of plant food materials. Health 1:220-230.

Wijngaard HH, Roble C, Brunton N (2009). A survey of Irish fruit and vegetable waste and by products as a source of polyphenolic antioxidants. Food Chem. 116:202-207.

Xiao-Lan C, Jin-Yi W, Ping L, Lian-Wen Q (2011). Ultrasonic-microwave assisted extraction and diagnostic ion filtering strategy by liquid chromatography-quadrupole time-of-flight mass spectrometry for rapid characterization of flavonoids in *Spatholobus suberectus*. J. Chromatogr. A. 1218:5774-5786.

Zhang H - Yu (2005). Structure - activity relationships and rational design Strategies for radical scavenging antioxidants. Curr. Comput. Aided Drug Des. 1:257-273.

20

In vitro effects of gibberellic acid and sucrose concentration on micropropagation of two elite sweet potato cultivars in Rwanda

Valery Ndagijimana[1], Jane Kahia[3] , Theodore Asiimwe[2], Peter Yao Sallah[1], Bancy Waweru[2], Isidore Mushimiyimana[2], Jean Ndirigwe[2], Sindi Kirimi[4], Damien Shumbusha[2], Peter Njenga[5], Modeste Kouassi[6] and Edmond Koffi[6]

[1]Faculty of Agriculture, National University of Rwanda (NUR), P. O. Box117, Huye, Rwanda.
[2]Rwanda Agriculture Board (RAB), P. O. Box 5016. Kigali, Rwanda.
[3]World Agroforestry Centre (ICRAF) Cote d' Ivoire Country Program Cocody Mermoz, Abidjan, Côte d'Ivoire | 08 BP 2823 ABIDJAN 08.
[4]International Potato Center (CIP), Sub-Saharan Africa Region, P. O. Box 25171, Nairobi, Kenya.
[5]Jomo Kenyatta University of Agriculture and Technology, Box 62000, Nairobi, Kenya.
[6]Centre National de Recherche Agronomique (CNRA), Laboratoire Central de Biotechnologies (LCB), 01 BP 1740 Abidjan 01, Côte d'Ivoire.

The current study aimed at evaluating the effect of gibberellic acid (GA$_3$) and sucrose on *in vitro* propagation of two elite sweet potato cultivars (Ukerewe and Gihingamukungu). Nodal explants from *in vitro* growing plantlets were harvested and cultured on Murashige and Skoog media supplemented with 2.5, 5, 10, 20 and 40 µM, GA$_3$. In a separate experiment, sucrose was evaluated at 30, 60, 90, 120, 150, 180 and 210 mM. For Ukerewe, the explants cultured on medium supplemented with 10 µM GA$_3$ recorded the longest (2.78 ± 0.36 cm) microshoots. On the other hand, cultivar Gihingamukungu explants cultured on media supplemented with 2.5 GA$_3$ µM produced the longest ((3.23 ± 0.40 cm) microshoots. Nodal explants from the two cultivars cultured on media supplemented with sucrose 150 mM yielded the longest microshoots (2.51 ± 0.26 and 2.34 ± 0.24 cm, respectively). From the results of the current study, it can be concluded that for micropropagation of the cultivar Ukerewe 10 µM GA$_3$ should be used while 2.5 GA$_3$ µM should be used for micropropagtion of cultivar Gihingamukungu. The regenerated plantlets were successfully weaned in the greenhouse. The protocol developed in this research will open new prospects for massive propagation of the elite sweet potato cultivars in Rwanda.

Key words: Ukerewe, Gihingamukungu, nodal explants, microshoot.

INTRODUCTION

Sweet potato (*Ipomoea batatas*) is a high yielding crop which is ranked second in the world after potatoes (Deng et al., 2012). It belongs to the family *Convolvulacea* (Xiansong, 2010) and it originated in America (Burden,

2005). Sweet potato is a major food; feed and industrial raw material in China whose total output in the world is estimated to be more than 80% (Farmer et al., 2007; Islam, 2006; Liu, 2011). Studies by Islam (2006) have revealed that sweet potato leaf extracts contains, antimutagenic, anticancer and antibacterial properties. Sweet potato is propagated by stem cuttings in Rwanda. This method of propagation is associated with increase in viral load over time on the planting materials and bacterial diseases that affect sweet potato in the major production zones of the country (ISAR, 2008). To eradicate these constraints, there is a need to develop and transfer new techniques for producing pathogen-free clonal planting materials which can help to significantly increase the potential yield of sweet potato (Zhang, 1995).

Multiplication by tissue culture techniques provides a viable alternative to the traditional methods of sweet potato propagation (Bachou, 2002) and could permit the production of relatively uniform plants on a massive scale in a shorter period of time (Mutandwa, 2008). In-vitro propagation of clonally propagated crops offers promise for rapid multiplication of quality planting materials and sustained optimal agricultural productivity. The production of plants in vitro is independent of season and can continue throughout the year. Sweet potato plants propagated by tissue culture mature earlier are more robust; leading to accelerated growth than the plants propagated through conventional methods (ASARECA, 2008).

Nodal explants are occasionally cultured on media supplemented with GA_3 to increase the length of shoots during multiplication or prior to rooting (Moshkov et al., 2008).

The most characteristic effects of GA_3 on shoot growth are increased inter-node extension, increased leaf growth and enhance apical dominance. The elongated shoots are then subdivided to serve as starting mother stock culture for another multiplication cycle.

The concentration of sucrose is one of the factors controlling the induction and growth of in vitro shoots (Gibson, 2000; Gurel and Gulsen, 1998). The optimum sucrose level for shoot development may vary among species and genotypes (Nowak et al., 2004). The concentration at which sugar is used has a great impact on the photosynthetic abilities of plantlets (Desjardins et al., 1995) and the relative success of subsequent acclimatization process. The optimum sucrose concentration as an efficient carbon source has been examined in tissue cultures systems of some plant species, such as Coffea Arabica cultivar Ruiru 11 (Kahia, 1999), Paederiafoetida (Amin et al., 2003) and Elaeocarpus robustus (Rahman et al., 2004). The current study aimed at evaluating the effect of different concentrations of gibberellic acid (GA_3) and sucrose on microshoots proliferation in two elite sweet potato cultivars.

MATERIALS AND METHODS

Plant materials

The study was carried out at the plant tissue culture laboratory of Rwanda Agriculture Board (RAB) located in Rubona, Southern Province of Rwanda (Altitude: 1630 m 2°29'07''S, 29°47'49''E). The two sweet potato cultivars were initially propagated in vitro by nodal culture at the Kenya Agricultural Research Institute, Muguga Plant Quarantine Services in Kenya and distributed to Rwanda through the Rwanda Agriculture Board.

Preparation of media

In the first experiment, nodal explants were cultured in Murashige and Skoog (MS) (1962) media supplemented with GA3 evaluated at 2.5, 5, 10, 20 and 40 µM, ascorbic acid (100 µM), calcium nitrate (50 µM), L-arginine (50 µM), 100 mg/l myo-inositol and 90 mM sucrose. In the second experiment, MS media was supplemented with 30, 60, 90, 120, 150, 180 and 210 mM sucrose. The medium pH was adjusted to 5.8 before gelrite was added and media heated to dissolve it. Ten (10) ml MS medium with supplements was dispensed into 25 x125 mm test tubes and steam sterilized in an autoclave at 1.06 kg cm^2 and 121ºC for 15 min.

Inoculation and incubation

Inoculation was carried out under aseptic conditions in a laminar airflow hood in the laboratory in Rubona. Explants with two nodes were dissected from in vitro growing cultures using sterile blade and forceps and the leaves were cut off. They were cultured into test tubes containing 10 ml medium under evaluation. Twenty (20) test tubes were used per treatment and these were sealed with parafilm before incubating them in a growth room maintained at 25 ± 2°C under the cool white fluorescent lights and 16 h photoperiod with a photon flux density of about 60 µ mol m^{-2} s^{-1} and 70-80% relative humidity.

Transplanting

The in vitro regenerated sweet potato plantlets were carefully removed from the test tubes and the roots gently cleaned with running tap water to remove the gelrite. The plantlets were then taken to the green house where they were soaked with 2% fungicide (Redomil) for 20 min. A weaning pot was filled with sterile potting mixture consisting of top soil, sand and manure mixed in the ratio of 3:2:1(w/w). The vessel was placed in a basin containing water to allow the potting mixture to take up water until the top became moist. The pot was then removed from the basin and the plantlets carefully planted using sharp wooden sticks. The plantlets were irrigated once a week with tap water for the first two weeks and twice a week thereafter.

Data collection

Collection of data on the number of microshoots, roots and their lengths was carried out one week after inoculation and on a weekly basis for four weeks during incubation. While in the glasshouse the number of surviving plantlets was observed.

Experimental design and data analysis

The trials were laid out in a Completely Randomized Design. The number of shoots and roots was counted while the length was

Table 1. Effect of different GA_3 concentrations (µM) on *in vitro* shoots proliferation and roots regeneration of Ukerewe sweet potato.

Concentration	Number of microshoots	Length of shoots (cm)	Number of roots	Length of roots (cm)
2.5	5.03 ± 0.62^a	1.65 ± 0.22^b	4.60 ± 0.58^b	5.50 ± 0.62^a
5	4.53 ± 0.51^a	1.82 ± 0.21^b	3.83 ± 0.33^b	3.96 ± 0.43^b
10	5.10 ± 0.68^a	2.78 ± 0.36^a	4.73 ± 0.37^b	4.24 ± 0.47^b
20	4.77 ± 0.64^a	1.52 ± 0.19^b	7.43 ± 0.69^a	3.57 ± 0.32^b
40	5.40 ± 0.73^a	1.58 ± 0.18^b	7.03 ± 0.61^a	3.81 ± 0.30^b
P value	0.8988	0.0013	<.0001	0.0256
LSD	1.7899	0.6714	1.51	1.2549

Values represent means ± SE. Means within a column followed by different letters are significantly different at $P = 0.05$. LSD: least significant difference test (LSD).

Table 2. Effect of different GA_3 concentrations (µM) on *in vitro* shoots proliferation and roots regeneration of Gihingamukungu sweet potato.

Concentration	Number of microshoots	length of shoots (cm)	Number of roots	length of roots (cm)
2.5	5.33 ± 0.59^a	3.23 ± 0.40^a	3.83 ± 0.30^a	4.15 ± 0.31^a
5	5.23 ± 0.54^a	2.08 ± 0.26^b	2.70 ± 0.25^b	4.10 ± 0.21^a
10	5.07 ± 0.53^a	2.18 ± 0.26^b	3.83 ± 0.39^a	4.51 ± 0.26^a
20	5.57 ± 0.69^a	1.74 ± 0.19^b	4.26 ± 0.27^a	3.23 ± 0.24^b
40	4.93 ± 0.57^a	1.49 ± 0.16^b	4.36 ± 0.39^a	4.05 ± 0.30^a
P value	0.9521	0.0001	0.0040	0.0198
LSD	1.6431	0.7432	0.9222	0.7586

Values represent means ± SE. Means within a column followed by different letters are significantly different at $P = 0.05$. LSD: least significant difference test (LSD).

measured in centimeter. The collected parameters were analyzed using SAS software (SAS Institute, 2001). Analyses of variance (ANOVA) were computed for each parameter and the data were summarized as mean ± SE of each parameter and presented in tables. Means were separated using least significant difference test (LSD) with 5% of level of significance

RESULTS

The effects of GA_3 on shoot proliferation and root growth from Ukerewe nodal explants is presented in Table 1. GA_3 at all the concentrations evaluated did not have a significant difference in the number of microshoots per explant. However, GA_3 evaluated at a concentration of 10 µM yielded the highest mean shoot length (2.78 ± 0.36) which was significantly different (P<.0001) from all other concentrations evaluated. The highest mean number (7.43 ± 0.69) of roots was observed on medium supplemented with 20 µM GA_3.

The effects of GA_3 on shoot proliferation and root growth from Gihingamukungu nodal explants is presented in Table 2. The media supplemented with 20 µM GA_3 produced the highest (5.57 ± 0.69) mean microshoot which was not significantly different from all other GA_3 concentrations evaluated. Explants cultured on medium supplemented with 2.5 µM GA_3 produced

microshoots with the highest (3.23 ± 0.40) mean length. On the other hand, the highest (4.36 ± 0.39) mean number of roots was achieved on medium supplemented with 40 µM GA_3 which was not significantly different from the numbers obtained with 2.5, 10 and 20 µM. Plate 1A shows the regenerated plantlets from explants cultured on medium supplemented with different GA_3 concentrations.

The effects of different concentrations of sucrose on shoot proliferation and root growth from Ukerewe sweet potato nodal explant is presented in Table 3. Increasing the concentration of sucrose from 30 to 150 mM increased the number of microshoots fivefold. The media supplemented with 180 mM sucrose produced the highest (5.93 ± 0.62) mean number of microshoots per explant which was not significantly different from the numbers produced on medium supplemented with sucrose 120, 150 and 210 mM. Nodal explants cultured on media supplemented with 150 mM sucrose produced the highest (2.51 ± 0.26) mean shoot length which was significantly higher at P <.0001 than the length obtained using the lower sucrose concentrations (30, 50 and 90 mM). The highest (7.47 ± 0.74) mean number of roots was produced on the medium supplemented with 210 mM sucrose.

The effects of sucrose concentration on shoot

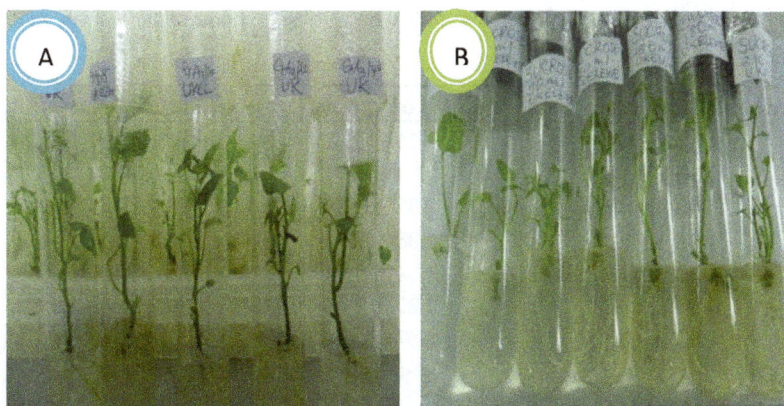

Plate 1. A: Regenerated sweet potato plantlets from nodal explants cultured on 2.5, 5, 10, 20 and 40 µM gibberellic acid **B:** *In vitro* regenerated plantlets showing profuse rooting on media supplemented with sucrose 120, 150 and 210 mM (from left to right).

Table 3. Effect of different sucrose concentrations (mM) on *in vitro* shoots proliferation and roots regeneration of Ukerewe sweet potato.

Concentration	Number of microshoots	Length of shoots (cm)	Number of roots	Length of roots (cm)
30	1.07 ± 0.08^d	0.600 ± 0.03^c	0.30 ± 0.09^f	0.22 ± 0.12^e
60	2.60 ± 0.31^c	1.35 ± 0.11^b	2.87 ± 0.27^e	3.05 ± 0.26^d
90	4.43 ± 0.47^b	1.67 ± 0.17^b	4.83 ± 0.44^{dc}	4.09 ± 0.40^c
120	5.23 ± 0.48^{ba}	2.45 ± 0.28^a	4.47 ± 0.39^d	4.61 ± 0.34^{bc}
150	5.90 ± 0.55^a	2.51 ± 0.26^a	7.03 ± 0.60^{ba}	5.74 ± 0.33^a
180	5.93 ± 0.62^a	2.41 ± 0.24^a	6.10 ± 0.42^{bc}	5.00 ± 0.38^{ba}
210	5.67 ± 0.47^{ba}	2.33 ± 0.23^a	7.47 ± 0.74^a	5.15 ± 0.34^{ba}
P value	<.0001	<.0001	<.0001	<.0001
LSD	1.2759	0.5715	1.3014	0.903

Values represent means ± SE. Means within a column followed by different letters are significantly different at $P = 0.05$. LSD: least significant difference test (LSD).

proliferation and root growth from Gihingamukungu nodal explants is presented in Table 4. The media supplemented with 210 mM sucrose produced the highest (4.93 ± 0.36) mean number of microshoot per explant. On the other hand, nodal explant cultured on media supplemented with 150 mM sucrose produced the highest (2.34 ± 0.24) mean shoot length and highest (5.30 ± 0.42) mean number of roots. Rooting was observed in all the cultures (Plate 1B).

The effect of GA_3 and sucrose on regeneration efficiency in the two cultivars is presented in Table 5. There were no significant difference in the responses of two cultivars to the gibberellic acid concentrations evaluated in terms of the number and length of microshoots. The effect of sucrose was significantly higher in cultivar Ukerewe compared to Gihingamukungu for all the parameters evaluated. The plantlets were successful weaned in the greenhouse with an average 60% survival rate (data not shown)

DISCUSSION

The production of plants from nodal explants has proven to be the most generally applicable and reliable method of regenerating true-to-type *in vitro* plantlets (George et al., 2008). The elongation of microshoot is one of the crucial aspects in developing protocols for regeneration of sweet potato. In order to promote elongation and accelerate microshoot development, and gibberellic acid (GA3) is sometimes added to the culture medium. In previous studies on micropropagation of sweet potato, the effect of GA_3 on elongation of microshoot has been evaluated and it was used at various concentrations e.g. 40 mg/L (Dagnino et al., 1991) and 0.02 g/L (Luo et al., 2006). During the current study, GA_3 promoted induction and elongation of microshoots in both the cultivars evaluated. These results were interesting as Dagnino et al. (1991) reported that GA_3 had no influence on culture of sweet potato meristem of cultivar curacao Alado

Table 4. Effect of different sucrose concentrations (mM) on *in vitro* shoots proliferation and roots regeneration of Gihingamukungu sweet potato

Concentration	Number of microshoots	Length of shoots (cm)	Number of roots	Length of roots (cm)
30	0.33 ± 0.09^c	0.11 ± 0.03^b	1.46 ± 0.32^c	1.41 ± 0.21^d
60	0.63 ± 0.10^c	0.51 ± 0.11^b	1.80 ± 0.24^c	1.62 ± 0.18^d
90	3.60 ± 0.45^b	1.83 ± 0.25^a	2.36 ± 0.20^c	2.25 ± 0.18^c
120	4.87 ± 0.54^a	1.98 ± 0.19^a	3.60 ± 0.30^b	2.81 ± 0.09^b
150	4.60 ± 0.39^{ba}	2.34 ± 0.24^a	5.30 ± 0.42^a	4.26 ± 0.25^a
180	4.90 ± 0.45^a	2.27 ± 0.23^a	4.46 ± 0.42^{ba}	4.80 ± 0.21^a
210	4.93 ± 0.36^a	1.87 ± 0.25^a	5.13 ± 0.38^a	3.03 ± 0.16^b
P value	<.0001	<.0001	<.0001	<.0001
LSD	1.0319	0.5619	0.9505	0.5396

Values represent means ± SE. Means within a column followed by different letters are significantly different at $P = 0.05$. LSD: least significant difference test (LSD).

Table 5. Comparing the effect of GA_3 and sucrose on shoot proliferation and root Regeneration of Ukerewe and Gihingamukungu sweet potato cultivars

Variety	GA_3 and sucrose	Number of shoots	Length of shoots (cm)	Number of roots	Length of roots (cm)
Ukerewe	GA_3	4.97 ± 0.28^a	1.87 ± 0.11^a	5.53 ± 0.26^a	4.22 ± 0.21^a
Gihingamukungu	GA_3	5.23 ± 0.26^a	2.14 ± 0.13^a	3.80 ± 0.15^b	4.01 ± 0.12^a
P value		0.4996	0.1080	<.0001	0.3874
LSD		0.757	0.3343	0.6037	0.4734
Ukerewe	Sucrose	4.40 ± 0.21^a	1.90 ± 0.09^a	4.72 ± 0.23^a	3.98 ± 0.17^a
Gihingamukungu	Sucrose	3.40 ± 0.19^b	1.56 ± 0.09^b	3.44 ± 0.16^b	2.89 ± 0.11^b
P value		0.0007	0.0101	<.0001	<.0001
LSD		0.5555	0.2548	0.5648	0.3965

GA_3: gibberellic acid, LSD: least significant difference test (LSD).

whereas meristem of cultivar Mae de Familai cultured on medium supplemented with GA_3 formed multiple shoots. In cassava, Villaluz (2005) reported that when used singly, GA_3 did not elicit any growth response from nodal explants however, Mushiyimana et al. (2011) reported that nodal explants cultured on MS medium supplemented with 40 µM GA_3 produced the highest mean number of microshoots and length. A possible explanation for such disparity seems to be genotypic difference. During the current study, prolific rooting was achieved in all the cultures. The reason for this could be the fact that GA_3 and sucrose are known to induce roots (Kochba et al., 1973; Calamar and De klerk, 2002). The presence of roots is of paramount importance because a good root system is essential for successful acclimatization of the plantlets and subsequent growth in the field since roots facilitate the absorption of nutrients and water from the soil (Xiansong, 2010).

In the current study, increasing the concentration of sucrose from the 90 mM (the concentration that is routinely used) resulted in increased mean number of microshoots per explant for both sweet potato cultivars.

The results of the current work agree with earlier reports that indicate that there are cases where higher concentrations > 3% of sucrose may be beneficial (Boggetti, 1997; Kahia, 1999; Van Huylenbroeck and Debergh, 1996). However, it contradicts other reports which have shown that high sucrose concentration was detrimental to shoot formation. These authors have suggested that the osmotic level in the medium with high sucrose concentration may be inhibitory to shoot growth and development (Karimet al., 2007; Nowak et al., 2004).

A genotype dependent one step protocol for the micropropagation of elite sweet potato cultivar Ukerewe, and Gihingamukungu, was developed. This protocol will provide the basis for the mass production of studied cultivars through *in vitro* techniques. This is the first report on evaluating the effect of different concentrations of sucrose to regenerate sweet potato plantlets.

Conflict of interests

The author(s) have not declared any conflict of interests.

ACKNOWLEDGEMENTS

The authors would like to thank the Rwanda Agriculture Board (RAB) Management for allowing them to use their facilities to carry out this work. The assistance rendered by the Tissue culture laboratory staff at RAB Rubona is highly appreciated.

REFERENCES

Amin MN, Rahman MM, Manik MS (2003). *In vitro* clonal propagation of *Paederiafoetida* L. A medicinal plant of Bangladesh. Plant Tissue Cult.13:117-123.

Association for Strengthening Agriculture Research in Eastern and Central Africa (ASARECA) (2008). Enhancement of cassava and sweet potato tissue culture and conservation technologies in Eastern and Central African region. Proceedings of Tissue culture workshop, Bujumbura.

Bachou H (2002). The Nutrition Situation in Uganda. Nutrition. 18(4):356-358.

Boggetti B (1997). Development of micropropagation and possible genetic transformation system for cashew (*Anacardium occidentale*). PhD Thesis University of London.

Burden D (2005). Sweet potato profile, agriculture marketing and resource center (AgMRC). A National information resource for value added agriculture. Iowa State University.

Calamar A, Geert-Jan-de K (2002). Effect of sucrose on root regeneration in apple. Plant Cell Tissue Org. Cult. 70:207-212.

Dagnino DS, Carelli MD, Arrabal RF, Esquibel MA (1991). Effect of Gibberelic acid on *Ipomoea batatas* regeneration from meristem culture. Presquisa Agropecuaria Brasilia 26:259-262.

Deng XP, Cheng YJ, Wu XB, Kwak SS, Chen W, Egrinya A (2012). Exogenous hydrogen peroxide positively influences root growth and exogenous hydrogen peroxide positively influences root growth and metabolism in leaves of sweet potato seedlings. Australian J. Crop Sci. 6(11):1572-1578.

Desjardins Y, Hdider C, de Riek J (1995). Carbon nutrition *in vitro*: regulation and manipulation of carbon assimilation in micropropagated system. In: *Automation and Enviromental Control in Plant Tissue Culture* (Aitken-Christie, J., Kozai, T. and Smith, M. A.,eds), Kluwer Academic Press. pp. 441-471.

Farmer M, Li X, Feng G, Zhao B, Chatagnier O, Gianinazzi S, Gianinazzi-Pearson V, Van Tuinen D (2007). Molecular monitoring of field-inoculated AMF to evaluate persistence in sweet potato crops in China. Appl. Soil Ecol. 35:599-609.

George EF, Hall MA, De Klerk GJ (2008). The background, Plant propagation by tissue culture Springer Verlag, Dordrecht, The Netherlands

Gibson SI (2000). Plant sugar response pathway part of a complex regulatory web. Plant Physiol. 124:1532-1539.

Gurel S, Gulsen Y (1998). The effects of different sucrose, agar and pH levels on *in vitro* shoot production of Almond (*Amygdaluscommunis* L.). Turk. J. Bot. 22:363-373.

Institute of Agronomic Sciences of Rwanda (ISAR) Sweet Potato Program (2008).

Islam S (2006). Sweet potato (*Ipomoea batatas* L.) Leaf its potential effect on human health and nutrition. J. Food Sci. 71(2):R13-R121.

Kahia WJ (1999). *In vitro* propagation of the Disease resistant cultivar – Ruiru 11. PhD thesis, University of London.

Karim MZ, Yokota S, Rahman MM, Eizawa J, Saito Y, Azad MAK, Ishiguri F, Iizuka K, Yoshizawa N (2007). Effects of the Sucrose Concentration and pH Level on Shoot Regeneration from Callus in *Arariaelata* Seem. Asian J. Plant Sci. 6:715-717.

Kochba JB, Spiegel- Roy P, Kochba M (1973). Stimulation of roots of citrus embryoids by Gibberelllic acid and adenine sulphate. Ann. Bot. 38:795-802.

Liu Q (2011). Sweet potato omics and biotechnology in China. Plant Omics J. 4(6):295-301.

Luo HR, Santa Maria M, Benavides J, Zhang DP, Zhang YZ (2006). Rapid genetic transformation of sweet potato (*Ipomoea batatas* (L.) Lam) via organogenesis. Afr. J. Biotechnol. 5(20):1851-1857.

Moshkov GI, Novikova EV, Hall MA (2008). Plant Growth Regulators III: Gibberellins, ethylene, abscisic acid, their analogues and inhibitors; miscellaneous compounds. In: *Plant propagation by tissue culture* (Edwin, M. A.J. and George, F., 3rd Edition), The Netherlands: Springer. p. 22.

Murashige T, Skoog F (1962). A revised medium for rapid growth and bioassays with tobacco tissue cultures. Plant Physiol. 15:473-497.

Mushiyimana I, Emannuel H, Gervais G, Peter Yao KS, Safia K, Felix G, Theodore A, Jane K, Daphrose G (2011). Micro-Propagation of Disease Resistant Cassava Variety in Rwanda. Rwanda J. 24:49-57.

Mutandwa E (2008). Performance of Tissue cultured sweet potatoes among smallholders in Zimbabwe. J. Agrobiotechnol. Manag. Econ. 11(1).

Nowak B, Miczynski K, Hudy L (2004). Sugar uptake and utilization during adventitious bud differentiation on *in vitro* leaf explant of WegierkaZwykla plum (*Prunusdomestica*). Plant Cell Tissue Org. Cult. 76:255-260.

Rahman MM, Amin MN, Ahmed R (2004). *In vitro* rapid regeneration from cotyledon explant of native olive (*Elaeocarpusrobustus*Roxb). Asian J. Plant Sci. 3:31-35.

SAS Institute (2001). SAS / STAT user's guide. Version 8.2. SAS Institute, Cary, USA

Van Huylenbroeck JM, Debergy PC (1996). Impact of sugar concentration *in vitro* photosynthesis and carbon metabolism during *ex vitro* rooting acclimatization of *Spathiphyllum* plantlets. Plant Physiol. 96:298-304.

Villaluz ZA (2005). Improvement of *in vitro* techniques for rapid meristem development and mass propagation of Philippine cassava (*Manihot esculenta* Crantz). Plant Cell Reports 9:356-359.

Xiansong Y (2010). Rapid production of virus-free plantlets by shoot tip culture *in vitro* of purple-coloured sweet potato (*Ipomoea batatas (L.) Lam.*). Pak. J. Biol. 42(3):2069-2075.

Zhang L (1995). Progress of Research and application of virus free sweet potato seeds in Shandong. Proceedings of the first Chinese-Japanese symposium of sweet potato and potato. Beijing Agriculture University.Press, Beijing.

21

A new method for the detection of oil degrading genes in *Pseudomonas aeruginosa* based on transformation and PCR hybridization

Shiju Mathew and Yahya Hasan Hobani

Department of Medical Lab Technology, College of Applied Medical Sciences, Jazan University, P.O. Box No. 114, Jazan, Kingdom of Saudi Arabia.

Biodegradation is the chemical breakdown of materials by a physiological environment. The term is often used in relation to ecology, waste management and environmental remediation. A specific gene from bacteria is identified and sequenced which has the capacity of oil degradation without any obvious strain specific discrimination using a combination of PCR and hybridization. The parameters of biodegradation that is culturing and PCR technique provide useful information for an assessment of the intrinsic biodegradation potential that is present at a site. PCR amplification products in the plasmid DNA of *Pseudomonas aeruginosa* was transformed into competent *Escherichia coli* cells. Thus the *E. coli* cells were conferred with oil degrading property and this was confirmed by growing them in Bushnell Hass medium along with petroleum oil. The *E. coli* cells were found to be catabolizing the oil. Results show that the capability for alkane degradation is a common trait in microbial communities. The method can be a very useful tool for the fast estimation of the biodegradation potential at polluted sites.

Key words: Detection, hydrocarbon biodegradation, PCR-hybridization, transformation.

INTRODUCTION

The use of enormous amounts of petroleum products contributes highly to environmental pollution. Spills of hydrocarbons occur from several causes, including blowouts, leakage from tanks, and dumping of waste petroleum products. The elevated loading of petroleum hydrocarbons in soil causes a significant decline in soil quality, and these soils have become unusable. Aliphatic alkanes are a group of hydrocarbons that are present in crude and refined oils. They were formed by reduction of organic material during the geochemical formation of oil. However, alkanes are also produced by plants and microorganisms and form part of the biomass (Bird and Lynch, 1974; Taylor and Calvin, 1987; Kunst and Samuels, 2003; Kloos et al., 2006).

Geogenic and biogenic alkane fractions differ in the complexity of the mixture and the mean chain length found (Hellmann, 1991). Introduced in greater amounts into the environment, for example by oil spills, aliphatic alkanes may become environmental pollutants. The bio-availability and toxicity of n-alkanes depends on their chain length (Gill and Ratledge, 1972). Only short chain n-alkanes are directly toxic, acting as solvents for cellular fats and membranes (Sikkema et al., 1995). However, long chain n-alkanes can contribute to the formation of oil films and slicks (Leahy and Colwell, 1990). These are hazardous to the macro- and microflora of the contaminated site blocking the exchange of water, water soluble nutrients and gases.

A wide range of non-related bacteria and fungi can use n-alkanes as sole carbon and energy source (Rehm and Reiff, 1981; Watkinson and Morgan, 1990; van Beilen et al., 2003). Bacterial degradation of n-alkanes is possible under aerobic and anaerobic conditions (Widdel and Rabus, 2001).

However, activation of the otherwise chemically inert aliphates with molecular oxygen allows much faster degradation rates. Although various mechanisms of aerobic activation have been described (Rehm and Reiff, 1981; Maeng et al., 1997; van Beilen et al., 2003), only the terminal oxidation pathway that involves a key process of degradation has been investigated in greater detail so far.

Hybridization probes derived from various organisms have been used for the detection of microbial communities after isolation of the bacteria (Sotzsky et al., 1994; Whyte et al., 1995; Vomberg and Klinner, 2000). Investigations with PCR-based methods were also mostly performed with cultured isolates (Smits et al., 1999; Vomberg and Klinner, 2000; van Beilen et al., 2002). The high sequence divergence found in *Pseudomonas Aeruginosa* bacteria from different taxonomic groups (Smits et al., 1999; van Beilen et al., 2003) caused a group-specificity in the detection of alkane degraders with the PCR and hybridization methods described in the literature. The big genetic material of the *P. aeruginosa* support the idea of using this microbes in biotechnological applications

The diversity of *P. aerginosa* different strains and that each strain should be study as a single case were highlighted. Therefore, comprehensive analysis of environmental samples required the use of multiple primer and probe sets targeting the respective subgroups (Luz et al., 2004; Heiss-Blanquet et al., 2005; Kloos et al., 2006).

Here, an improved PCR based method is described that in combination with hybridization allowed a specific and sensitive detection of the unknown gene in environmental samples without obvious discrimination of any of the known bacterial groups possessing this gene.

MATERIALS AND METHODS

Reference strains and media

Strains used as references were *Bacillus subtilis, Pseudomonas aeruginosa* (ATCC 27853), *Staphylococcus aureus* and *Escherichia coli.* They were grown in NB medium (8 g l^{-1} nutrient broth No. 4, Fluka, Buchs, Switzerland).

HC medium contained per l : 2g NH_4NO_3, 4g KH_2PO_4, 6 g $Na_2HPO_4 \cdot 2H_2O$, 200 mg $MgSO_4$, 50mg $CaCl_2 \cdot 2H_2O$, 136.3 µg $ZnCl_2$, 3.2 mg $FeCl_3$, 2.0 mg $MnCl_2 \cdot 4H_2O$, 170.5 µg $CuCl_2 \cdot 2H_2O$, 475.9 µg $CoCl_2 \cdot 6H_2O$, 61.8µg HBO_3, 3.9 µg $NaMoO_4 \cdot 2H_2O$. The Ph of the medium was adjusted to 7.0 with KOH before autoclaving. The appropriate C-source was autoclaved or filter sterilized separately before addition to the medium

Molecular biological methods

Preparation of genomic DNA

For preparation of genomic DNA from pure cultures, cells were grown over night and harvested by centrifugation. Cells were resuspended in 320 µl 1×TE (10 mM Tris pH 7.5, 1 mM EDTA) and incubated for 1 h. After addition of 80 µl 10% SDS, samples were incubated at 65°C for 2 h. The final DNA extraction was done with the Mini Kit (Qiagen, Germany) starting with the addition of buffer AP2 according to the manufacturer's protocol. The collection site for soil sample was randomly selected followed by the procedure of DNA isolation using Genei Kit, Bangalore

Estimation of genomic DNA

DNA concentration and purity were determined using ULTROSPEC 2000 spectrophotometer at an absorbance of 260 and 280 nm. Quality of DNA can be calculated using the formula; Quality of DNA = A_{260nm} / A_{280nm}. If the value ranges from: 1.75 - 1.9 Good quality DNA; ≤ 1.75 Protein contamination; ≥ 1.9 RNA contamination. Quantity of DNA can be calculated using the formula; Quantity of DNA = A_{260nm} x 50 x dilution factor / 1000.

Detection of oil degrading gene in the genomic DNA

PCR primers are responsible for identifying the polymorphism or specific DNA sequence presence for oil degradation. So, along with the sample, control strains are also used and analyzed the DNA sample. The primer has been specially designed using the PubMed software of NCBI. nahC F -5'-AAG GCG CAG GCT TGC AAG TG-3'; nahC R -5'-TCG TCG CTT TCC CAG AAG CC-3'. The PCR mix contained in a final volume of 50 µl: 5 µl buffer (provided with Taq polymerase), 1.5 µl $MgCl_2$ (50 mM), 5 µl dNTP-mix (2.5 mM each nucleotide), 5 µl each primer (10 µM), 10 ng purified DNA of cultured strains or 5 ng soil DNA and 2.5 U Taq-DNA polymerase (Biorad, USA). Cycling was performed with initial denaturation for 3 min at 40°C, 34 cycles with 30 s at 94°C, 45 s at 53°C, 60s 72°C, and final elongation for 5min at 72°C.

PCR products were separated in 1.5% agarose gels. Gels were blotted on positively charged nylon membrane by capillary transfer with 0.4 M NaOH for hybridization. Hybridization was performed with the oligonucleotide. The oligonucleotide was labeled with DigddUTP using the 3'-end labeling kit (Genei, Bangalore, India) according to the manufacturer's protocol. Five hundred picomoles of oligonucleotide were used per 50 ml hybridization buffer containing 5×SSC (20×SSC: 3 M NaCl, 0.3 M Na_3-citrate), 0.1% Na-lauroylsulfate, 0.02% Na-N-lauroylsarcosine, 0.5% blocking reagent. Hybridization was performed at 42°C over night and was followed by two washes with 2×SSC/0.1% SDS for 5min at room temperature, and two washes with 0.5×SSC/0.1% SDS at 42°C. The colour detection kit was used according to the manufacturer's instructions to detect hybrids (Kloos et al., 2006).

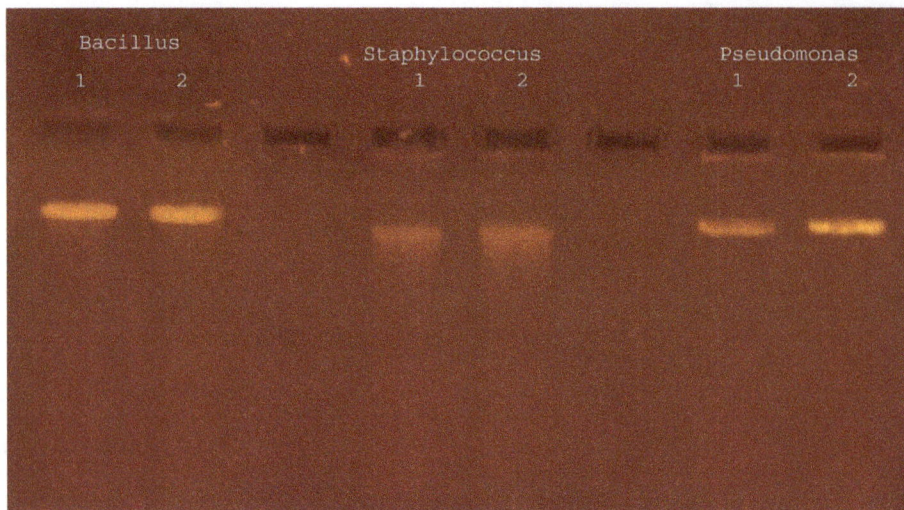

Figure 1. Clear genomic DNA bands obtained for each of the sample in the agarose gel when viewed under UV transilluminator. Lane 1 controlled Genomic DNA and Lane 2 collected Genomic DNA samples of each microorganism DNA that is *Bacillus*, *Stapyllococcus* and *Pseudomonas*.

Transformation and cloning

The amplified specific DNA fragments were cloned to competent *E. coli* using the Novagen Kit, Germany. Plasmids from transformants were prepared using the method of Birnboim and Doly (1979) and checked for the presence of an insert of the expected size. A fast initial screening of the transformants was performed by colony hybridization according to the method of Grunstein and Hogness (1975). Plasmids used for sequencing were further purified with the Plasmid Mini Kit (Qiagen, Germany). Both strands were read from double stranded plasmid with the opposing vector primers. Sequences were compared to Genbank with BLASTN (Altschul et al., 1997). Trees were calculated with NTSYS software (Dubey et al., 2002; Boyer, 2006; Walker, 2007).

RESULTS AND DISCUSSION

Detection of oil degrading gene by PCR and hybridization

Specific detection of gene was achieved combining PCR amplification with oligonucleotide hybridization. To confirm the presence of DNA and to separate it from protein and RNA, agarose gel electrophoresis (AGE) was done (Figure 1). The PCR primers target essentially the same regions as the primers described by Smits et al. (1999). However, the reverse primer was shifted 6 bases, and both primers used here were more degenerate. The expected band of 500bp was amplified from DNA of the reference strains *P. aeruginosa*. Sequences of these PCR products differed only in the primer sequences from those published. Unspecific PCR products of various sizes were obtained with the nondegrading strains Bacillus subtilis and Escherichia coli strain. Hybridization with an oligonucleotide probe binding within the amplicon

allowed to distinguish specific and non-specific products (Figure 2). Hybridization signals were obtained only for the expected products of the degraders. The detection limit of the combined PCR/hybridization assay was estimated with chromosomal DNA of the reference strains *P. aeruginosa* to be 0.1ng DNA. Assuming a mean bacterial genome size of 3.6 Mb (Fogel et al., 1999; Kloos *et al.,* 2006) this detection limit corresponded to 2.6×10^4 gene copies.

Evaluation of the detection method with the reference isolates

The PCR/hybridization method was used to screen soil isolates for the occurrence of alkB by colony-PCR. Isolates were obtained under non-selective conditions from a reference strains. Fifty randomly picked isolates were screened for each of the two independent samples. A single PCR product of the expected size was obtained for 8 and 10% of the isolates. None or unspecific products were observed for all other isolates. Again, only PCR products of the expected size hybridized with the internal probe (Figures 3 and 4). Sequencing of these PCR products after cloning confirmed their homology to alkB. Derived protein sequences showed highest homologies to AlkB from other bacterial gene (Smits et al., 1999; Khalameyzer et al., 1999; Andreoni et al., 2000; Kloos et al., 2006)

Transformationtion of oil degrading gene by PCR and hybridization

The results have confirmed that an oil degrading gene is

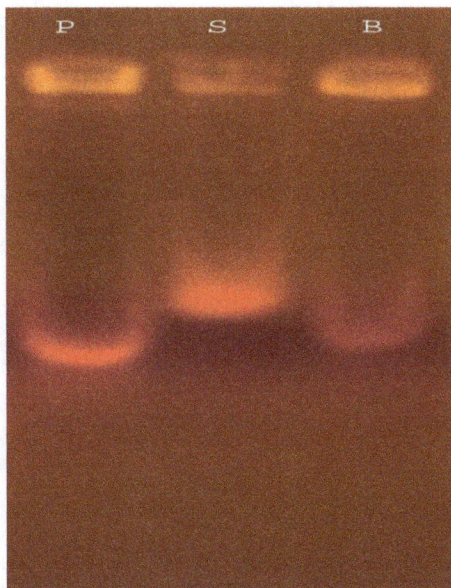

Figure 2. The confirmation of amplified DNA product is only present in Pseudomonas whereas in Bacillus and Stapyllococcus it is absent as shown in agarose gel.

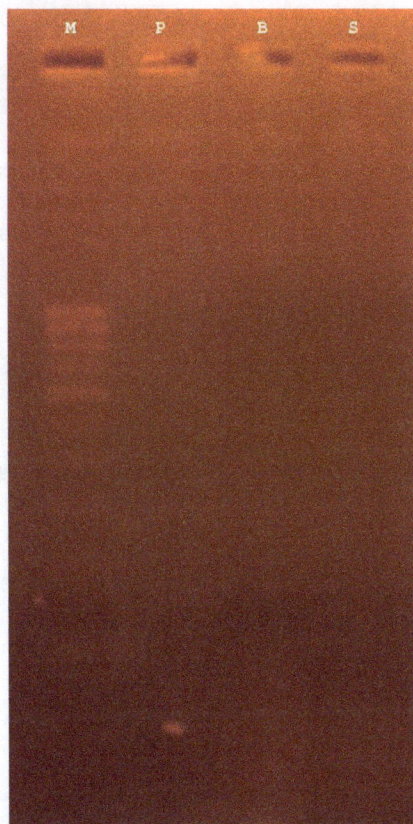

Figure 3. Figure shows that there was no amplification of DNA in any of the bacterial samples. This infers that the genomic DNA of these bacteria lacks any oil degrading genes used along with a 100 bp marker.

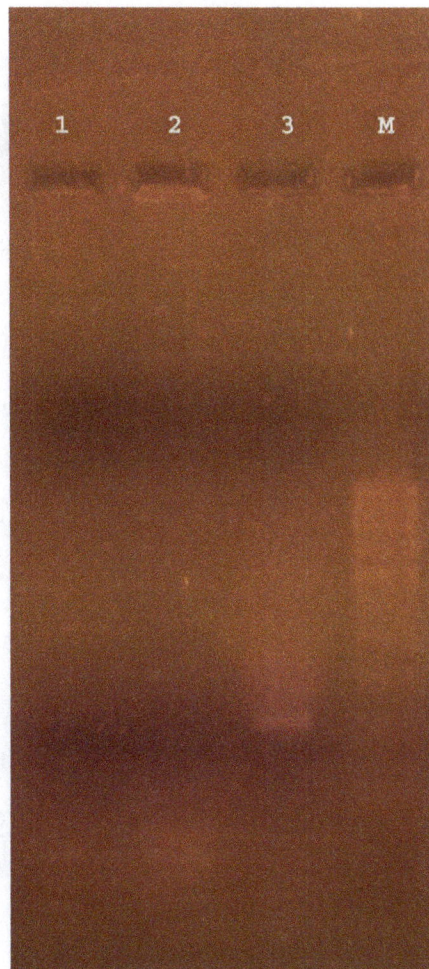

Figure 4. Figure showing the confirmation of plasmid DNA of *Pseudomonas aeruginosa* has oil degrading genes. The band appeared has a size of about 200bp. All other strains show a negative result and had no amplification in response to the oil degrading primer.

present in the *P. aeruginosa*. An annex to this work was concentrated on the transfer this particular oil degrading gene into a non oil degrading bacteria (Figure 5). The non-oil degrading bacteria were selected. *E. coli* cells were selected which were made competent using calcium chloride and were transformed using Bushnell Hass (BH) medium along with petroleum oil layered on top of the medium and further showed that a normally non-oil degrading bacteria has been successfully transformed to oil degrading *E. coli* (Figure 6).

Conclusion

Biodegradation is the chemical breakdown of materials by a physiological environment. Oily wastewater, especially from oil field, has posed a great hazard for

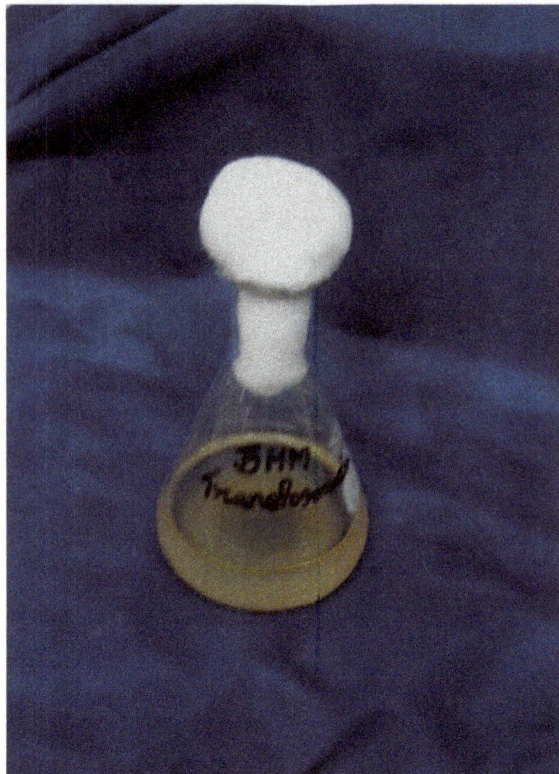

Figure 5. The transformed *E. coli* cell which can degrade the oil that is *E. coli* cells were selected which were made competent using calcium chloride and were transformed using Bushnell Hass (BH) medium.

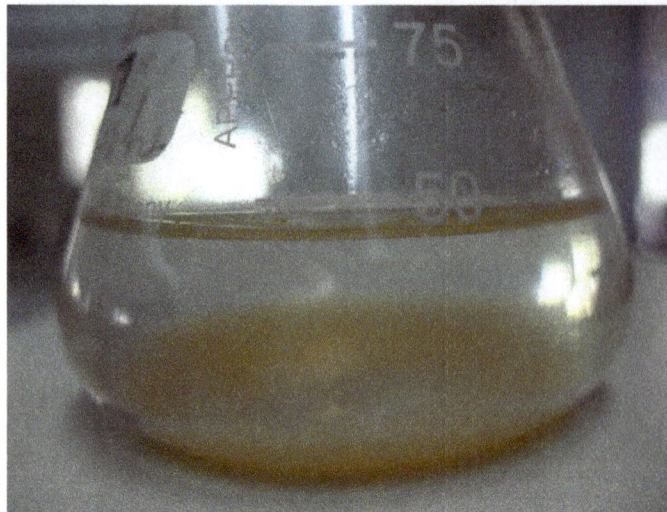

Figure 6. The transformed *E. coli* cells have degraded the petroleum oil present in the medium which could be seen as small bubbles on the surface of the medium.

Conflict of Interests

The author(s) have not declared any conflict of interests.

ACKNOWLEDGEMENT

I thank our lab colleagues for their assistance with this project and valuable comments on this manuscript. I also thank Dr. Gowher Nabi for their continuous support in research. The work was supported by the university research funding.

terrestrial and marine ecosystems. During biodegradation, crude oil is used as an organic carbon source by a microbial process, resulting in the breakdown of crude oil components to low molecular weight compounds. The focus of the research is identifying novel oil degrading gene in the cosmopolitan available *Pseudomonas* and also to evaluate the highly sophisticated PCR technique to detect the oil degrading gene in *Pseudomonas* species. Though the target of the work is to concentrate on *Pseudomonas* the other two strains are used as controls. It is observed after PCR amplification (Agarose gel) that *Pseudomonas* DNA contain oil degrading gene. Resulting into the plasmid DNA of *Pseudomonas* was transformed into competent *E. coli* cells. Thus the *E. coli* cells were conferred with oil degrading property and this was confirmed by growing them in Bushnell Hass medium along with petroleum oil. The *E. coli* cells were found to be catabolizing the oil. Molecular data were in accordance with physiological experiments for detection and enumeration of alkane degrading bacteria. Results show that the capability for alkane degradation is a common trait in soil microbial communities. Thus above results can be concluded that the PCR mediated detection and identification of oil degrading gene in *Pseudomonas aeruginosa*.

REFERENCES

Altschul SF, Madden TL, Schaffer AA, Zhang J, Zhang Z, Miller W, Lipman DJ (1997). Gapped BLAST and PSI-BLAST: a new generation of protein database search programs. Nucleic Acids Res. 25:3389-3402.

Andreoni V, Bernasconi S, Colombo M, Van Beilen JB, Cavalca L (2000). Detection of genes for alkane and naphthalene catabolism in Rhodococcus sp. strain 1BN. Environ. Microbiol. 2:572-577.

Bird CW, Lynch JM (1974). Formation of hydrocarbons by microorganisms. Chem. Soc. Rev. 3:309-328.

Birnboim HC, Doly JA (1979). Rapid alkaline extraction procedure for screening recombinant plasmid DNA. Nucleic Acids Res. 7:1513-1523.

Boyer R (2006). Biochemistry Laboratory: Modern Theory and Techniques. Mod. Exp. Biochem. 2:140-144.

Dubey RC, Gupta CP, Maheshwari DK (2002). Plant growth enhancement and suppression of *Macrophomina phaseolina* causing charcoal rot of peanut by fluorescent Pseudomonas. Biol. Fertil. Soils. 35:399-405.

Fogel GB, Collins CR, Li J, Brunk CF (1999). Prokaryotic genome size and SSU rDNA copy number: estimation of microbial relative abundance from a mixed population. Microb. Ecol. 38:93-113.

Gill CO, Ratledge C (1972). Toxicity of n-alkanes, n-alk-1-enes, nalkan-1-ols and n-alkyl-1-bromides towards yeasts. J. Gen. Microbiol. 72:165-172.

Grunstein M, Hogness DS (1975). Colony hybridization: a method for the isolation of cloned DNAs that contain a specific gene. Proc. Natl. Acad. Sci. 72:3961-3965.

Heiss-Blanquet S, Benoit Y, Maréchaux C, Monot F (2005). Assessing the role of alkane hydroxylase genotypes in environmental samples by competitive PCR. J. Appl. Microbiol. 99:1392-1403.

Hellmann H (1991). IR-spectroscopic analysis of alkanes in soil, water and sediment—differenciation of mineral oil and biogene fractions (German). Z. Wasser- und Abwasser-Forsch. Appl. Environ. Microbiol. 24:226-232.

Khalameyzer V, Fischer I, Bornscheuer UT, Altenbuchner J (1999). Screening, nucleotide sequence, and biochemical characterization of an esterase from Pseudomonas fluorescens with high activity towards lactones. Appl. Environ. Microbiol. 65:477-482.

Kloos K, Munch JC, Schloter M (2006). new method for the detection of alkane- onooxygenase homologous genes (alkB) in soils based on PCR-hybridization. J. Microbiol. Meth. 66:486-496.

Kunst L, Samuels AL (2003). Biosynthesis and secretion of plant cuticular wax. Prog. Lipid Res. 42:51-80.

Leahy JG, Colwell RR (1990). Microbial degradation of hydrocarbons in the environment. Microbiol. Rev. 54:305-315.

Luz AP, Pellizari VH, Whyte LG, Greer CW (2004). A survey of indigenous microbial hydrocarbon degradation genes in soils from Antarctica and Brazil. Can. J. Microbiol. 50:323-333.

Maeng JH, Sakai Y, Tani Y, Kato N (1997). Isolation and characterization of a novel oxygenase that catalyzes the first step of n-alkane oxidation in Acinetobacter sp. strain M-1. J. Bacteriol. 178:3695-3700.

Rehm HJ, Reiff I (1981). Mechanisms and occurrence of microbial oxidation of long-chain alkanes. Adv. Biochem. Eng. 19:175-215.

Sikkema J, De Bont JA, Poolman B (1995). Mechanisms of membrane toxicity of hydrocarbons. Microbiol. Rev. 59:201-222.

Smits TH, Röthlisberger M, Witholt B, van Beilen JB (1999). Molecular screening for alkane hydroxylase genes in Gramnegative and Gram-positive strains. Environ. Microbiol. 1:307-317.

Sotzsky JB, Greer CW, Atlas RM (1994). Frequency of genes in aromatic and aliphatic hydrocarbon biodegradation pathways within bacterial populations from Alaskan sediments. Can. J. Microbiol. 40:981-985.

Taylor SE, Calvin M (1987). Hydrocarbons from plants: biosynthesis and utilization. Commun. Agric. Food Chem. 1:1-26.

Van Beilen JB, Li Z, DuetzWA, Smits THM, Witholt B (2003). Diversity of alkane hydroxylase systems in the environment. Oil Gas Sci. Technol. 4:427-440.

Van Beilen JB, Smits THM, Whyte LG, Schorcht S, Röthlisberger M, Plaggenmeier T, Engesser KH, Witholt B (2002). Alkane hydroxylase homologues in Gram-positive strains. Environ. Microbiol. 4:676-682.

Vomberg A, Klinner U (2000). Distribution of alkB genes within nalkane-degrading bacteria. J. Appl. Microbiol. 89:339-348.

Walker J, Wilson K (2007). The Molecular Evolution of species in the Presence of Slightly Deleterious Mutations and Population Size Change. Princ. Tech. Biochem. Mol. Biol. 5:454-455.

Watkinson RJ, Morgan P (1990). Physiology of aliphatic hydrocarbon-degrading microorganisms. Biodegrad. 1:79-92.

Whyte LG, Greer CW, Inniss WE (1995). Assessment of the biodegradation potential of psychrotrophic microorganisms. Can. J. Microbiol. 42:99-106.

Widdel F, Rabus R (2001). Anaerobic biodegradation of saturated and aromatic hydrocarbons. Curr. Opin. Biotechnol. 12:259-276.

22

Molecular characterization of resistance to Russian wheat aphid *(Diuraphis noxia* Kurdjumov) in bread wheat (*Triticum aestivum* L.) line KRWA9

E. A. Masinde[1,2] , J. N. Malinga[1], W. A. Ngenya[1,2], R. M. S. Mulwa[2] and M. Cakir[3]

[1]Kenya Agricultural Research Institute, P.O Box Private Bag - 20107 Njoro, Kenya.
[2]Crops Horticulture and Soils Department, Egerton University P.O Box 523, Egerton, Kenya.
[3]WA State Agricultural Biotechnology Center, School of Veterinary and Life Sciences, Murdoch University 90 South St., Murdoch WA 6150, Australia

The Russian wheat aphid (RWA), *Diuraphis noxia* (Kurdjumov) causes extensive economic damage to wheat (*Triticum aestivum* L.) in most wheat growing regions of the world. Control of RWA using systemic insecticides is expensive and pollutes the environment therefore the most effective method of RWA control is the development of RWA resistant cultivars. This study was initiated to determine inheritance of RWA resistance in a wheat resistance source KRWA9, and identify the chromosome location of the resistance gene. Inheritance was studied in parent materials, F_1 populations, F_2 populations and $F_{2:3}$ families of a cross between resistant line KRWA9 and a susceptible variety NjoroBW2. Seedlings were infested with RWA then scored for damage on a visual scale of 1 to 9 after 21 days of infestation. The segregation data from NjoroBW2 × KRWA9 population depicted monogenic dominant inheritance of the resistance gene with phenotypic ratios of 3:1 in F_2 populations and 1:2:1 in $F_{2:3}$ families. Bulk segregant analysis approach was used for the mapping of resistance. Nine simple sequence repeat (SSR) primers were tested between parental lines and bulks, and only chromosome 7DS SSR marker *Xgwm111* produced clear polymorphism between the parental lines and the resistant and susceptible bulks. Detailed analysis of this marker with the full population revealed very close linkage to resistance with a coefficient of determination (R^2) value of 85%. This marker provides good opportunities for the marker-assisted breeding towards improving Russian wheat aphid resistance.

Key words: Russian wheat aphid, resistance, susceptibility, simple sequence repeat (*SSR*) markers.

INTRODUCTION

The Russian wheat aphid (RWA), *Diuraphis noxia* (Kurdjumov), a pest of wheat and barley, is indigenous to southern Russia, Iran, Afghanistan and countries bordering the Mediterranean Sea (Hewitt et al., 1984). The pest has spread widely and is now found in all the continents except Australia (Ennahli et al., 2009), and causes economic damage to wheat in many parts of the world. In Ethiopia, Miller and Haile (1988) reported 68% yield loss in wheat. In South Africa, 21–92% yield losses were reported (Du Toit and Walters, 1984). In Kenya, it can cause losses of up to 90% in wheat (Malinga, 2007) and sometimes up to 100% due to prolonged drought conditions. RWA attacks the plant by infesting the young growing tip, deep in the leaf whorls where it feeds from the phloem of longitudinal veins. Symptoms of RWA attack appear as chlorotic spots that coalesce to form white, yellow or purple streaks running parallel to the mid rib of leaves (Botha and Matsiliza, 2006). In young plants, heavy infestation leads to prostate tillers while adult plants show trapped ears within the flag leaf looking like a fish hook. Severe infestation may lead to head sterility and death of host plant.

Insecticide use and particularly contact foliar applications are ineffective because of the feeding nature of the aphid. The aphid feeds within the rolled leaf whorl so cannot be easily reached by contact foliar sprays. This necessitates the use of more expensive systemic insecticides which apart from being harmful to the environment promote development of resistant biotypes and destroys biological agents. RWA resistant cultivars have been observed to have a yield advantage as compared to susceptible cultivars (Tolmay et al., 2000) and resistant cultivars have low cost as seed is usually the least expensive component in the production system besides being environment friendly. Host plant resistance is therefore, the most desirable alternative that could form part of an integrated pest management programme (IPM).

The first RWA resistant cultivar, TugelaDn (containing resistance gene *Dn1*), was released in South Africa in 1992 (Van Niekerk, 2001). A new biotype-designated RWASA2 was identified in 2005 virulent to *Dn1, Dn2, Dn3* and *Dn9* (Jankielsohn, 2011). Most of the RWA resistant cultivars available for commercial production in South Africa (Tolmay et al., 2007) were overcome by RWASA2. Similarly, resistant cultivar Halt (containing *Dn4*) was released in the United States in 1994 (Quick et al., 1996), but a new biotype, USARWA2 with virulence to resistance genes *Dn4* and *Dny* was reported in 2004 (Haley et al., 2004), also overcoming the majority of commercially available resistant cultivars. Although RWA resistance expression is known to be influenced by genetic background (Randolph et al., 2005; Tolmay and Van Deventer, 2005), it is nonetheless assumed to function on a gene-for-gene basis in terms of the resistance/biotype interaction (Ricciardi et al., 2010). Recently a third biotype, RWASA3 virulent to *Dn1, Dn2, Dn3, Dn4* and *Dn9* was reported in South Africa by Jankielsohn (2011). Notably, neither *Dn4* nor *Dny* had been deployed against RWA in South Africa. In Kenya, two biotypes with genetic differences have been discovered in the major wheat growing areas, that is, Njoro and Timau (Malinga et al., 2007a). Amplified fragment

length polymorphism markers used to detect genetic differences showed that the Njoro biotype may contain more virulent populations as compared to Timau biotype (Malinga et al., 2007a). This was the first confirmatory report on biotypes in Kenya and it raised great challenges to resistance breeding programs for Russian wheat aphid.

Breeding for RWA resistant cultivars requires a reliable method of selecting plants containing a resistant gene. While phenotype based selection method is straight-forward, it has several limitations like the environmental influence on symptoms of damage expression. It is therefore highly desirable to employ a screening technique that is based on molecular markers linked to the resistance genes. Aside from overcoming the problems associated with phenotypic screening, marker-assisted selection (MAS) would enable gene pyramiding which is the combination of two or more resistance genes efficiently. This will expedite the process of breeding for multiple and durable resistance.

Most of the known wheat genes conferring resistance to RWA, have been mapped using microsatellite markers. Nine of these resistance genes are located on the D genome of wheat and one on the 1RS/1BL translocation (McIntosh et al., 2003). A study by Liu et al. (2001) revealed that the locus for wheat microsatellite GWM111 (*Xgwm111*), located on wheat chromosome 7DS (short arm), is tightly linked to RWA resistance genes *Dn1, Dn2* and *Dn5*, as well as *Dnx* in wheat resistance source PI 220127. The segregation data indicated that RWA resistance in PI 220127 is also conferred by a single dominant resistance gene (*Dnx*) (Liu et al., 2001). These results by Liu et al. (2001) confirmed that *Dn1, Dn2* and *Dn5* are tightly linked to each other, and this provided new information about their location, being 7DS, near the centromere, instead of as previously reported on 7DL. According to Miller et al. (2001), the marker *Xgwm437* is closely linked to *Dn2* at 2.8cM. *Xgwm106* and *Xgwm337* flanked *Dn4* on chromosome 1DS at 7.4 and 12.9 cM, respectively (Liu et al., 2002). Nkongolo et al. (1991a) reported RWA resistance gene *dn3* in *Triticum tauschii*. *Dn5* is located on wheat chromosome 7DS rather than 7DL and microsatellite marker *Xgwm635* shows close linkage to the gene (Liu et al., 2001). The markers *Xgwm44* and *Xgwm111* are linked to *Dn6* near the centromere on chromosome 7DS at 14.6 and 3.0 cM, respectively (Liu et al., 2002). This was the first report of the chromosome location of *Dn6*, which is either allelic or tightly linked to *Dn1, Dn2, Dn5* and *Dnx*. *Xgwm635* (near the distal end of 7DS) clearly marked the location of a previously suggested resistance gene in PI 294994, which was designated as *Dn8* (Liu et al., 2001). *Xgwm642*, in a defense gene-rich region of chromosome 1DL, marked another new gene *Dn9* from PI 294994 (Liu et al., 2001). A third new gene *Dny* from the Chinese wheat Lin-Yuan207 was localized on chromosome 1DL between *Xgwm111* and *Xgwm337* (Liu et al., 2001). A study was carried out with PCR markers for Russian Wheat Aphid Resistance Gene $Dn7$ on Chromosome 1RS/1BL and two markers which amplified rye-specific fragments proved to be useful for MAS. $Xrems1303$ amplified a 320-bp band only in cultivars with high-level resistance to USA biotype 2 and was effective for MAS of $Dn7$. $Xib267$ was found to be linked to the susceptible locus and amplified a fragment specific for rye Petkus 1RS (Lapitan et al., 2007).

Most of the Kenyan commercial wheat varieties are susceptible to RWA (Kiplagat, 2005) and since breeding of RWA resistant cultivars is further complicated due to presence of RWA biotypes, rapid breeding for and deployment of additional wheat cultivars resistant to RWA is urgently needed to reduce further losses from RWA outbreaks. This study was carried out to determine the inheritance and chromosome location of RWA resistance gene in the wheat source KRWA9.

MATERIALS AND METHODS

Plant materials and population development

Seeds were obtained from the Kenya Agricultural Research Institute, Njoro and planted in the crossing block in a row spacing of 30 cm. Crossing was carried out between resistant line 'KRWA9' and susceptible commercial variety 'Njoro BW2' to obtain F_1 progeny. The F_1 progeny was planted the following season and selfed to obtain F_2 seeds. $F_{2:3}$ families were obtained by planting seeds harvested from individual F_2 plants. Plants grew under normal rainfall regime with occasional irrigation supplement.

Phenotyping

The parents, F_1 plants, 100 F_2 plants and $F_{2:3}$ families were screened for RWA resistance under greenhouse conditions. Parents, F_1 and F_2 seedlings were grown in 20-cm-diameter pots containing *sterilized forest soil and sand at a ratio of 3:1* mixed with 5 g Di-ammonium phosphate (18-46-0) fertilizer. Each pot contained two to four seedlings. Fifteen (15) seeds from each $F_{2:3}$ family were planted on evaluation flats (1.5 × 1.0 × 0.75 m) containing *sterilized forest soil and sand at a ratio of 3:1* mixed with 75 g Di-ammonium phosphate (18-46-0) fertilizer. Due to poor germination, screening data was collected from ten plants of each $F_{2:3}$ family. The plants were watered regularly to ensure that they did not suffer moisture stress.

The virulent RWA colony that had earlier been biotyped by Malinga et al. (2007b) was collected from symptomatic bread wheat in the screenhouse and multiplied in preparation for infestation. The aphid colony was established on 'Kenya Kwale', a wheat variety that is highly susceptible to RWA and maintained in the greenhouse with temperatures 25:18°C, photoperiod (LD 12:12) and relative humidity varying between 60-80%. The pots and evaluation flats were caged with a 60 cm high wire cage and covered with a polyester screen mesh (68 meshes per square cm) to prevent aphids from getting in or escaping. Five adult aphids (3 - 5 instar stage) were placed on the whorls of seedlings at the two leaf stage using a camel hair brush. Five aphids were used for each plant to ensure maximum infestation pressure was achieved. RWA infestation was rated at twenty one days after infestation and scoring done according to a modified 1 - 9 visual scale (Malinga, 2007). Plants showing damage scale of 1 - 5 were grouped as resistant

and 6 - 9 susceptible.

Statistical analysis

The data of RWA reaction for individual F_2 plants was tested against an expected phenotypic segregation ratio of 3:1 using the Chi square (χ^2) goodness of fit test, to confirm the mode of inheritance at probability level of P = 0.05. The data on RWA reaction for individual $F_{2:3}$ families was tested against an expected phenotypic segregation ratio of 1:2:1 using the Chi square (χ^2) test to also confirm the mode of inheritance at probability level of P = 0.05. The segregation of $F_{2:3}$ families was expected to confirm the segregation ratios observed in F_2 populations and aid in the classification of F_2 lines for the bulk segregant analysis.

Genotyping using microsatellite markers

DNA was isolated from parents and 100 F_2 plants following the protocol by Dellaporta and Woods (1983) with some modifications. Approximately 500 mg of leaf tissue was ground with liquid nitrogen before adding and mixing with 500 µl of extraction buffer (0.1 M Tris-HCl pH 8.0, 0.05 M ethylenediaminetetraacetic acid (EDTA), 0.5 M NaCl, 1% polyvinylpyrolidone, 1.6% sodium dodecyl sulphate (SDS). This was followed by the addition of 50 µl of 20% SDS, and after mixing by inversion the tubes were incubated for 15 min at 65°C. The samples were removed from incubator and 250 ml of potassium acetate (-20°C) followed by incubation in freezer for 10 min at -20°C. The samples were then centrifuged at 13,000 rpm for 5 min and 500 µl of isopropanol (at -20°C) was added to the supernatant in new tubes. The mixture was incubated for 10 min at -20°C followed by centrifugation at 13,000 rpm for 5 min. The supernatant was discarded, DNA pellet washed with 500 µl of 70% ethanol (at -20°C) followed by air-drying. The DNA pellet was resuspended in 100 ul of 10:1 TE (10 mM Tris:1 mM EDTA) buffer. The samples were RNase treated by adding 2.25 µL of 10 mg ml^{-1} RNase and incubating for 30 min at 65°C followed by storing at -20°C till further use.

DNA was quantified spectrophotometrically and quality checked by 1% agarose gel electrophoresis, against lambda DNA of known quantity. Presence of DNA was confirmed by visualizing the bands on the gel under a UV transilluminator (Alpha Innotech, Taiwan). Comparison of the concentration of DNA was done against known standards of 100, 125, 250 500 and 1000 ng/µl lambda DNA to determine quantity. DNA was diluted to a working stock of 30 ng/µl for PCR reactions.

Bulk segregant analysis (BSA) with microsatellite markers was used to identify DNA markers associated with RWA resistance. Nine primers for $Xgwm$ microsatellites were used in this study. These microsatellite markers have been mapped in wheat chromosome 7D. They included $Xgwm30$, $Xgwm44$, $Xgwm46$, $Xgwm56$, $Xgwm111$, $Xgwm297$, $Xgwm333$, $Xgwm437$ and $Xgwm644$ (Roder et al., 1998). BSA was done using DNA from KRWA9, NjoroBW2, resistant homozygous plants, resistant heterozygous (segregating) plants, homozygous susceptible plants and control resistance sources PI 137739 ($Dn1$), PI 262660 ($Dn2$), USA9 ($Dn7$) and PI 294994 ($Dn5$, $Dn8$ and $Dn9$). DNA solution was bulked into their respective resistant and susceptible bulks. The resistant bulk consisted of equal amounts of DNA 10 µl from eight homozygous resistant plants. The susceptible bulk contained DNA from eight susceptible plants. The third bulk contained DNA from segregating plants. There were two more bulks with equal amounts of DNA 10 µl from each parent NjoroBW2 and KRWA9. All PCR reactions were performed in 13 µl reaction volumes containing 1.25 µl of 10X PCR buffer, 8.5 µl of ddH$_2$O, 0.5 µl of 10 mM dNTPs, 0.75 µl of 50 mM MgCl$_2$, 0.25 µl of 10 mM each of forward and reverse primer and 0.05 µl of Invitrogen Taq DNA polymerase recombinant

Table 1. Chi-square values for seedling reaction to Russian wheat aphid in KRWA9, NjoroBW2, F_1, F_2 and $F_{2:3}$ populations of KRWA9 × NjoroBW2 cross.

Parents and crosses parents	Pop	Total	R	S	Observed R:S	Expected R:S	χ^2	P-value
KRWA9	P1	44	44	0	44:0	44:0	-	-
NjoroBW2	P2	45	0	45	0:45	0:45	-	-
Crosses								
KRWA9 × NjoroBW2	F_1	24	24	0	24:0	24:0 (1:0)	0.00	1.00
	F_2	100	77	23	77:23	75:25 (3:1)	0.21	0.644

KRWA9 × NjoroBW2	Pop	Total	R:Seg:S		Observed R:Seg :S	Expected R:Seg:S	χ^2	P-value
	$F_{2:3}$	100	28:49:23		28:49:23	25:50:25 (1:2:1)	0.53	0.767

R = Resistance, S = Susceptible, Pop = Population, χ^2 = Chi-square, Seg = Segregating, Significance at P = 0.05 level (df = 1, CV = 3.841 and df = 2, CV = 5.991).

(5 U/µl) and 1.5 µl template DNA. PCR amplifications were carried out on PCR machine (Applied Biosystems 2720 Thermal Cycler, Singapore). The microsatellite products were resolved on 2.0% agarose gels in TAE buffer. The bands were visualized under a UV transilluminator (Alpha Innotech, Taiwan). The electrophoresis products were captured on a camera and transferred to a computer.

Once a specific polymorphism between resistant and susceptible bulks had been identified by BSA screening, individual co-segregation analysis, based on the associations between marker genotype and RWA reaction phenotype, was carried out on the total F_2 segregating population to determine the genetic linkage between a RWA resistance gene and a marker.

Microsatellite marker, *Xgwm111* (linked to RWA resistance) and weighted at 210 bp was used to confirm the presence of RWA resistance gene in NjoroBW2 × KRWA9 F_2 population. The PCR profile was a follows: an initial denaturing step at 94°C for 3 min followed by 45 cycles at 94°C for 1 min, annealing for primer *Xgwm111* at 55°C for 1 min.

This was followed by primer elongation at 72°C for 2 min and final 10 min primer extension at 72°C. The simple sequence repeat (**SSR**) products were resolved on 2.0% agarose gels in TAE buffer and bands visualized under a UV transilluminator (Alpha Innotech, Taiwan). The electrophoresis products were captured on a camera and transferred to a computer.

Marker analysis

Informative bands were scored as present (+) or absent (-) and since SSRs are co-dominant markers, it was expected that alleles from both parents would be observed in some samples. Single marker analysis was done using the JoinMap software (Stam and Van Ooijen 1995) to detect QTL associated with *Xgwm111*. Linear regression was done to obtain coefficient of determination (R^2) that explains the phenotypic variation arising from QTL linked to a marker. Chi-square goodness-of-fit test was carried out to test conformity to Mendelian segregation patterns. The Chi square (χ^2) value and segregation ratios from gel data were later compared against Chi square (χ^2) value and phenotypic segregation ratios resulting from RWA reactions of individual F_2 populations and $F_{2:3}$ families.

RESULTS

Inheritance analysis

The resistant parent KRWA9 showed resistance reactions having minimal levels of chlorosis and rolling, with damage scores of 1 - 3. This indicated high levels of resistance in the resistant parent. The susceptible parent NjoroBW2 showed a susceptible reaction with damage scores of 7 - 9. Most NjoroBW2 seedlings had severe leaf chlorosis, streaking and rolling leading to death after 21 days of infestation. The F_1 population of cross NjoroBW2 × KRWA9 showed resistance reaction with damage scores of 1 - 4. The resistance reaction of F_1 population was not significantly different from the reaction of KRWA9 indicating that the resistance gene in KRWA9 is dominant. The χ^2 statistics for NjoroBW2 × KRWA9 F_1 population was significant at P<0.05 with a fit in ratio of 1:0 (Table 1). In NjoroBW2 × KRWA9 F_2 generation, the hybrids segregated and were classified into their respective phenotypic classes. The F_2 population showed both susceptible and resistant reactions with damage scores of 1 - 9. The χ^2 statistics was significant at P<0.05 with a fit in ratio of 3:1 (Table 1). The $F_{2:3}$ progenies were classified as homozygous resistant and heterozygous resistant (segregating) based on the seedling reactions to RWA. The $F_{2:3}$ homozygous resistant progenies showed damage scores of 1 - 5, indicating resistance. Heterozygous resistant progenies showed damage scores of 1 - 9 indicating both resistance and susceptible reactions. The χ^2 statistics for $F_{2:3}$ population of NjoroBW2 × KRWA9 was significant at P<0.05 (Table 1) with a fit in ratio of 1:2:1. These results confirmed the model of 3:1 at F_2 populations with a fit of 1:2:1 at $F_{2:3}$ families for monohybrid inheritance.

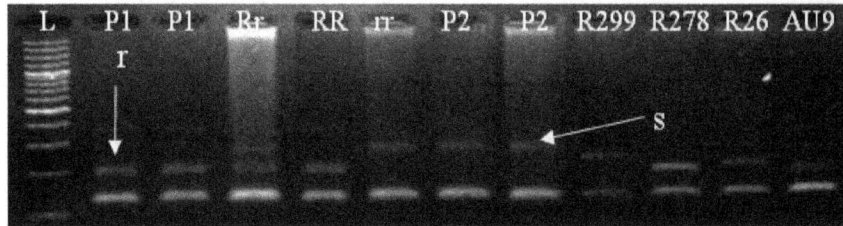

Figure 1. DNA bands amplified from F_2 DNA bulks using primer pair *Xgwm111* and electrophoresed in a 2% agarose gel. L = 100kb ladder, P1 = resistant parent bulk, P2 = susceptible parent bulk, RR = homozygous F_2 plant bulk, Rr = heterozygous F_2 plant bulk, rr = susceptible F_2 plant bulk, AU9 = resistance source having gene *Dn7*, R299 = (PI 294994) resistance source having genes *Dn5, Dn8, Dn9*, R26 = (PI 137739) resistance source having gene *Dn1*, R278 = (PI 262660) resistance source having gene *Dn2*, r = resistance band, s = susceptible band.

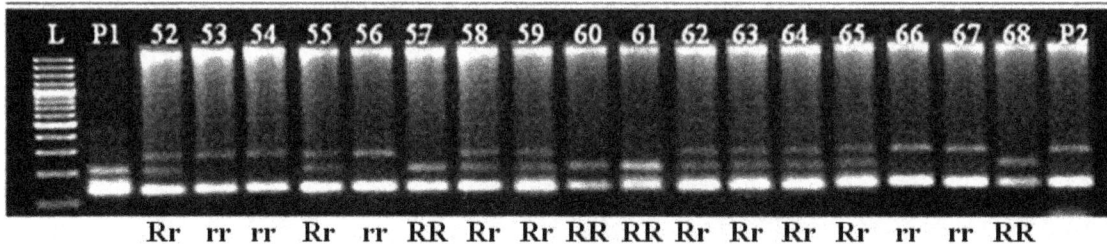

Figure 2. DNA bands amplified from F_2 progeny of NjoroBW2 × KRWA9 using primer pair *Xgwm111* and electrophoresed in a 2% agarose gel. P1 = resistant parent, P2 = susceptible parent, RR = Homozygous resistant, Rr = Homozygous susceptible, rr = Homozygous susceptible, L = 100 bp ladder.

Genotypic analysis

Nine primers (*Xgwm30, Xgwm44, Xgwm46, Xgwm56, Xgwm111, Xgwm297, Xgwm333, Xgwm437* and *Xgwm644*) were screened for polymorphism and only chromosome 7DS primer *Xgwm111* produced a distinguishing polymorphism. Primer *Xgwm111* produced a band that clearly and consistently differentiated the parents, resistant and susceptible bulks (Figure 1). A band was produced on control resistance source PI 137739 which was similar to the one on resistance source KRWA9. The band was approximately 210 bp and was subsequently tested on F_2 population individuals. Other bands were produced on resistance sources PI 262660 (*Dn2*), PI 294994 (*Dn5, Dn8* and *Dn9*) and AUS9 (*Dn7*). Figure 1 shows the banding patterns for KRWA9, NjoroBW2, homozygous resistant plants, heterozygous resistant plants, homozygous susceptible plants and control resistance sources "R299", "R278", "R26" and "AU9". KRWA9 showed two distinctive bands; one was 210 bp while the other was 160 bp. The susceptible parent NjoroBW2 showed two distinctive bands; one was 280 bp while the other was 160 bp (Figure 1). It was observed that both parents had a common 160 bp band. The 210 bp band was present in the resistant parent but absent in the susceptible parent. This band was

designated as the band of interest. The inclusion of different resistant sources helped to accurately identify the DNA markers for gene of interest. The primer *Xgwm111* also produced a 210 bp band that clearly and consistently differentiated the parents, resistant, heterozygous and susceptible plants in the F_2 population (Figure 2). Based on the banding patterns observed in the F_2 population, 28 plants were homozygous resistant, 49 heterozygous and 23 homozygous susceptible (Table 3). This ratio did not differ from the expected 1:2:1 segregation ratio (x^2 = 5.991, df = 2, $P \le 0.05$).

Linkage analysis

The F_2 population of NjoroBW2 × KRWA9 cross showed a wide range of segregation for response to infestation by RWA. The frequency distribution of RWA feeding damage on the F_2 population was somewhat bimodal, indicating the presence of one major resistance gene in KRWA9 (Figure 3). Simple regression analysis identified marker *Xgwm111 to be* highly significantly associated with resistance in KRWA9. The marker had an LOD score of 40.1 and high R^2 value of 85% indicating that it is a very significant marker for the resistance in KRWA9 (Table 2). Genetic data for *Xgwm111* marker showed a

Table 2. Statistical indicators for SSR marker *Xgwm111*.

Marker	LOD*	R^{2**}	P^{***}	Source of resistance
Xgwm111	40.1	85%	0.000	KRWA9

* = p ≤ 0.1, ** = p ≤ 0.05, *** = p ≤ 0.01

Table 3. Summary of primer *Xgwm111* F_2 gel data.

Genotype	Observed values	Expected values	Chi square (χ^2)	P value
A	28	25	0.53	0.767
B	23	25		
H	49	50		
Total	100	100		

A = Homozygous resistant, B = homozygous susceptible, H = heterozygous (Significance at P = 0.05 level, df = 2, CV = 5.991).

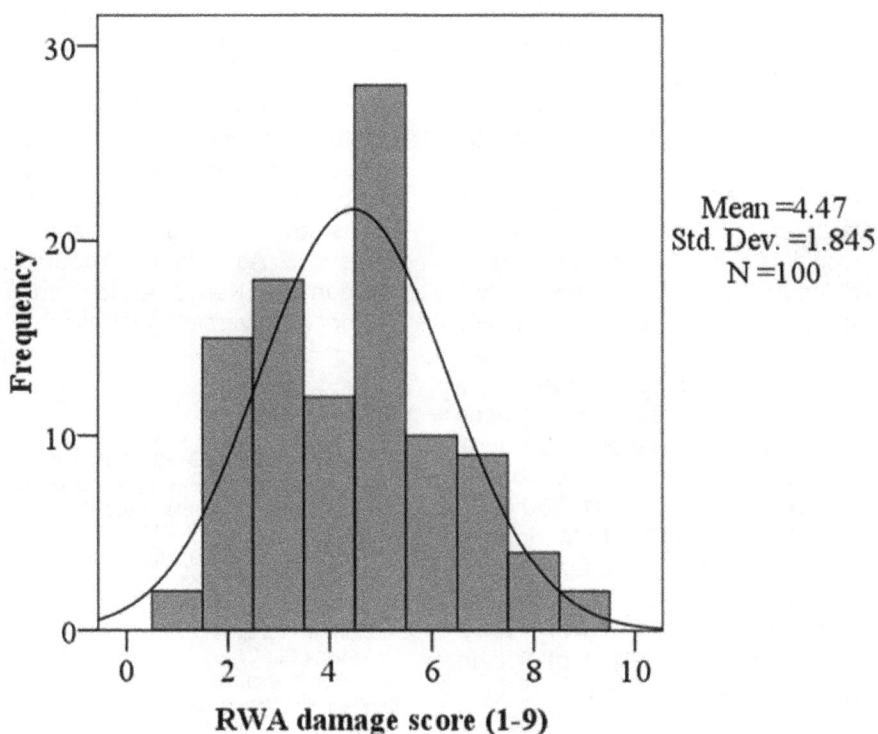

Figure 3. RWA damage distribution in F_2 population.

complete co-segregation with the disease data in the mapping population indicating a very tight linkage to the RWA resistance gene in KRWA9.

DISCUSSION

KRWA9 was selected for this study because visual observations of RWA feeding damage on it suggested that this source of resistance has high level resistance (Pathak et al., 2007; Malinga et al., 2008). This resistance could be transferred to NjoroBW2 a popular commercial wheat variety which is susceptible to RWA. The F_1 seedlings of the cross between NjoroBW2 and KRWA9 were all resistant indicating the resistance in KRWA9 is dominant. The segregation observed in the F_2 population and the $F_{2:3}$ families further confirmed the dominance of resistance in KRWA9. Most RWA resistant genotypes have single dominant genes located on chromosome 1D and 7D (Du toit, 1987; Nkongolo et al.,

1991b; Saidi and Quick, 1996; Liu et al., 2001; Liu, 2001). Resistance sources reported to have single dominant genes include PI137739 (Dn1), PI262660 (Dn2), PI372129 (Dn4) and PI243781 (Dn6) (Du Toit, 1989; Nkongolo et al., 1991b; Saidi and Quick, 1994). The dominant nature of RWA resistance gene could be easily identified in the segregating populations. However, the major problem with single gene inheritance is that insect can develop biotypes very fast if the resistant cultivar is grown on a large scale. Colorado State University has developed several commercially available RWA resistant varieties of winter wheat such as Halt, Prairie Red, Prowers 99 and Yuma (Thomas et al., 2002). All these varieties have the Dn4 resistance gene derived from PI 372129 (Turcikum 57). It was later reported that RWA resistant cultivars with the Dn4 gene were susceptible to a new biotype designated as "Biotype 2" (Haley et al., 2004). This led to sourcing of more resistant materials. Gene Dn7 that was previously transferred from rye to wheat background via a 1 RS/1BL translocation had been reported to be resistant biotype 1 and 2 and depicts high levels of resistance as compared to other Dn genes (Collins et al., 2005; Turanli et al., 2012). However, part of the rye chromosome containing Dn7 has detrimental genes resulting to poor bread making quality (Graybosch et al., 1990). Breeding for resistance with Dn7 gene is no longer a desirable strategy and identification of diverse sources of resistance would be a highly desirable to keep ahead of biotype development in RWA. Pyramiding two or more resistance genes in a single cultivar will also increase the longevity of resistance.

The marker Xgwm111 has previously been found to be linked to genes Dn1, Dn2 and Dn5 in resistance sources PI 137739, PI 262660 and PI 294994, respectively (Liu et al., 2005). In their study, the marker Xgwm111 produced band sizes 210 bp in PI 137739 for gene Dn1, 200 bp in PI 262660 for gene Dn2 and 200 bp in PI294994 for gene Dn5 (Liu et al., 2005). The results are in agreement with Liu et al. (2001, 2002), who reported that Xgwm111 amplifies functional fragments from DNA of RWA-resistant wheat sources with expected sizes of 200 to 225 bp that are associated with RWA resistance.

In the F_2 population, marker Xgwm111 followed the expected Mendelian segregation ratio of 3:1 or 1:2:1 (Table 3). These findings are consistent with Pathak et al. (2007) on a single dominant gene controlling resistance in KRWA9. The marker also completely co-segregated with the disease data and it is believed that the resistance gene in KRWA9 must be tightly linked to the marker. This offers a good opportunity for breeders to use this marker to select for resistance to RWA.

Conclusion

The usage of host plant resistance at the low cost is environmentally safe and is an ideal method to control the Russian wheat aphid. KRWA9 is a good source of

resistance to RWA biotypes in Kenya and marker Xgwm111 could be used for marker assisted selection of resistance associated with this line. Similarity exists between KRWA9 and PI 137739, therefore there is a need to screen more markers in order to find more polymorphic markers in this region of chromosome 7DS. Most RWA resistance sources are monogenic and the challenge is that insects can develop biotypes very fast which could overcome the resistant cultivars. Identification of many sources of RWA resistance would be highly desirable to keep ahead of biotype development in the RWA by way of deploying multiple resistance genes to new breeding lines.

Conflict of Interests

The author(s) have not declared any conflict of interests.

ACKNOWLEDGEMENTS

We would like to thank the Kenya Agricultural Research Institute for facilitating the development, screening and molecular analysis breeding populations. We are grateful to Egerton University for technical support in carrying out this study. Funding of this research was provided by Enhanced Agricultural Productivity Programme (EAPP) through the Kenya Agricultural Research Institute and Murdoch University, Australia.

REFERENCES

Botha CEJ, Matsiliza B (2006). Reduction in transport in wheat (Triticum aestivum L.) is caused by sustained phloem feeding by the Russian wheat aphid (Duraphis noxia Kudjumov). South Afr. J. Bot. 70:249-254.

Collins MB, Haley SD, Randolph TL, Peairs FB, Rudolph JB (2005). Comparison of Dn4- and Dn7-carrying spring wheat genotypes artificially infested with Russian wheat aphid (Homoptera: Aphididae) Biotype 1. J. Econ. Entomol. 98(5):1698-1703.

Dellaporta SL, Wood J, Hicks JB (1983). A plant DNA minipreparation: version II. Plant Mol. Biol. Rep. 1:19-21.

Du Toit F, Walters MC (1984). Damage assessment and economic threshold values for chemical control of the Russian wheat aphid, Diuraphis noxia (Mordvilko) on winter wheat, pp. 58-62. In M. C. Walters [ed.] Progress in Russian Wheat Aphid (Diuraphis noxia) research in the Republic of South Africa. Technical communication 191. Department of Agriculture, Republic of South Africa.

Du Toit F (1989). Inheritance of resistance in two Triticum aestivum lines to Russian wheat aphid (Homoptera: Aphididae). J. Econ. Entomol. 82:1251-1253.

Ennahli S, El Bouhssini M, Grando S, Anathakrishnan R, Niide T, Starkus L, Starkey S, Smith CM (2009). Comparison of categories of resistance in wheat and barley genotypes against biotype 2 of the Russian wheat aphid, Diuraphis noxia (Kurdjumov). Arthropod Plant Interact. 3:45-53.

Graybosch RA, Peterson CJ, Hansen LW, Mattern PJ (1990). Relationships between protein solubility characteristics, 1BL/1RS, high molecular weight glutenin composition and end use quality in winter wheat germplasm. Cereal chem. 67:342-349.

Haley SD, Peairs FB, Walker CB, Rudolph JB, Randolph TL (2004). Occurrence of a new Russian wheat aphid biotype in Colorado

Crop Sci. 44:1589-1592.

Hewitt PH, van Niekerk GJJ, Walters MC, Kriel CF, Fouche A (1984). Aspects of ecology of the Russian wheat aphid, *Diuraphis noxia*, in the Bloemfontein district. I. The colonization and infestation of sown wheat, identification of summer hosts and cause of infestation symptoms. In: M. C. Walters (eds) Progress in Russian wheat aphid. Research in the Republic of South Africa. Tech. Commun. Dept Agric Rep. S Africa 191:3-13.

Jankielsohn A (2011). Distribution and diversity of Russian wheat aphid (Hemiptera: Aphididae) biotypes in South Africa and Lesotho. J. Econ. Entomol. 104(5):1736-1741.

Kiplagat OK (2005). The Russian wheat aphid (*Diuraphis noxia* Mord.). Damage on Kenyan wheat (*Triticum aestivum* L.) varieties and possible control through resistance breeding. PhD Thesis Wageningen University. ISBN 90-8504-175-9.

Lapitan NLV, Peng J, Sharma V (2007). A high-density map and PCR markers for russian wheat aphid resistance gene *Dn7* on chromosome 1RS/1BL. Crop Sci. 47:811-820.

Liu XM, Smith CM, Friebe BR, Gill BS (2005). Molecular mapping and allelic relationships of Russian wheat aphid - resistance genes. Crop Sci. 45:2273-2280.

Liu XM, Smith CM, Gill BS (2002). Identification of microsatellite markers linked to Russian wheat aphid resistance genes *Dn4* and *Dn6*. Theor. Appl. Genet. 104:1042-1048.

Liu XM, Smith CM, Gill BS, Tolmay V (2001). Microsatellite markers linked to six Russian wheat aphid resistance genes in wheat. Theor. Appl. Genet. 102:504-510.

Malinga JN (2007). Studies on Russian wheat aphid (*Diuraphis noxia*: Kurdjumov; Homoptera) with special empasis to biotypes and host plant resistance in bread wheat (*Triticum aestivum*) in Kenya. PhD Thesis. Egerton University, Kenya.

Malinga JN, Kinyua M, Wanjama J, Kamau A, Awalla J (2007a). Differential Population Increase, Damage and Polymorphism within Kenyan Russian wheat aphid Populations. 10th KARI Biennial Scientific Conference. 13-17 November, 2006. Nairobi, Kenya

Malinga JN, Kinyua MG, Kamau AW, Wanjama JK, Awalla JO, Pathak RS (2007b). Biotyping and Genetic Variation within Tropical Population of Russian Wheat Aphid, *Duraphis noxia* Kurdjumov (Homoptera: Aphididae) in Kenya. J. Entomol. 4:350-361.

Malinga JN, Kinyua MG, Kamau AW, Wanjama JK, Pathak RS (2008). Characterisation of Bread Wheat Genotypes Resistant To Russian Wheat Aphid in Kenya. E. Afr. Agric. For. J. 74(1-2):51-58.

McIntosh RA, Yamazaki Y, Devos K, Dubcovsky J, Rogers WJ, Appels R (2003). Catalogue of gene symbols for wheat. In: Pogna NE, Romano M, Pogna EA, Galterio G (eds) Proceedings of the 10th International Wheat Genetics Symposium. 4:1-34.

Miller CA, Altinkut A, Lapitan NLV (2001). A microsatellite marker for tagging *Dn2*, a wheat gene conferring resistance to the Russian wheat aphid. Crop Sci. 41:1584-1589.

Miller RH, Haile A (1988). Russian wheat aphid on barley in Ethiopia. Rachis 7:51-53.

Nkongolo KK, Quick JS, Limin AE, Fowler DB (1991a). Sources and inheritance of resistance to Russian wheat aphid in Triticum species amphiploids and *Triticum tauschii*. Can. J. Plant. Sci. 71:703-708.

Nkongolo KK, Quick JS, Peairs FB, Meyer, WL (1991b). Inheritance of resistance of PI 372129 to the Russian wheat aphid. Crop Sci. 31:905-907.

Quick JS, Ellis GE, Normann RM, Stromberger JA, Shanahan JF, Peairs FB, Rudolph JB, Lorenz K (1996). Registration of Halt wheat. Crop Sci. 36(1):210-210.

Ricciardi M, Tocho E, Tacaliti MS, Vasicek A, Gime DO, Paglione A, Simmonds J, Snape JW, Cakir M, Castro AM (2010). Mapping quantitative trait loci for resistance against Russian wheat aphid (*Diuraphis noxia*) in wheat (*Triticum aestivum* L.) Crop Pasture Sci. 61:970-977.

Roder MS, Korzun V, Wendehake K, Plaschke J, Tixier MH, Leroy P, Ganal MW (1998). A microsatellite map of wheat. Genet. 149(4):2007-2023.

Saidi A, Quick JS (1994). Inheritance of Russian wheat aphid resistance in four winter wheats. In F.B. Peairs, M.K. Kroening and C.L. Simmons (comps.) Proceedings of the Sixth Russian Wheat Aphid Workshop, Colorado State University, Ft. Collins, CO. pp.126-132.

Saidi A, Quick JS (1996). Inheritance and allelic relationships among Russian wheat aphid resistance genes in winter wheat. Crop Sci. 36:256-258.

Stam P, Van Ooijen JW (1995). JOINMAP version 2.0: software for the calculation of genetic linkage maps. CPRO-DLO, Wageningen.

Thomas J, Hein G, Baltensperger D, Nelson L, Haley S (2002). Managing the Russian wheat aphid with resistant wheat varieties. NebFacts (September 2002) Nebraska Cooperative Extension NF96-307. Publ. of Cooperative Extension Institute of agriculture and Natural Resources, University of Nebraska, Lincoln.

Tolmay VL, Lindeque RC Prinsloo GJ (2007). Preliminary evidence of a resistance-breaking biotype of the Russian wheat aphid, *Diuraphis noxia* (Kurdjumov) (Homoptera: Aphididae), in South Africa. Afr. Entomol. 15:228-230.

Tolmay VL, Prinsloo G, Hatting J (2000). Russian wheat resistant wheat cultivars as the main component of an integrated control program. In: Proceedings of the eleventh regional Wheat workshop for Eastern, Central, and Southern Africa. Addis Ababa, Ethiopia: CIMMYT pp. 190-194.

Tolmay VL, Van Deventer CW (2005). Yield retention of resistant wheat cultivars, severely infested with Russian wheat aphid, *Diuraphis noxia* (Kurdjumov), in South Africa. S. Afr. J. Plant Soil. 22:246-250.

Turanli F, Ilker E, Ersin Dogan F, Askan L, Istipliler D (2012). Inheritance of Resistance to Russian wheat aphid (*Diuraphis noxia* Kurdjumov) in bread wheat (*Triticum aestivum* L.). Turk J. Field Crops. 17(2):171-176.

Van Niekerk HA (2001). Southern Africa wheat pool. In: The world wheat book: the history of wheat breeding. Ed. by AP B, WJ A. Lavoisier Publishing, Paris, FR, pp. 923-936.

23

Molecular identification of *Lactobacillus plantarum* isolated from fermenting cereals

Adeyemo, S. M.[1] **and Onilude, A. A.**[2]

[1]Department of Microbiology, Obafemi Awolowo University, Ile-Ife, Osun State, Nigeria.
[2]Department of Microbiology, University of Ibadan, Oyo State, Nigeria.

The identification of a microbial isolate to genus level only amounts to a partial characterization of the isolate, but this can tell us a lot about that organism. Knowing the species allows the laboratory access to the body of knowledge that exists on that species. Identification schemes using phenotypic characteristics such as colony and cell morphology, Gram reaction and other staining characteristics, nutritional and physiological requirements for growth and metabolic characteristics have been developed and improved over many decades to a point where laboratories are able to identify isolates to species level using simple conventional methods. This phenotypic method however have some limitations apart from being laborious and time consuming, some organisms may however be misidentified either at genus or species level. This work aims at looking directly at the genome of lactic acid bacteria (LAB) and from this identifies some species using its genotypic and phenotypic characteristics. These bacteria species were identified by sequencing specific sections of ribosomal DNA - the 16S rRNA gene, after amplification by PCR, and then comparing the results to sequences stored on a related database. The results from both conventional and molecular methods were then compared. Twenty (20) *Lactobacillus plantarum* were isolated from spontaneously fermented cereals made into *"Ogi"* and identified using classical methods. They were further characterized using molecular methods by polymerase chain reaction (PCR) amplification of 16S rDNA genes to confirm their identities. The genotypic characterization however showed that 85% of the organisms identified using conventional method as *L. plantarum* correlated, while 15% did not correlate; 2 were identified as *Lactobacillus pentosus* and one unidentified *Lactobacillus* sp. The method is a rapid and reliable way of producing a large number of copies of a specific DNA sequence for the identification of LAB. This method is however, able to solve the problem of poor identification that is usually associated with the identification of this fastidious organism that is regularly used as probiotics, starter culture and bio-preservatives in fermented foods that are consumed and in biotechnology because they are generally regarded as safe.

Key words: Molecular methods, conventional, *Lactobacillus plantarum* identification, fermented foods, species and genera level, rapid, reliable.

INTRODUCTION

Microorganisms have been isolated from different sources especially from different food samples and grown in pure cultures over the centuries. A major aspect of microbiology and the work of food microbiologists and various microbiology laboratories is the ability to identify and characterize various isolates so that they can be differentiated from one another. Different schemes that can be used to describe the characteristics and properties of microbial isolates are essential in every branch of microbiology. These schemes have been undergoing different forms of development and refinement over the years. The various methods are not static; but have been improved from time to time and proper identification is very essential when it has to do with foods that are consumed (Lucke, 2000; Olaoye and Onilude, 2009). The advent of molecular biology in the 1980s contributed a set of powerful new tools that have helped microbiologists to detect the smallest variations within microbial species and even within individual strains (Olaoye and Onilude, 2009). This is because different organisms have different genetic combination.

In fact, the technology has progressed far beyond the level needed by most routine laboratories, where identifying the species of any isolate is likely to be sufficient. Distinguishing between different strains of the same species (typing) is more likely to be of value in a research laboratory. Nevertheless, methods and equipment designed to help with both species identification and typing are commercially available for a range of applications (Lucke, 2000).

There are different molecular characterization techniques namely genotyping, multilocus sequence typing (MLST), pulsed-field gel electrophoresis (PFGE), ribotyping, repetitive sequence-based PCR (rep-PCR) and the use of 16S rDNA genes which relies on the relative stability of the 16S and 23S rRNA genes coding for ribosomal-RNA and so on (Ogier et al., 2002; Gomes et al., 2008; Paula et al., 2012).

Molecular characterization of microorganisms however has some distinct advantages over the known conventional methods. The molecular method of identification and characterization of microorganisms have been preferred over the classical ones which make use of the biochemical reactions and proteolytic activities of the organisms (Morgan et al., 2009). The classical and conventional method of identification is slow, laborious, time consuming and may not be 100% specific and accurate. It is also problematic and subjective due to ambiguous biochemical or physiological traits.

Bulut et al. (2005) reported that identification of lactic acid bacteria (LAB) by phenotypic methods such as sugar fermentation may be uncertain and complicated owing to the increase in species that vary with few characters. The commercially available system based on this technology is a valuable complementary tool to other routine identification technologies. However, identification based on the 16S rRNA gene is by no means infallible as the sequence stretch analysed is a reduced section of the full genome and the variability of this marker is low.

The development of molecular typing methods has offered the possibility of accelerating a great deal of bacterial identification which avoid so many biases that are related to the classical methods. The polymerase chain reaction (PCR) has however provided a method to detect DNA sequences with high speed and sensitivity. This technique is emerging as a new tool in identifying and selecting bacteria with specific and desirable functions (Bulut et al., 2005). A combination of different approaches in the identification of different organisms offer a solution to the use of the conventional method that makes use of the ability of LAB to produce acid from carbohydrate and other metabolic activities only (Morgan et al., 2009).

According to Merien et al. (2013), the nucleotide base sequences of Lactobacillus spp. 16S ribosomal DNA also provides accurate basis for phylogenetic identification of organisms that are slow growing, fastidious and are therefore poorly identified by conventional methods. These small ribosomal units exist universally among bacteria and include regions with species-specific variability which makes it possible to identify bacteria to species level.

The use of Lactobacillus sp. as probiotics in man has been found to enhance their immunity and increase their ability to fight and survive against food related pathogens. Also, nursing mothers prefer natural products with fewer artificial preservatives in foods that are used for weaning infants with natural fortification or supplements. They have also been found to be consumed in fermented foods that contain them for their health benefits (Adeyemo and Onilude, 2013).

Lactobacillus plantarum particularly has also been implicated in the reduction of raffinose- family of oligosaccharide content of soybeans used in the formulation of a weaning food blend by their ability to hydrolyse the raffinose to simple sugars and hence improve the weaning food (Adeyemo and Onilude, 2014). Fermentation with cultures containing LAB is able to produce healthy, safe, high quality and nutritious beneficial food products such as fermented milk, meat, vegetables, grains, cereals, legumes, meat, beverages, etc. These organisms produce lactic acid which has a way of preserving such fermented foods and also improve the flavour, texture and nutritional compounds of such foods through the metabolic activities of LAB during fermentation. Also, the metabolism and physiology of LAB is used in different biotechnological processes in industries to formulate LAB starters with useful metabolic activities and capabilities so as to ensure a wide range of quality fermented products with consistent characteristics (Adeyemo and Onilude, 2013).

Being used as probiotics and starter culture in many

food industries and in fermentation technology, a prompt and rapid identification of *L. plantarum* is of utmost importance so as not to confuse this very important organism with other organisms of the same genus or species that are closely related. As a result of this, there is need for accurate identification of this organism, the importance of which cannot be over emphasized.

MATERIALS AND METHODS

Sample collection

Local varieties (LV) of sorghum (*Sorghum bicolor*) were obtained from a market and typed varieties (TV) from Institute of Agricultural Research & Training, Ibadan, Nigeria. They were all processed to *ogi* in the laboratory using the traditional method of Banigo and Muller (1972). *Ogi* was also obtained from traditional sellers within Ibadan (CO) and used for comparative studies. The samples were collected in clean polythene bags and transported to the laboratory.

Isolation of lactic acid bacteria

One gram each of the samples listed above was subjected to ten-fold serial dilutions using the method of Harrigan and MacCance (1976). Isolation of organisms was done with the pour plate method using molten MRS agar. After solidification, they were incubated anaerobically in an anaerobic jar at 30°C for 48-72 h. Pure cultures were selected and stored on slant overlaid with sterile glycerol.

Identification of the isolates

Morphological and macroscopic characteristics

For proper identification of the isolates, the cultural, morphological, biochemical and physiological characterization including microscopic and macroscopic examinations of the various isolates were carried out according to Sneath et al. (2009). Gram positive and catalase negative organisms were subjected to further biochemical tests.

Biochemical characteristics

Isolates were identified phenotypically on the basis of the following biochemical test after Gram's staining, catalase, oxidase, methyl red test, Voges Proskaeur, nitrate reduction, starch, casein and gelatin hydrolysis, growth at different pH and temperature and NaCl ranges and the ability to produce CO_2 from glucose and production of acid from carbohydrates such as fructose, lactose, maltose, galactose, arabinose, mannose, xylose, dulcitol, inositol, mannitol, raffinose, trehalose, rhamnose, etc.(Sneath et al., 2009).

Genetic characterization of isolates

Extraction of genomic DNA of LAB isolates

DNA extraction from the LAB isolates was carried out using a modified GES (5M guanidine thiocyanate (Fisher scientific, England), 0.1 N EDTA (Sigma, England) and 0.5% N-lauroyl - sarcosine sodium salt (Sigma, England) (w/v) DNA extraction method (Pitcher et al., 1989). Aliquots of 1.5 ml of overnight cultures grown in appropriate broth were centrifuged (Biofuge,

Heraeus, Germany) in Eppendorf tubes at 13,000 g for 1 min. Pellets obtained were washed in 1 ml of ice cold lysis buffer (25 mM Tris-HCl (Sigma, England), 10 mM EDTA, 50 mM sucrose (BOH GPR 303997J), pH 8). The pellets were re-suspended in 100 μl of lysis buffer in addition to 50 mgml^{-1} lysozyme (Sigma, England.) and incubated at 37°C for 30 min. 0.5 ml of the GES solution were added and mixed thoroughly. This was incubated at room temperature for 15 min. The lysate was then placed on ice for 2 min and 0.25 ml of 7.5 M ammonium acetate (Fisher scientific, England). Cooled ice was also added, vortexed and incubated on ice for 10 min. Aliquots (0.5 ml) of 24:1 chloroform : isoamyalcohol (Sigma, England) were added, vortexed and centrifuged for 10 min at 13,000 g. Aliquots of 800 ml of the upper phase were removed quantitively and placed in a clean Eppendorf tube. Cold isopropanol (Fisher scientific, England) was added and mixed for 1 min. This was then centrifuged at 13,000 g for 5 min and the supernatant removed from the pellet. The pellet was washed three times in 500 μl of 70% ethanol and dried at 37°C for 15 min. Aliquots (50 μl) of TE buffer were added and 5 μl of the DNA were checked on 1% agarose (Biogene, Kimbolton, UK) gels in 200 ml 1X TAE buffer and the DNA samples were then stored at -20°C for future use.

Polymerase chain reaction (PCR) amplification of 16S rDNA gene

The method of Bulut et al. (2005) was used. Amplification of 16S rDNA gene - ITS region, was performed by using the following primer pairs. Forward (16S ITS For), 5'-AGAGTTTGATCCTGGCCTCAG-3$^/$ and reverse (16S - ITS Rev), 5' - CAAGGCATCCACCGT - 3$^/$, 16S rDNA V3, forward 5$^/$ - CCTAGGGGAGGCAGCAG - 3$^/$ and 16S rDNA V3, reverse, 5' - ARRACCGCGCTGCTGC-3$^/$. The forward 5'-CCTACGGGAGGCAGCAG-3' and reverse, 5'-ATTACCGCGGCTGCTGG-3', primers used occupied positions 341-358 and 518-534, respectively of the V3 region in the 16S ribosomal DNA of *Escherichia coli*. The primers specify about 200 bp of the PCR products (as could be seen on the gel after electrophoresis).

The V3 primer pair was used for ease of sequencing of the gene, using the variable region 3 (V3), for the genetic identification of the isolates.

Each of the polymerase chain reactions (PCR) was performed in a 50 μl reaction volume containing 50 μg genomic DNA as the template. 10 μl of 0.2 mM deoxynucleoside triphospates, dNTPs (Promega UI20A - UI23A, Madison, WI, USA), 10 μl of 2.5 mM $MgCl_2$, 10 pmol each (0.1 μl volume) of the DNA primer in PCR buffer (Promega, UK), and 10 μl of 1.25 units Taq DNA polymerase (Promega, UK) and 18.9 μl distilled water. Amplification conditions were as follows: an initial denaturation step of 5 min at 94°C, 40 amplification cycles, each consisting of 1 min denaturation at 94°C, 1 min annealing at 42°C, and 1 min elongation at 72°C. Reactions were terminated with a final extension step for 10 min at 72°C. PCR amplification was performed in a Thermocycler (Techne- Progene, Cambridge, UK).

Gel electrophoresis of 16S rDNA PCR Products

Electrophoresis of the amplified 16s rDNA PCR products were performed on the Bio-Rad contour - clamped homogenous electric field (CHEF) DRII electrophoresis cell. This was done through 1.5% (w/v) agarose gel (Biogene, Germany) in 0.5 X TAE buffer at 84 V for 1.5-2 h. This was prepared by boiling 1.5 g of agarose powder in 100 ml of 0.5X TAE buffer. A 100 bp ladder (Promega, U.K) and 1 Kb DNA ladder (Promega, U.K) were used as molecular size markers.

Sequencing and analysis Of 16S rDNA gene

Purification of PCR 16S rDNA gene

75 µl of the PCR 16S rDNA amplified products (obtained above) were resolved in 1% agarose gels with the conditions earlier described. PCR products were resolved by gel electrophoresis, using an agarose gel (1.5%; Biogene) that was stained with of 0.5 µg/ml ethidium bromide, in 1xTAE buffer at 84 V for 1.5 - 2 h.

The DNA bands were then visualised using a UV transilluminator (Amersham Pharmacia Biotech, UK) with 313 nm emission and pictures were taken using Fuji Film Imaging system FT1-500 (Amersham Pharmacia Biotech, UK).

The resulting bands in agarose gel were carefully excised with sterile scalpels and then purified the Wizard PCR preps DNA purification kit (Promega, USA). The purified DNA was kept at 4°C until used.

Drying of the purified 16S rDNA genes

To a 50 µl of the purified DNA, 0.1 µl of sodium acetate buffer (3M, pH 5.0) and 2.0 µl of 100% ethanol were added. This was then incubated at -20°C for 1 h. It was brought out and left to stand at room temperature for 5 min, and then centrifuged at 13,000 g at 4°C for 45 min. The liquid was removed, leaving only the DNA in the Eppendorf tubes. The DNA was dried in an incubator at 37°C for 30 min.

Sequencing of 16S rDNA gene

The dry DNA samples (obtained using V3 primers) were sequenced using a computer analytical sequencer (MGW - Biotech, Germany) with the V3 and V5 primer Rev, acting as the basis according to manufacturer's instructions. The generated nucleotide sequences were subjected to analysis. Sequencing of the purified 16S rDNA DNA products was performed using the sequencing unit of the University of Nottingham; a 373 DNA sequence (Perkin-Elmer Applied Biosystems) was used with the Taq Dye Deoxy terminator cycle sequencing kit (Perkin-Elmer Applied Biosystems). The full identities of the isolates were then obtained by subjecting the nucleotide sequences to searches in the Gene Bank (http://www.ncbi.nlm.nih.gov/blast/) with the Blast search program.

Analysis of the 16S rDNA gene sequence

The generated sequences of the 16s rDNA genes were subjected to alignment in the databases at the BLAST, Basic Local Alignment and Search Tool, Website: http://www.ncbi.nih.gov/blast/.igi. The isolates were then identified based on the result of the analysis.

RESULTS

Table 1 shows the result of the conventional method of identification of LAB, the carbohydrate utilization pattern and biochemical characteristics of the isolates. All the 20 isolates were identified as L. plantarum. The result obtained agrees with the characterization pattern of other authors (Sneath et al., 2009).

Table 2 shows the comparison between the phenotypic method and the genotypic method using the 16S rDNA gene sequence of the 20 isolates that were initially identified

as L. plantarum. The topmost sequences producing significant alignments when the nucleotide sequences were subjected to Basic Local Alignment Search Tool (BLAST) in the gene bank Database (http://www.ncbi.nlm.nih.gov/blast/Blast.igi) for L. plantarum isolates.

Altogether, seventeen L. plantarum isolates that have been identified before showed a significant alignment in the gene database. The result of the PCR sequencing correlated in 17 out of 20 isolates while there was no correlation in 3 out of 20. The names and accession numbers of these seventeen isolates have significant alignments with the L. plantarum. All the seventeen topmost species was shown to produce significant alignment with the marker and have expected value (E value) of between 1e - 73 and 5e - 7 and maximum identification (Max identity) of between 95 and 100%. They were all L. plantarum. Three out of the twenty isolates did not have significant alignment with the others. They were identified as L. pentosus and one unidentified Lactobacillus sp. There was significant difference in the molecular method and the conventional methods. The result however did not correlate but a divergent view was presented which shows a difference in their gene sequence.

Table 3 shows the qualities and quantities of the 16S rDNA genes of the L. plantarum obtained by PCR using V3 primer, after purification.

The 16S rDNA of the 17 species after amplification with primers was found to belong to the L. plantarum group as they were identified as L. plantarum by partial gene sequencing. The 16S rDNA genes of the other of the three organisms were not shown because a different gene sequence was presented.

Figure 1 shows the L. plantarum strain 16S ribosomal RNA gene, the partial sequence alignment of 16S rDNA after amplification of the gene by PCR in the gene bank data base. Molecular characterisation of the isolates was done by extracting the DNA gene sequence using universal primers and when compared, it was identified as L. plantarum with alignment.

Figure 2 shows the nucleotide sizes in base pairs (bp) of the plasmids of the selected seventeen L. plantarum isolate that were used for further work after their identities have been confirmed by 16S rDNA. This base sequence provides significant information on the 16S rDNA gene sequence of the L. plantarum. The nucleotide base sequence of the 16S rDNA has provided a basis for phylogenetic identification and analysis.

DISCUSSION

Accurate and definitive microorganism identification is essential for a wide variety of application including biotechnological, industrial, biomedical, pharmaceutical and environmental studies. The 16S rDNA sequence based analysis is a central method to understand not only

Table 1. Physiological and biochemical characteristics of isolates.

Isolate code	Gram reaction	Cell morphology	Catalase	Oxidase	Casein hydrolysis	Gel HND	M.R	V.P	H₂SP	Growth at 15°C	45°C	pH at 3.9	pH at 9.2	pH at 5	4% NaCl	CIT.UTI	Glucose	Xylose	Rhamnnose	Triammonium citrate	Raffinose	Sucrose	Lactose	Maltose	Galactose	Fructose	Arabinnose	Mannose	Dulcitol	Mannitol	Inositol	Motility	Indole	NH₃Arg	Nitrate red	Probable identity
1	+	R	-	-	-	-	-	-	+	+	-	+	+	+	+	-	+	D	-	+	+	+	+	+	+	+	W	+	-	+	-	-	-	-	-	*Lactobacillus plantarum*
2	+	R	-	-	-	-	-	-	+	+	-	+	+	+	+	-	+	D	-	+	+	+	+	+	+	+	W	+	-	+	-	-	-	-	-	*L. plantarum*
3	+	R	-	-	-	-	-	-	+	+	-	+	+	+	+	-	+	D	-	+	+	+	+	+	+	+	W	+	-	+	-	-	-	-	-	*L. plantarum*
4	+	R	-	-	-	-	-	-	+	+	-	+	+	+	+	-	+	D	-	+	+	+	+	+	+	+	W	+	-	+	-	-	-	-	-	*L. plantarum*
5	+	R	-	-	-	-	-	-	+	+	-	+	+	+	+	-	+	D	-	+	+	+	+	+	+	+	W	+	-	+	-	-	-	-	-	*L. plantarum*
6	+	R	-	-	-	-	-	-	+	+	-	+	+	+	+	-	+	D	-	+	+	+	+	+	+	+	W	+	-	+	-	-	-	-	-	*L. plantarum*
7	+	R	-	-	-	-	-	-	+	+	-	+	+	+	+	-	+	D	-	+	+	+	+	+	+	+	W	+	-	+	-	-	-	-	-	*L. plantarum*
8	+	R	-	-	-	-	-	-	+	+	-	+	+	+	+	-	+	D	-	+	+	+	+	+	+	+	W	+	-	+	-	-	-	-	-	*L. plantarum*
9	+	R	-	-	-	-	-	-	+	+	-	+	+	+	+	-	+	D	-	+	+	+	+	+	+	+	W	+	-	+	-	-	-	-	-	*L. plantarum*
10	+	R	-	-	-	-	-	-	+	+	-	+	+	+	+	-	+	D	-	+	+	+	+	+	+	+	W	+	-	+	-	-	-	-	-	*L. plantarum*
11	+	R	-	-	-	-	-	-	+	+	-	+	+	+	+	-	+	D	-	+	+	+	+	+	+	+	W	+	-	+	-	-	-	-	-	*L. plantarum*
12	+	R	-	-	-	-	-	-	+	+	-	+	+	+	+	-	+	D	-	+	+	+	+	+	+	+	W	+	-	+	-	-	-	-	-	*L. plantarum*
13	+	R	-	-	-	-	-	-	+	+	-	+	+	+	+	-	+	D	-	+	+	+	+	+	+	+	W	+	-	+	-	-	-	-	-	*L. plantarum*
14	+	R	-	-	-	-	-	-	+	+	-	+	+	+	+	-	+	D	-	+	+	+	+	+	+	+	W	+	-	+	-	-	-	-	-	*L. plantarum*
15	+	R	-	-	-	-	-	-	+	+	-	+	+	+	+	-	+	D	-	+	+	+	+	+	+	+	W	+	-	+	-	-	-	-	-	*L. plantarum*
16	+	R	-	-	-	-	-	-	+	+	-	+	+	+	+	-	+	D	-	+	+	+	+	+	+	+	W	+	-	+	-	-	-	-	-	*L. plantarum*
17	+	R	-	-	-	-	-	-	+	+	-	+	+	+	+	-	+	D	-	+	+	+	+	+	+	+	W	+	-	+	-	-	-	-	-	*L. plantarum*
18	+	R	-	-	-	-	-	-	+	+	-	+	+	+	+	-	+	D	-	+	+	+	+	+	+	+	W	+	-	+	-	-	-	-	-	*L. plantarum*
19	+	R	-	-	-	-	-	-	+	+	-	+	+	+	+	-	+	D	-	+	+	+	+	+	+	+	W	+	-	+	-	-	-	-	-	*L. plantarum*
20	+	R	-	-	-	-	-	-	+	+	-	+	+	+	+	-	+	D	-	+	+	+	+	+	+	+	W	+	+	+	-	-	-	-	-	*L. plantarum*

R = Rod; + = A positive reaction; - = A negative reaction; D = A delayed reaction; W = A weakly positive reaction; M.R = methyl red test, V.P = Voges Proskaeur

Table 2. Comparison of phenotypic and genotypic methods of identification of *L. plantarum*.

Isolate code	Conventional identity	Closest relative (using 16srDNA gene sequencing)	Identity	Gene bank accession no
L. plantarum CO1	*L. plantarum*	*L. plantarum*	95%	GQ180906.1
L. plantarum CO2	*L. plantarum*	*L. plantarum*	95%	GQ166663.1
L. plantarum CO3	*L. plantarum*	*L. plantarum*	95%	GQ166662.1
L. plantarum CO4	*L. plantarum*	*L. plantarum*	95%	GQ166661.1
L. plantarum CO5	*L. plantarum*	*L. pentosus*	91%	GQ180915.1
L. plantarum CO6	*L. plantarum*	*L. plantarum*	95%	GQ180902.1
L. plantarum LV1	*L. plantarum*	*L. plantarum*	95%	FJ861114.1
L. plantarum LV2	*L. plantarum*	*L. plantarum*	95%	FJ861113.1
L. plantarum LV3	*L. plantarum*	*L. plantarum*	95%	FJ861112.1
L. plantarum LV4	*L. plantarum*	*L. plantarum*	95%	FJ861111.1
L. plantarum LV5	*L. plantarum*	*L. plantarum*	95%	FJ851111.1
L. plantarum LV6	*L. plantarum*	*L. pentosus*	91%	FJ851122.1
L. plantarum LV7	*L. plantarum*	*L. plantarum*	95%	FJ851116.1
L. plantarum LV8	*L. plantarum*	*L. plantarum*	95%	FJ851113.1
L. plantarum TV1	*L. plantarum*	*L. plantarum*	95%	FJ84495.1
L. plantarum TV2	*L. plantarum*	*L. plantarum*	95%	FJ844955.1
L. plantarum TV3	*L. plantarum*	*L. plantarum*	95%	FJ844949.1
L. plantarum TV4	*L. plantarum*	*L. plantarum*	95%	FJ844954.1
L. plantarum TV5	*L. plantarum*	*Lactobacillus* sp.	90%	FJ843956.1
L. plantarum TV6	*L. plantarum*	*L. plantarum*	95%	FJ844953.1

Table 3. Qualities and quantities of the 16S rDNA genes of the *L. plantarum* obtained by PCR using V3 primer, after purification.

S/N	Sample ID	16S rDNA			
		Conc. (ug/L)	A260nm	A260/280	0.0260/230
5	H101	18.34	0.367	1.82	0.02

the microbial diversity within and across the group but also to identify new strains. Bacterial species have at least one copy of the 16S rDNA gene containing highly conserved regions together with hyper variable regions, which is used for identification of new strains. However, a considerable variation can occur between species in both the length and the sequence of 16S rDNA ITS region, therefore this region is useful in characterization of bacterial species (Mohammed et al., 2011). The 16S rDNA gene is very useful because the genome of all bacteria contains this conserved gene and any small variability in this region is unique and specific to each species. This characteristic is usually harnessed in their identification (Mohania et al., 2008).

Considering the conventional method for identifying LAB isolates, the objective of this study was to compare the phenotypic method and the 16SrDNA sequencing which is a species-specific PCR reaction for the proper identification of the twenty *Lactobacillus* sp. The genus level was however the same for all the isolates, they were

further characterized using PCR reactions to perform complete identification. The results obtained with 95% reliability and higher were considered; those lower than this were not considered because their gene sequences were identified as different organisms. Considering that species-specific PCR reactions target specific genes of genera and species, the molecular method was considered reliable. Molecular bacteria identification is based on the full length of 16S rDNA gene sequence by several studies have shown that the initial few base pair sequence provides sufficient discrimination between strains because this region shows a high genetic diversity.

Of the 20 isolates used in this work, three presented divergent results as compared to 16S rDNA sequencing and species-specific PCR reaction. This confirmed the result of 17 out of 20 isolates tested (17/20), that is, 85% and divergent result were obtained in 3 out of 20 (15%) isolates that were screened (3/20). Out of these, 2 were identified as *L. pentosus* while the last was a

|GQ180905.1|*Lactobacillus plantarum* strain TJ2 16S ribosomal RNA gene, partial sequence, Length=182, Score = 283 bits (153), Expect = 1e-73,

```
Identities = 153/153 (100%), Gaps = 0/153 (0%) Strand=Plus/Plus
```

```
Query
GTCTGATGGAGCAACGCCGCGTGAGTGAAGAAGGGTTTCGGCTCGTAAAACTCTGTTGTT

| | | | | | | | | | | | | | | | | | | | | | | | | | | | | | | | | | | | | | | | | | | | | | | | | | | | | | | | | | | |
Sbjct
GTCTGATGGAGCAACGCCGCGTGAGTGAAGAAGGGTTTCGGCTCGTAAAACTCTGTTGTT

Query
AAAGAAGAACATATCTGAGAGTAACTGTTCAGGTATTGACGGTATTTAACCAGAAAGCCA

| | | | | | | | | | | | | | | | | | | | | | | | | | | | | | | | | | | | | | | | | | | | | | | | | | | | | | | | | | | |
Sbjct
AAAGAAGAACATATCTGAGAGTAACTGTTCAGGTATTGACGGTATTTAACCAGAAAGCCA

Query           CGGCTAACTACGTGCCAGCAGCCGCGGTAATAA
                | | | | | | | | | | | | | | | | | | | | | | | | | | | | | | | | |
Sbjct           CGGCTAACTACGTGCCAGCAGCCGCGGTAATAA
```

Figure 1. Alignment of 16S rDNA nucleotide sequences of *L. plantarum* against *L. plantarum* strain LpT2 (accession no GQ166663.1) and *L. plantarum* strain LpT1 (accession no GQ166662.1) in the gene bank data base.

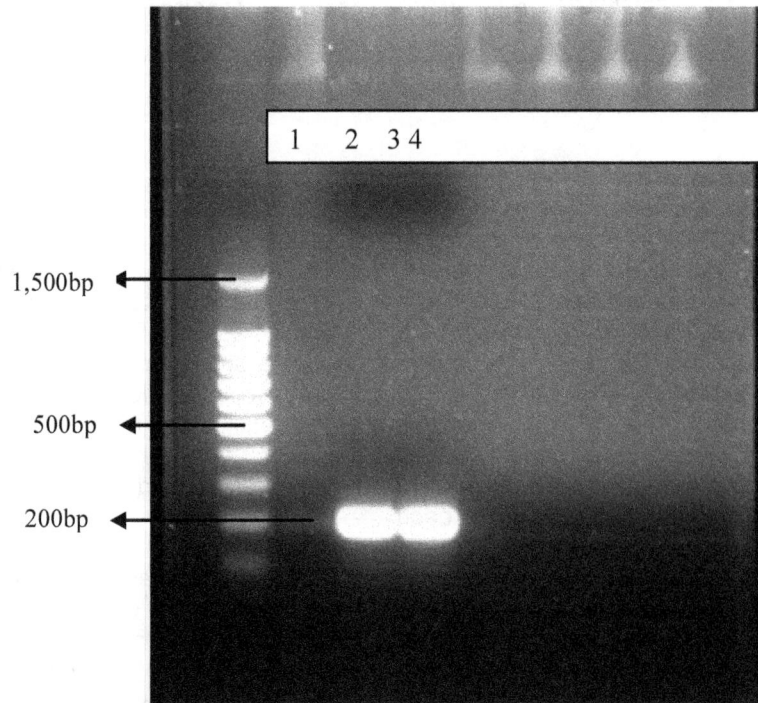

Figure 2. The nucleotide sizes of the plasmids of the selected nine *L. plantarum* isolate.

Lactobacillus sp. that could not be identified. This result agrees with the report of Marroki et al. (2011) who reported a similar view stating that *L. plantarum* and *L. pentosus* have very similar 16S rDNA sequences that only differ by 2 base pair. Other authors also reported that both organisms belong to the same phylogenetic group and they can only be differentiated when analysis of 16S-23S larger spacer is done (Ennahar et al., 2003). This may also be the same reason for the other *Lactobacillus* sp. that was not identified by this method presenting a result that did not correlate with those obtained earlier by phenotypic method. However, the result of the conventional method cannot be discarded completely but it can be regarded as giving a clue or presumptive result which can then be confirmed by molecular method.

Differences between genotypic and phenotypic tests have been identified previously not just for LAB but also for many other bacteria (Gomes et al., 2008; Paula et al., 2012). They also noted that this tool is useful for identifying microorganisms at sub species level which cannot easily be identified by other common technique. Phenotypic method may also have poor reproducibility as a result of changes that occur during the growth and metabolism of different organisms. This also agrees with the report of Mohania et al. (2008) who reported that bacterial isolates do not express their genes at the same time or they may lose some characteristics such as plasmids during culturing. This may however be responsible for the inconsistencies that are usually identified in sugar fermentation patterns and other biochemical tests that rely on physiological characteristics of different organisms for identification.

Gill et al. (2006) also stressed another importance of this molecular method being a desirable advantage of 16S rDNA over the conventional one. Apart from being rapid, the sequence could also be performed not only on bacterial culture but also on the sample so as to study the diversity of the organisms without culturing. The efficacy and efficiency of this method was clearly demonstrated in this work by differentiating strains belonging to the same species and it has been clearly identified by various authors such as Gill et al. (2006) and Morgan et al. (2009) because the results are not subjective.

The molecular method used in this work further confirmed the real identities of *L. plantarum* that were used for further work in the fermentation pattern for the formulation of a weaning food blend as earlier reported by Adeyemo and Onilude (2013). The real identities of the organisms are usually revealed by molecular methods and the results can be reproduced at any time and in different places without environmental variations. Based on the result of this study, the 16S rDNA sequencing method is specific for the gene of target and broader strategies that can characterize lactic acid bacteria without prior knowledge of genetic targets, this is however a desirable characteristics of this method, it is

thus recommended for proper identification of organisms to be used in fermented foods as starter culture or bio-preservative.

The result obtained in this work agrees with the result obtained by Parker et al. (2001). They opined that several PCR methods have subsequently been developed to overcome difficulties experienced with phenotypic methods. The method described in this work allows the amplification of specific PCR products. This enables direct sequencing of unknown regions without the need for DNA cloning but makes use of analysis of microbial genetic elements. Shittu et al. (2006) also noted the accuracy of the molecular diagnostic method in the ability to rapidly identify microorganisms isolated from clinical samples from genus level to species level using automated systems. Reduction of analysis time and reproducibility would be advantageous, especially for organisms that are fastidious, slow-growing and of medical and industrial importance.

The result obtained also solves the problem of misidentification. This agrees with the work of Woo et al. (2008) who reported that some LAB species are closely related to *Lactobacillus* sp. The importance of accurate identification need to be emphasized in LAB obtained from fermented foods that are used as probiotics or starter cultures. This is because some LAB are also involved in clinical infections such as *Leuconostoc* sp., *Pediococcus* sp. *and Enterococcus* sp. These organisms are of medical importance and should not be misidentified with other *Lactobacillus* sp. The use of 16S rDNA will lower the risk of inaccurate or poor identification of these pathogens that are also similar to other *Lactobacillus* sp.

However, in industrial microbiology for example, there are various importance of rapid methods of identification of microorganisms. First, it is of paramount importance to food/industrial microbiologists for screening and identification of organisms that are of great industrial and biotechnological purposes. Rapid detection and identification of microorganisms also allows for continuous monitoring of microbial growth in relation to various metabolites that are produced by them especially in pharmaceutical industries such as enzymes, vaccines, antibiotics, organic acids etc. Also, the ease of producing a large number of copies of a specific DNA sequence can be applied in the industry for the production of many important products from microorganisms using some specific genes from them.

Finally, the advantage of genotyping is that it is an accurate method for the identification of *L. plantarum* in that the genome is stable; the genetic composition of the organism is independent of cultural conditions and method of isolation; it can easily be subjected to auto-mation and the results can be analysed statistically with ease. LAB are referred to as "probiotics" and it belongs to the group of organisms that are generally regarded as safe (GRAS). Its prompt and quick identification is a useful tool in distinguishing between these probiotics and other opportunistic pathogens that may also be present as contaminant in fermented foods.

Conflict of Interests

The author(s) have not declared any conflict of interests.

ACKNOWLEDGEMENT

The author wishes to acknowledge the contribution of Dr. Olusegun Olaoye of Michael Okpara University of Agriculture, Umudike, Abia State, Nigeria towards the molecular aspect of this work.

REFERENCES

Adeyemo SM, Onilude AA (2013). Enzymatic Reduction of Anti-nutritional Factors In soybeans by *Lactobacillus plantarum* Isolated from fermenting cereals. Nig. Food J. 13:71-79.

Adeyemo SM, Onilude AA (2014). Reduction of Oligosaccharide content of soybeans by the action of *L. plantarum* isolated from fermented cereals. Afr. J. Biotechnol.13:3790-3796.

Banigo EOI, Muller HG (1972). Manufacture of *ogi* (Nigerian fermented cereal porridge): Comparative evaluation of corn sorghum and millet. Can. Inst. Food Sci. Technol. J. 5:217-221.

Bulut C, Gunes H, Okuklu B, Harsa S, Killic S, Coban HS, Yenidinya AF (2005). Homofermentative lactic acid bacteria of a traditional cheese, *Comlek peyniri* from cypadocia region. J. Diary Res. 72:19-24.

Ennahar S, Cai Y, Fujita Y (2003). Phylogenetic diversity of lactic acid bacteria associated with paddy rice silage as determined by 16S ribosomal DNA analysis. Appl. Environ. Microbiol. 69:444-451.

Gill SR, Pop M, Beboy RT, Eckburg PB, Tambaugh PJ, Samuel BS, Gordon JI, Relman DA, Frazer LC, Nelson KE (2008). Metagenomic analysis of the human distal gut microbiome. Sci. 312:1355-1359.

Gomes BC, Esteves CT, Palazzo IC, Darini AL, Felis GE, Sechi LA, Francho BD, de Martinis EC (2008). Prevalence and characterization of *Enterococcus* spp. isolated from Brazilllian foods. Food Microbiol. 25:668-675.

Harrigan WF, Mc Cance ME (1976). Laboratory Methods in Food and Dairy products. Academy Press, London.

Lucke FK (2000). Utilization of Microbes to process and preserve meat. Meat Sci. 56:105-115.

Marroki A, Zuniga M, Kihal M, Martinez PG (2010). Characterization of *Lactobacillus* from Algerian Goat's milk based on Phenotypic, 16S rDNA sequencing and their technological properties. Braz. J. Microbiol. 42:158-171.

Merien EB, Imane C, Mimoune Z, Marouane M, Abdelhay A, Elmostsfa E, Mohammed EM, Amin L (2013). Comparison of the conventional method and 16S rDNA gene sequencing method in identification of clinical and hospital environmental isolates in Morocco. Afr. J. Microbiol. Res. 7:5637-5644.

Mohammed SU, Magray D, Kumar A, Rawat A, Srivastava S (2011). Identification of E. *coli* through analysis of 16S rRNA and 16S-23S rRNA internal transcribed spacer region sequences. Bioinform. 6:370-371 (2011 Biomedical Informatics).

Mohania D, Nagpal R, Kumar M, Bhardwaj A, Yadav M, Jain S, Marotta F, Singh V, Parkash O, Yadav H (2008). Molecular approaches for identification and characterization of Lactic acid bacteria. J. Dig. Dis. 9:190-198.

Morgan MC, Boyette M, Goforth C, Sperry KV, Shermalyn R (2009). Comparison of the Biolog OmniLog Identification System and 16S rDNA gene sequence for accuracy in identification of atypical bacteria of clinical origin. J. Med. Microbiol. 79:336-343.

Ogier JC, Son O, Gruss A, Tailliez P, Delacroix-Buchet A (2002). Identification of the bacterial microflora in dairy products by temporal temperature gradient gel electrophoresis. Appl. Environ. Microbiol. 68:3691-3701.

Olaoye OA, Onilude AA (2009). A study on isolation of presumption technological important microorganisms from Nigerian beef. American-Eurasian J. Sustain. Agric. (Accepted, In Press).

Parker JD, Rabinovitch PS, Burmer GC (2001). Targeted gene walking polymerase chain reaction. Nucleic Acids Res. 19:3055-3060.

Paula MM, Luana MP, Abelardo SJ, Luis AN (2011). Comparison of phenotypic and molecular tests to identify lactic acid bacteria. Braz. J. Microbiol. 44:109-112.

Pitcher DG, Saunders NAT, Slowen RJ (1989). Rapid extraction of bacteria genomic DNA with guanidium thiocyanate. Lett. Appl. Microbiol. 8:192-198.

Shittu A, Lin J, Morrison D, Kolawole D (2006). Identification and molecular characterization of mannitol salt positive, coagulase-negative staphylococci from nasal samples of medical personnel and students. J. Med. Microbiol. 55:317-324.

Sneath PHA, Mair NS, Sharpe ME, Holt JG (2009). Bergey's Manual of Systematic Bacteriology. Baltimore: in Kleins and Wilkins.

Woo PC, Lau SK, Teng JL, Tse H, Yuen KY (2008). Then and now:Use of 16S rDNA gene sequencing for bacterial identification and discovery of novel bacteria in clinical microbiology laboratories. J. Clin. Microbiol. Infect.14:908-934.

Permissions

All chapters in this book were first published in IJBMBR, by Academic Journals; hereby published with permission under the Creative Commons Attribution License or equivalent. Every chapter published in this book has been scrutinized by our experts. Their significance has been extensively debated. The topics covered herein carry significant findings which will fuel the growth of the discipline. They may even be implemented as practical applications or may be referred to as a beginning point for another development.

The contributors of this book come from diverse backgrounds, making this book a truly international effort. This book will bring forth new frontiers with its revolutionizing research information and detailed analysis of the nascent developments around the world.

We would like to thank all the contributing authors for lending their expertise to make the book truly unique. They have played a crucial role in the development of this book. Without their invaluable contributions this book wouldn't have been possible. They have made vital efforts to compile up to date information on the varied aspects of this subject to make this book a valuable addition to the collection of many professionals and students.

This book was conceptualized with the vision of imparting up-to-date information and advanced data in this field. To ensure the same, a matchless editorial board was set up. Every individual on the board went through rigorous rounds of assessment to prove their worth. After which they invested a large part of their time researching and compiling the most relevant data for our readers.

The editorial board has been involved in producing this book since its inception. They have spent rigorous hours researching and exploring the diverse topics which have resulted in the successful publishing of this book. They have passed on their knowledge of decades through this book. To expedite this challenging task, the publisher supported the team at every step. A small team of assistant editors was also appointed to further simplify the editing procedure and attain best results for the readers.

Apart from the editorial board, the designing team has also invested a significant amount of their time in understanding the subject and creating the most relevant covers. They scrutinized every image to scout for the most suitable representation of the subject and create an appropriate cover for the book.

The publishing team has been an ardent support to the editorial, designing and production team. Their endless efforts to recruit the best for this project, has resulted in the accomplishment of this book. They are a veteran in the field of academics and their pool of knowledge is as vast as their experience in printing. Their expertise and guidance has proved useful at every step. Their uncompromising quality standards have made this book an exceptional effort. Their encouragement from time to time has been an inspiration for everyone.

The publisher and the editorial board hope that this book will prove to be a valuable piece of knowledge for researchers, students, practitioners and scholars across the globe.

List of Contributors

Okiemute Emmanuel Idise
Department of Microbiology, Delta State University, Abraka, Nigeria

Seyed Alireza Valadabadi
Faculty of Agriculture, Islamic Azad University, Shahr-e-Qods Branch, Tehran, Iran

Hossein Aliabadi Farahani
Faculty of Agriculture, Islamic Azad University, Shahr-e-Qods Branch, Tehran, Iran

Poosakkannu Anbu
Department of Plant Molecular Biology and Biotechnology, Centre for Plant Molecular Biology, Tamil Nadu Agricultural University, Coimbatore-641 003, India
Department of Biological and Environmental Sciences, University of Jyväskylä, P.O. Box, 35, FIN-40014, Finland

Loganathan Arul
Department of Biological and Environmental Sciences, University of Jyväskylä, P.O. Box, 35, FIN-40014, Finland

Daniel Anyika
Institute for Biotechnology Research, Jomo Kenyatta University of Agriculture and Technology (JKUAT), P.O. Box 62000, Nairobi, 00200, Kenya

Hamadi Boga
Department of Botany, Faculty of Science, Jomo Kenyatta University of Agriculture and Technology (JKUAT), P.O. Box 62000, Nairobi, 00200, Kenya

Romano Mwirichia
Institute for Biotechnology Research, Jomo Kenyatta University of Agriculture and Technology (JKUAT), P.O. Box 62000, Nairobi, 00200, Kenya

Abdeen Mustafa Omer
Energy Research Institute, Khartoum, Sudan

Shilpa Penugonda
Department of Microbiology, Kakatiya University, Warangal-506009, Andhra Pradesh, India

S. Girisham
Department of Microbiology, Kakatiya University, Warangal-506009, Andhra Pradesh, India

S. M. Reddy
Department of Microbiology, Kakatiya University, Warangal-506009, Andhra Pradesh, India

Ahmad Ebrahimi
Islamic Azad University, Iranshahr Branch, Iran

Payam Moaveni
Islamic Azad University, Shahr-e-Qods Branch, Iran

Hossein Aliabadi Farahani
Member of Young Researchers Club, Islamic Azad University, Shahr-e Qods Branch, Iran

S. E. Agarry
Biochemical Engineering Research Laboratory, Department of Chemical Engineering, Ladoke Akintola University of Technology, Ogbomoso, Oyo State, Nigeria

B. O. Solomon
Biochemical Engineering Research Laboratory, Department of Chemical Engineering, Obafemi Awolowo University, Ile-Ife, Osun State, Nigeria
National Biotechnology Development Agency, Abuja, Nigeria

T. O. K. Audu
Department of Chemical Engineering, University of Benin, Benin-City, Edo State, Nigeria

Isaac Kofi Bimpong
Africa Rice Centre, BP 96, St Louis, Senegal, West Africa
International Rice Research Institute (IRRI), DAPO Box 7777, Metro Manila, Philippines

Joong Hyoun Chin
International Rice Research Institute (IRRI), DAPO Box 7777, Metro Manila, Philippines

Joie Ramos
International Rice Research Institute (IRRI), DAPO Box 7777, Metro Manila, Philippines

Hee-Jong Koh
Dept of Plant Science, College of Agriculture and Life Sciences, Seoul National University, Seoul, 151-921, Korea

S. O. P. Urunmatsoma
Department of Chemistry, Geochemical Research Laboratory, University of Benin, Benin City, Nigeria

E. U. Ikhuoria
Department of Chemistry, Geochemical Research Laboratory, University of Benin, Benin City, Nigeria

F. E. Okieimen
Department of Chemistry, Geochemical Research Laboratory, University of Benin, Benin City, Nigeria

E. U. Ikhuoria
Department of Chemistry, University of Benin, Benin City, Nigeria

A. S. Folayan
Department of Chemistry, University of Benin, Benin City, Nigeria

F. E. Okieimen
Department of Chemistry, University of Benin, Benin City, Nigeria

Dargie Tsegay
Montpellier SupAgro_Centre International d'études Supérieures en Sciences Agronomiques, 2 Place Pierre Viala, 34060 Cedex 2, Montpellier, FRANCE

Bizuayehu Tesfaye
Montpellier SupAgro_Centre International d'études Supérieures en Sciences Agronomiques, 2 Place Pierre Viala, 34060 Cedex 2, Montpellier, FRANCE

Ali Mohamme
Montpellier SupAgro_Centre International d'études Supérieures en Sciences Agronomiques, 2 Place Pierre Viala, 34060 Cedex 2, Montpellier, FRANCE

Haddis Yirga
Montpellier SupAgro_Centre International d'études Supérieures en Sciences Agronomiques, 2 Place Pierre Viala, 34060 Cedex 2, Montpellier, FRANCE

Andnet Bayleyegn
Montpellier SupAgro_Centre International d'études Supérieures en Sciences Agronomiques, 2 Place Pierre Viala, 34060 Cedex 2, Montpellier, FRANCE

Edward Ikenna Odum
Department of Microbiology, Delta State University, Abraka, Delta State, Nigeria

Ifat Bashir
Additional Directorate of Sericulture Development Department, Tulsi Bagh, Srinagar- 190 001 (J&K), India

S. D. Sharma
Central Sericultural Research and Training Institute Srirampura Mysore- 570008, India

Shabir A. Bhat
Division of Sericulture, Mirgund, Sher-e-Kashmir University of Agricultural Sciences and Technology of Kashmir, Post Box: 674,GPO Srinagar- 190001, India

Godliving Y. S. Mtui
Department of Molecular Biology and Biotechnology, University of Dar es Salaam, P. O. Box 35179, Dar es Salaam, Tanzania

Surekha
Department of Botany, Government National Post-Graduate College, Sirsa-125005, India

Joginder Singh Duhan
Department of Biotechnology, Chaudhary Devi Lal University, Sirsa-125055, India

Hailay Gebremedhin
Debre Birhan University, College of Agriculture and Natural Resource Science, Department of Plant Science, Debre Birhan, Ethiopia

Bizuayehu Tesfaye
Debre Birhan University, College of Agriculture and Natural Resource Science, Department of Plant Science, Debre Birhan, Ethiopia

Ali Mohammed
Debre Birhan University, College of Agriculture and Natural Resource Science, Department of Plant Science, Debre Birhan, Ethiopia

Dargie Tsegay
Debre Birhan University, College of Agriculture and Natural Resource Science, Department of Plant Science, Debre Birhan, Ethiopia

Manas Denre
Department of Agricultural Biochemistry, Bidhan Chandra Krishi Viswavidyalaya, Mohanpur, Nadia-741252, West Bengal, India
Department of Soil Science and Agricultural Chemistry, Birsa Agricultural University, Kanke, Ranchi-834006, Jharkhand, India

Soumya Ghanti
Department of Spices and Plantation Crops, Bidhan Chandra Krishi Viswavidyalaya, Mohanpur, Nadia-741252, West Bengal, India

Kheyali Sarkar
Department of Botany, Raniganj Girls' College, Raniganj, Burdwan-713347, West Bengal, India

B. Daramola
Department of Food Technology, Federal Polytechnic, PMB 5351, Ado-Ekiti, Ekiti State, Nigeria

Valery Ndagijimana
Faculty of Agriculture, National University of Rwanda (NUR), P. O. Box117, Huye, Rwanda

Jane Kahia
World Agroforestry Centre (ICRAF) Cote d' Ivoire
Country Program Cocody Mermoz, Abidjan, Côte
d'Ivoire | 08 BP 2823 ABIDJAN 08

Theodore Asiimwe
Rwanda Agriculture Board (RAB), P. O. Box 5016. Kigali,
Rwanda

Peter Yao Sallah
Faculty of Agriculture, National University of Rwanda
(NUR), P. O. Box117, Huye, Rwanda

Bancy Waweru
Rwanda Agriculture Board (RAB), P. O. Box 5016. Kigali,
Rwanda

Isidore Mushimiyimana
Rwanda Agriculture Board (RAB), P. O. Box 5016. Kigali,
Rwanda

Jean Ndirigwe
Rwanda Agriculture Board (RAB), P. O. Box 5016. Kigali,
Rwanda

Sindi Kirimi
International Potato Center (CIP), Sub-Saharan Africa
Region, P. O. Box 25171, Nairobi, Kenya

Damien Shumbusha
Rwanda Agriculture Board (RAB), P. O. Box 5016. Kigali,
Rwanda

Peter Njenga
Jomo Kenyatta University of Agriculture and Technology,
Box 62000, Nairobi, Kenya

Modeste Kouassi
Centre National de Recherche Agronomique (CNRA),
Laboratoire Central de Biotechnologies (LCB), 01 BP
1740Abidjan 01, Côte d'Ivoire.Edmond Koffi6

Shiju Mathew
Department of Medical Lab Technology, College of
Applied Medical Sciences, Jazan University, P.O. Box No.
114, Jazan, Kingdom of Saudi Arabia

Yahya Hasan Hobani
Department of Medical Lab Technology, College of
Applied Medical Sciences, Jazan University, P.O. Box No.
114, Jazan, Kingdom of Saudi Arabia

E. A. Masinde
Kenya Agricultural Research Institute, P.O Box Private
Bag - 20107 Njoro, Kenya
Crops Horticulture and Soils Department, Egerton
University P.O Box 523, Egerton, Kenya

J. N. Malinga
Kenya Agricultural Research Institute, P.O Box Private
Bag - 20107 Njoro, Kenya

W. A. Ngenya
Kenya Agricultural Research Institute, P.O Box Private
Bag - 20107 Njoro, Kenya
Crops Horticulture and Soils Department, Egerton
University P.O Box 523, Egerton, Kenya

R. M. S Mulwa
Crops Horticulture and Soils Department, Egerton
University P.O Box 523, Egerton, Kenya

M. Cakir
WA State Agricultural Biotechnology Center, School of
Veterinary and Life Sciences, Murdoch University 90
South St.,Murdoch WA 6150, Australia

S. M. Adeyemo
Department of Microbiology, Obafemi Awolowo
University, Ile-Ife, Osun State, Nigeria

A. A. Onilude
Department of Microbiology, University of Ibadan, Oyo
State, Nigeria

www.ingramcontent.com/pod-product-compliance
Lightning Source LLC
Chambersburg PA
CBHW050449200326
41458CB00014B/5116